Psychopharmacology in Oncology and Palliative Care

Luigi Grassi • Michelle Riba
Editors

Psychopharmacology in Oncology and Palliative Care

A Practical Manual

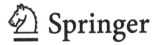 Springer

Editors
Luigi Grassi
Institute of Psychiatry
Department of Biomedical & Specialty
    Surgical Sciences
University of Ferrara
Ferrara, Italy

Michelle Riba
Department of Psychiatry
University of Michigan
Ann Arbor, Michigan
USA

ISBN 978-3-642-40133-6   ISBN 978-3-642-40134-3 (eBook)
DOI 10.1007/978-3-642-40134-3
Springer Heidelberg New York Dordrecht London

Library of Congress Control Number: 2014943454

Foreword

The editors of *Psychopharmacology in Oncology and Palliative Care: A Practical Manual*, published by the World Psychiatric Association, have graciously invited me to write the foreword. The attention to psychopharmacology comes after the first book in the series covering the general principles on which psycho-oncology is based. It is a tribute to the field that sufficient information exists today with an evidence base and that a textbook can be published focusing on the pharmacologic interventions alone. It is going to serve as a benchmark in the field internationally.

The book represents the continuing collaboration between the World Psychiatric Association and the International Psycho-Oncology Society to make available the most recent clinical and research approaches to psychiatric care of patients with cancer. Drs. Grassi and Riba have called on global experts in specific areas to provide updates relevant to the psychiatric, psychosocial, and ethical care of children, elders, and those receiving palliative care for cancer. Such topics as delirium, depression, anxiety, sleep, substance abuse, pain, fatigue, and sexual disorders are often neglected by treating physicians and their teams due to lack of knowledge about the range of evidence-based interventions available.

This book, written largely by psychiatrists and psychologists, outlines the information needed to improve care, outlined in succinct and readable language. Patients around the world will experience a better quality of life as they go through the cancer journey because of the information made available to their physicians through the chapters in this book.

New York, NY   Jimmie Holland
February 4, 2014   Wayne E. Chapman Chair in Psychiatric Oncology,
                                                         Memorial Sloan Kettering Cancer Center
                                        Professor of Psychiatry, Weill Cornell Medical College

Preface

Psycho-oncology has grown exponentially over the last years, with a mandatory indication for multidisciplinary intervention and inclusion of psycho-oncology programs within many national cancer plan acts. The need for psychosocial training of all healthcare professionals working in oncology is now considered essential for good quality of cancer care.

Psychopharmacology has a central specific role both because of the efficacy of psychotropic drugs in the treatment of psychiatric disorders secondary to cancer and because of the new data derived by psychopharmacological research in psychiatry that, when applied in oncology and palliative care, may be of extreme help in relieving cancer patients from their suffering. A manual or practical text on psychopharmacology in oncology has been lacking, and for this reason, the idea of this book originated with the intention to fill this gap, by giving clinicians practical indications and suggestions relative to the efficacy and safety of psychotropic drugs in the treatment of psychiatric disorders in cancer patients across the trajectory of disease. One of the main aims of the book is in fact to present the main issues involved in psychopharmacological management of psychiatric disorders in cancer and palliative care, according to the different possible psychiatric diagnoses, with special attention to have psychopharmacological intervention within a broad framework of an integrative psychosocial, patient-centered approach. A second aim is to illustrate the significant and challenging problems clinicians may encounter (e.g., drugs, pharmacological characteristics, side effects, drug–drug interaction, doses, and route of administration) including the emerging theme of adjuvant use of psychotropic drugs for the treatment of symptoms/syndromes not mainly related to psychiatric disorders (e.g., pain, hot-flashes, fatigue). A third aim is to examine the needs of special populations, including children and adolescents, as well as the elderly, affected by cancer, when psychopharmacology treatment is indicated.

The book consists of three parts. In Part I, the general aspects in psychopharmacological treatment, with specific reference to oncology and palliative care, are examined. Chapter 1, by Grassi and Riba, serves to delineate the changes in the use of psychotropic drugs as a pillar of intervention for psychiatric disorders in cancer care and the need for reconceptualizing *psychopharmoncology* as an integration of psychosocial and psychopharmacological treatments in clinical practice. In Chap. 2, Roth and Alici provide an overview of the general principles of pharmacokinetics and pharmacodynamics with a focus on psychotropic medications commonly used for patients with cancer and in palliative care settings. The most significant diagnostic issues in terms of need for a comprehensive psychiatric interview and mental status examination when conducted in oncology and palliative care settings and a proper use of psychiatric taxonomic systems are discussed by Grassi, Nanni, and Riba in Chap. 3. Mitchell and Bultz discuss, in Chap. 4, the need for a proper psychosocial assessment of cancer patients when planning for psychopharmacological intervention. Screening for anxiety and depression, distress, cognitive decline, adaptation to illness, as well as unmet needs and well-being are comprehensively described by the authors. Chapter 5, by Grassi, Caruso and Baile, deals with the importance of communication and interpersonal relationships in the diagnostic phase and in the shared decision making in planning a psychopharmacological intervention, with particular reference to the problem of adherence. In Chap. 6, Kogon and Spiegel underline the importance of a careful integration of psychosocial and psychopharmacological treatment in cancer care. The authors discuss the need for attention to the symbolic communication when clinicians propose psychopharmacological treatment and the benefit of combining and integrating psychotropic medication and psychosocial interventions. Tang and Fielding in Chap. 7 examine the important theme of complementary and nonconventional treatments. More specifically, the role of traditional Chinese medicine, including herbal formulations, acupuncture, and activity-based interventions (Qigong and Tai Chi Chuane), and yoga is described with reference to integration with psychopharmacology, and as a practice that more and more frequently is provided in cancer settings.

Part II of this book is dedicated to the use of psychotropic drugs for the treatment of the specific psychiatric disorders in clinical oncology and palliative care settings. In Chap. 8, Shimizu, Yosiuchi, and Onishi offer an overview of the treatment of anxiety disorders and trauma- and stressor-related disorders, according to the most recent changes provided by the DSM-5, and present the role of medications with anti-anxiety properties and their adverse effects and drug interactions. The extremely debated area of depression and depressive disorders is the focus of Chap. 9 by Fitzgerald, Li, Grassi, and Rodin, who comprehensively discuss the need for appropriate diagnosis of depression, including a careful examination of the patient's medical condition, for a correct prescription of antidepressant medications, which takes into account both the profile of action and the potential adverse effects and drug–drug interactions. Chaturvedi, Torta, and Ieraci summarize in Chap. 10 the complex problem of pharmacological treatment of somatoform disorders and other somatic symptom conditions (e.g., pain, fatigue, hot-flashes, pruritus, anorexia and weight loss, and nausea and vomiting). The importance of sensitive exploration of somatic symptoms, examination of possible biological and neurotransmitter mechanisms, and appropriate intervention are highlighted by the authors. In Chap. 11, the significant, though underestimated, area of bipolar disorders, as a particular challenge for the oncology team, is reviewed by Ellingrod, Hertz, and McInnis, who discuss psychopharmacological clinical strategies for these disorders and, in general, unstable mood in patients with cancer, emphasizing the need for regular monitoring of clinical mood symptoms, medication levels, and physical health. In Chap. 12, the correct approach to delirium, as one of the most common neuropsychiatric complications, associated with significant morbidity and mortality, is provided by Breitbart and Alici, who present a detailed overview of the pharmacological management options for the disorder in cancer patients and in palliative care settings. The role of multidisciplinary team intervention for psychotic disorders is presented in Chap. 13 by Kim and Fang who discuss how to integrate proper psychopharmacotherapy (e.g., choice of drugs, dosages, side effects, drug–drug interactions) and communication strategies when treating both patients with severe mental illness who have developed cancer and those who developed psychotic disorders as a consequence of cancer. In Chap. 14, Monteiro, Ribeiro, and Xavier review the vast and important area relative to the treatment of sleep disorders, as a significant, yet underestimated problem to be addressed in cancer and palliative care settings. Screening of sleep complaints, classification of the several expression of sleep disorders, evaluation of the possible etiologic factors, and correct treatment are comprehensively discussed. The significant problem of substance and alcohol abuse in cancer is reviewed in Chap. 15 by Passik, Miller, Ruhele, and Kirsh who discuss the impact of these behaviors on potentially life-saving and life-extending cancer treatments and the need for the application of addiction medicine techniques and interventions in cancer care. In Chap. 16, Benedict and Nelson focus attention on cancer-related changes in sexual function by reviewing the possible interventions for both male and female cancer patients, including the use of medical, educational, and psychological strategies, to facilitate sexual recovery and promote satisfying sexual experiences for patients and their partners.

In the third part of the book, some special issues relative to psychopharmacology in oncology and palliative care are taken into consideration. In Chap. 17, Lynn and Valentine alert clinicians to the possible emergencies or dangers arising from pharmacologic management, including serotonin syndrome, neuroleptic malignant syndrome, and overdose of psychotropic drugs commonly utilized in oncology and palliative care. Forgey and Bursch, in Chap. 18, offer a thorough description of the very important area of childhood cancer, with specific reference to psychopharmacological treatment recommendations for children with cancer, within a larger framework of behavioral and family-based interventions management. The age-related physiological changes that may affect the response to psychotropic medication and their clinical implications for the use of psychopharmacologic treatments in elderly patients with cancer are the aims of Chap. 19 by Iaboni, Fitzgerald, and Rodin. In the following Chap. 20, Ferrari and Caraceni offer an in-depth insight regarding end-of-life care, with specific reference to palliative sedation therapy (PST). Evidence-based use of some psychotropic drugs is described by the authors to help cancer and palliative care physicians when dealing with refractory symptoms (e.g., delirium, dyspnea, pain, nausea and vomiting) at the end of life. In Chap. 21, Alici and Dunn point out the topic of psychopharmacology research in oncology and palliative care, considering the problems and urgent needs to be addressed (e.g., limited number of studies, methodological limitations, the challenges in establishing psychiatric diagnoses, the validity of measures and instruments used as outcome measures). Chapter 22, by Levin and Kissane, is dedicated to the ethical framework that informs the practice of oncology and palliative care. The autonomy, dignity, and vulnerability of the cancer patient, the nature of informed consent in treatment decisions, and challenging ethical domains (e.g., use of unproven therapies, invasive treatments and complex decisions in end-of-life care) are discussed with specific reference to psychopharmacology.

The book, written by experts in the field, is designed to be easy to read and to reference, with information displayed in concise tables and boxes accompanied by further detail within the text and some clinical cases exemplifying the themes discussed in each chapter. We hope that it may ensure interest for all those working with cancer patients, including oncologists, surgeons, pediatricians, geriatricians, radiotherapy oncologists, palliative care physicians, and general practitioners. We also hope to sensitize more mental health professionals, including psychiatrists, psychologists, and behavioral scientists, to the psychopharmacological treatment of psychiatric disorders and/or syndromes in cancer patients.

We are deeply grateful to all the authors who graciously accepted to share their experience. Without their enthusiasm, commitment, and expertise this book would not have been possible. We owe a debt of gratitude to the board of the World Psychiatric Association (WPA), with special mention to Jimmie Holland, founding chair of the WPA Section on Psycho-Oncology, and Rodolfo Fahrer, founding chair of the WPA Section on Psychiatry, Medicine and Primary Care. We also appreciate the support of the leaders of the World Psychiatric Association (WPA) and the opportunity to serve as cochairs of the WPA section on Psycho-Oncology and Palliative Care. The encouragement we have received from our friends and colleagues of the International Psycho-Oncology Society (IPOS) with whom we have collaborated in many projects over the last years is extremely worth mentioning. We thank our colleagues and staff at the Unit of Psychiatry, University of Ferrara, Italy, and at the Department of Psychiatry and Comprehensive Cancer Center, University of Michigan, USA. We also extend our acknowledgments to the staff of Springer for their help and guidance. We are deeply indebted to our teachers and mentors who also supported us in the difficult journey of psychosocial care in oncology and psychosomatic medicine. Our families who constantly encouraged us deserve special mention, as well as all the patients and their families who taught us so much.

Ferrara, Italy   Luigi Grassi
Ann Arbor, MI, USA   Michelle Riba
February 2014

Contents

Part I General Aspects in Psychopharmacological Treatment

**1 Psychopharmacology in Oncology and Palliative Care:
General Issues**   3
Luigi Grassi and Michelle Riba

**2 General Principles of Psychopharmacological Treatment
in Psycho-Oncology**   13
Andrew J. Roth and Yesne Alici

3 Diagnostic Issues   31
Luigi Grassi, Maria Giulia Nanni, and Michelle Riba

4 Psychological Assessment in Psychopharmacology   49
Alex J. Mitchell and Barry D. Bultz

5 Interpersonal Relationship Issues in Psychopharmacology   69
Luigi Grassi, Rosangela Caruso, and Walter Baile

**6 Integration of Psychopharmacotherapy with Psychotherapy
and Other Psychosocial Treatment**   81
Manuela Kogon and David Spiegel

**7 Psychopharmacology and Complementary and Nonconventional
Treatments in Oncology** 101
Lili Tang and Richard Fielding

**Part II Psychotropic Drug Use in Clinical Oncology and Palliative
Care Settings**

8 Treatment of Anxiety and Stress-Related Disorders 129
Ken Shimizu, Kazuhiro Yoshiuchi, and Hideki Onishi

9 Pharmacotherapy of Depression in Cancer Patients 145
Peter Fitzgerald, Madeline Li, Luigi Grassi, and Gary Rodin

10 Treatment of Somatoform Disorders and Other Somatic Symptom
    Conditions (Pain, Fatigue, Hot Flashes, and Pruritus). 163
    Santosh K. Chaturvedi, Valentina Ieraci, and Riccardo Torta

11 Bipolar Disorder in the Cancer Patient. 189
    Daniel L. Hertz, Vicki L. Ellingrod, and Melvin G. McInnis

12 Treatment of Delirium and Confusional States in Oncology
    and Palliative Care Settings. 203
    William S. Breitbart and Yesne Alici

13 Pharmacological Treatment of Psychotic Disorders. 229
    Jong-Heun Kim and Chun-Kai Fang

14 Treatment of Sleep Disorders. 239
    Lúcia Monteiro, Andreia Ribeiro, and Salomé Xavier

15 Substance Abuse in Oncology. 267
    Steven D. Passik, Nicholas Miller, Matthew Ruehle,
    and Kenneth L. Kirsh

16 Treatment of Sexual Disorders Following Cancer Treatments. . . . 295
    Catherine Benedict and Christian J. Nelson

Part III   Special Issues

17 Psychiatric Emergencies. 317
    Rachel Y. Lynn and Alan D. Valentine

18 Psychopharmacology in Palliative Care and Oncology:
    Childhood and Adolescence. 331
    Marcy Forgey and Brenda Bursch

19 Special Issues in Psychopharmacology: The Elderly. 349
    Andrea Iaboni, Peter Fitzgerald, and Gary Rodin

20 Sedation for Psychological Distress at the End of Life. 369
    Laura Ferrari and Augusto Caraceni

21 Research Issues in Psychopharmacology in Oncology
    and Palliative Care Settings. 381
    Yesne Alici and Laura B. Dunn

22 Ethics of Psychopharmacological and Biological Treatments
    in Psycho-oncology. 393
    Tomer T. Levin and David W. Kissane

Index. 407

List of Contributors

Yesne Alici Department of Psychiatry and Behavioral Sciences, Memorial Sloan Kettering Cancer Center, New York, NY, USA

Walter Baile Program for Interpersonal Communication and Relationship Enhancement (I*CARE), Department of Faculty and Academic Development, University of Texas, M.D. Anderson Cancer Center, Houston, TX, USA

Catherine Benedict Department of Psychiatry and Behavioral Sciences, Memorial Sloan-Kettering Cancer Center, New York, NY, USA

William S. Breitbart Department of Psychiatry and Behavioral Sciences, Memorial Sloan Kettering Cancer Center, New York, NY, USA

Barry D. Bultz Department of Psychosocial Oncology, Tom Baker Cancer Centre, University of Calgary, Calgary, AB, Canada

Brenda Bursch Pediatric C/L Psychiatry Service Division of Child Psychiatry, Department of Psychiatry and Biobehavioral Sciences, UCLA Semel Institute for Neuroscience and Human Behavior, David Geffen School of Medicine at UCLA, Semel, Los Angeles, CA, USA

Department of Pediatrics, UCLA Semel Institute for Neuroscience and Human Behavior, David Geffen School of Medicine at UCLA, Semel, Los Angeles, CA, USA

Augusto Caraceni Palliative Care, Pain Therapy and Rehabilitation Fondazione IRCCS Istituto Nazionale dei Tumori, Milan, Italy

Rosangela Caruso Institute of Psychiatry, Department of Biomedical and Specialty Surgical Sciences, University of Ferrara, Ferrara, Italy

Santosh K. Chaturvedi Psychiatric Rehabilitation Services, National Institute of Mental Health and Neurosciences, Bangalore, India

Laura B. Dunn Department of Psychiatry, University of California, San Francisco, San Francisco, CA, USA

Vicki L. Ellingrod John Gideon Serle Professor of Clinical and Translational Pharmacy, University of Michigan College of Pharmacy and School of Medicine, Ann Arbor, MI, USA

Chun-Kai Fang Department of Psychiatry, Mackay Memorial Hospital, Taipei, Taiwan, ROC

Hospice and Palliative Care Center (HPCC) & Suicide Prevention Center (SPC), Mackay Memorial Hospital, Taipei, Taiwan, ROC

Laura Ferrari Palliative Care, Pain Therapy and Rehabilitation Fondazione IRCCS Istituto Nazionale dei Tumori, Milan, Italy

Richard Fielding Centre for Psycho-Oncology Research and Training, School of Public Health, The University of Hong Kong, Hong Kong, China

Peter Fitzgerald Psychosocial Oncology and Palliative Care, Princess Margaret Cancer Centre, University Health Network, Toronto, ON, Canada

Marcy Forgey Pediatric C/L Psychiatry Service Division of Child Psychiatry, Department of Psychiatry and Biobehavioral Sciences, UCLA Semel Institute for Neuroscience and Human Behavior, David Geffen School of Medicine at UCLA, Semel, Los Angeles, CA, USA

Luigi Grassi Institute of Psychiatry, Department of Biomedical and Speciality Surgical Sciences, University of Ferrara, Ferrara, Italy

Daniel L. Hertz University of Michigan College of Pharmacy, Ann Arbor, MI, USA

Andrea Iaboni Department of Psychiatry, Toronto Rehabilitation Institute, University Health Network, Toronto, ON, Canada

Valentina Ieraci Department of Neuroscience, University of Turin, Turin, Italy

Jong-Heun Kim Mental Health Clinic, National Cancer Center, Goyang, Gyeonggi-do, Republic of Korea

Kenneth L. Kirsh Millennium Laboratories, San Diego, CA, USA

David W. Kissane Department of Psychiatry, Monash Medical Centre, Monash University, Clayton, VIC, Australia

Manuela Kogon Stanford Center for Integrative Medicine, Stanford University, Stanford, CA, USA

Tomer T. Levin Department of Psychiatry and Behavioral Sciences, Memorial Sloan Kettering Cancer Center, New York, NY, USA

Madeline Li Department of Psychosocial Oncology and Palliative Care, Princess Margaret Cancer Centre, University Health Network, Toronto, ON, Canada

Rachel Y. Lynn Department of Psychiatry, The University of Texas MD Anderson Cancer Center, Houston, TX, USA

Melvin G. McInnis Thomas B and Nancy Upjohn Woodworth Professor of Bipolar Disorder and Depression, University of Michigan School of Medicine, Ann Arbor, MI, USA

Nicholas Miller Millenium Laboratories, San Diego, CA, USA

Alex J. Mitchell Department of Psycho-oncology, Cancer Studies and Molecular Medicine, University of Leicester, Leicester, UK

Lúcia Monteiro Psychiatry Service, Psychosocial Department, Instituto Português de Oncologia Lisboa, Lisbon, Portugal

Maria Giulia Nanni Institute of Psychiatry, Department of Biomedical and Specialty Surgical Sciences, University of Ferrara, Ferrara, Italy

Christian J. Nelson Department of Psychiatry and Behavioral Sciences, Memorial Sloan-Kettering Cancer Center, New York, NY, USA

Hideki Onishi Department of Psycho-Oncology, Saitama Medical University International Medical Center, Hidaka City, Saitama, Japan

Steven D. Passik Millenium Laboratories, San Diego, CA, USA

Michelle Riba Department of Psychiatry, University of Michigan, Ann Arbor, MI, USA

Director, Psycho-Oncology Program, University of Michigan Comprehensive Cancer Center, Ann Arbor, MI, USA

Andreia Ribeiro Psychiatry Unit, Psychosocial Department, Instituto Português de Oncologia de Lisboa, Lisbon, Portugal

Gary Rodin Psychosocial Oncology and Palliative Care, Princess Margaret Cancer Centre, University Health Network, Toronto, ON, Canada

Andrew J. Roth Weill Cornell Medical College, New York, NY, USA

Department of Psychiatry and Behavioral Sciences, Memorial Sloan Kettering Cancer Center, New York, NY, USA

Matthew Ruehle Millennium Laboratories, San Diego, CA, USA

Ken Shimizu Psycho-oncology Division, National Cancer Center Hospital, Chuou-ku, Tokyo, Japan

David Spiegel Department of Psychiatry and Behavioral Sciences, Stanford University, Stanford, CA, USA

Lili Tang Department of Psycho-Oncology, Peking University Cancer Hospital, Beijing, China

Riccardo Torta Department of Neuroscience, University of Turin, Turin, Italy

Alan D. Valentine Department of Psychiatry, The University of Texas MD Anderson Cancer Center, Houston, TX, USA

Salomé Xavier Psychiatry Service, Hospital Prof. Dr. Fernando Fonseca, Amadora, Portugal

Kazuhiro Yoshiuchi Department of Stress Sciences and Psychosomatic Medicine, Graduate School of Medicine, University of Tokyo, Bunkyo-ku, Tokyo, Japan

About the Editors

Luigi Grassi, M.D., is Professor and Chair of Psychiatry and Chair of the Department of Biomedical and Specialty Surgical Sciences of the University of Ferrara, Italy, and Head of the University Unit of Hospital Psychiatry, S. Anna Hospital, and Local Health Agency in Ferrara. He is the author of about 200 scientific papers, chapters of books, and books, including *Clinical Psycho-Oncology: An International Perspective* (Wiley, Chichester, 2012), with Michelle Riba. He has been the President of the International Psycho-Oncology Society (IPOS) (2006–2008) and the Italian Society of Psycho-Oncology (SIPO) (2003–2011). He is currently Chair of the IPOS Federation of Psycho-Oncology Societies and of the World Psychiatric Association Section on Psycho-Oncology & Palliative Care. Dr. Grassi's clinical and research interests are in the area of psycho-oncology, consultation-liaison psychiatry and psychosomatic medicine, and psychosocial and psychiatry rehabilitation.

Michelle B. Riba, M.D., M.S., is Professor and Associate Chair for Integrated Medicine and Psychiatric Services and Associate Director of the University of Michigan Depression Center, Director of the PsychOncology Program at the University of Michigan Comprehensive, and Director of the Psychosomatic Medicine Fellowship. She has served on numerous editorial boards and is the author or editor of over 200 scientific articles, books, including *Clinical Psycho-Oncology: An International Perspective* (Wiley, Chichester, 2012), with Luigi Grassi, chapters, and scientific abstracts. Dr. Riba is Past President of the American Psychiatric Association, Association for Academic Psychiatry, and American Association of Directors of Psychiatric Residency Training. She is currently on the Executive Committee of the World Psychiatric Association and Secretary for Scientific Publications. As a psychosomatic medicine psychiatrist, Dr. Riba's clinical and research interests include primary care psychiatry, psycho-oncology, depression and cardiovascular disease, and screening for distress in patients with medical illness.

Part I

General Aspects in Psychopharmacological Treatment

Psychopharmacology in Oncology and Palliative Care: General Issues

1

Luigi Grassi and Michelle Riba

τὸν αὐτὸν δὲ λόγον ἔχει ἥ τε τοῦ λόγου δύναμις πρὸς τὴν τῆς ψυχῆς τάξιν ἥ τε τῶν φαρμάκων τάξις πρὸς τὴν τῶν σωμάτων φύσιν. ὥσπερ γὰρ τῶν φαρμάκων ἄλλους ἄλλα χυμοὺς ἐκ τοῦ σώματος ἐξάγει, καὶ τὰ μὲν νόσου τὰ δὲ βίου παύει, οὕτω καὶ τῶν λόγων οἱ μὲν ἐλύπησαν, οἱ δὲ ἔτερψαν, οἱ δὲ ἐφόβησαν, οἱ δὲ εἰς θάρσος κατέστησαν τοὺς ἀκούοντας, οἱ δὲ πειθοῖ τινι κακῇι τὴν ψυχὴν ἐφαρμάκευσαν καὶ ἐξεγοήτευσαν.

The power of discourse stands in the same relation to the soul's organization as the pharmacopoeia does to the physiology of bodies. For just as different drugs draw off different humors from the body, and some put an end to disease and others to life, so too of discourses: some give pain, others delight, others terrify, others rouse the hearers to courage, and yet others by a certain vile persuasion drug and trick the soul.
(Gorgias from Leontini, c. 485 – c. 380 BC, Encomium of Helena)

Abstract

At least 25–30 % of patients with cancer and even a higher percentage of those in an advanced phase of illness meet the criteria for a psychiatric diagnosis, including depression, anxiety, stress-related syndromes, including severe adjustment disorders, sleep disorders, and delirium. A number of studies in psycho-oncology have accumulated over the last 35 years on the use of psychotropic

L. Grassi (✉)
Institute of Psychiatry, Department of Biomedical and Specialty Surgical Sciences, University of Ferrara, Ferrara, Italy
e-mail: luigi.grassi@unife.it

M. Riba
Department of Psychiatry, University of Michigan, Ann Arbor, MI, USA

Director, Psycho-Onclology Program, University of Michigan Comprehensive Cancer Center, Ann Arbor, MI, USA
e-mail: mriba@med.umich.edu

L. Grassi and M. Riba (eds.), *Psychopharmacology in Oncology and Palliative Care*, DOI 10.1007/978-3-642-40134-3_1, © Springer-Verlag Berlin Heidelberg 2014

drugs as a pillar in the treatment of psychiatric disorders. Major advances in research have also shown the efficacy of psychotropic drugs as adjuvant treatment of cancer-related symptoms, such as pain, hot flashes, pruritus, nausea and vomiting, fatigue, and cognitive impairment. The knowledge about pharmacokinetics and pharmacodynamics, clinical use, safety, side effects, and efficacy of drugs in cancer care is essential. The aims of this chapter are to consider the need for an integrated psychological and psychopharmacological intervention, as the concept of *psychopharmoncology* specifies, favoring the vision of an integrated and multidimensional approach in oncology, and palliative care services as well as in community-based cancer centers.

1.1   Introduction

Cancer is a devastating disease with profound psychological and behavioral implications on patients and family members. There are significant changes in the body and body image, including physical mutilations, stomas, pain, nausea and vomiting, hair loss, and fatigue (physical level); there are the loss of certainties, the change of perspective regarding the future, the instability of one's own emotional state, such as fears, anxiety, worries, sadness, and the threat of possible death and dying (psychological level); there are changes in the sense of meaning, including one's own personal values, the meaning of time and being, transcendence (spiritual level); there are issues regarding the sense of belonging ("to be with") in the family, in the microcosm of close social bonds and in the macrocosm of society, including work and social activities (interpersonal level). These very complicated shifts are some of the most significant dimensions determined by cancer and its treatment (Grassi and Riba 2012). All the different possible phases of the cancer trajectory, from diagnosis to long-term survival, from recurrence to advanced phases and end of life, are foci for the development of psychological problems or more specific psychiatric disorders.

Psycho-oncology literature has, for the last 50 years, examined these aspects and indicated the need for a comprehensive approach to cancer in order to treat maladaptive reactions to the disease or frank psychiatric disorders with the aim to improve patients' quality of life. The first psychiatric diagnostic approach can be traced to the observations of Sutherland (1956, 1957) who, as a pioneer in the field of psycho-oncology, described and underlined the several clinical types of psychological or psychopathological reactions commonly seen after cancer diagnosis and treatment: dependency, anxiety, postoperative depression, hypochondriac response, obsessive-compulsive reactions, and paranoid reactions. He also pointed out that patients affected by cancer are persons under a special and severe form of stress, during which many fundamental underlying convictions, based on their life history and experiences (e.g., pattern of relationship with attachment figures) are brought to the surface.

Subsequently, other studies confirmed the importance of diagnosing psychosocial disorders, especially anxiety and depression, among cancer patients in the different stages of illness (Plumb and Holland 1977; Maguire et al. 1978; Plumb and Holland 1981). When the Diagnostic Statistical Manual for Mental Disorders in its 3rd edition (DSM-III) was available in clinical settings, giving clinicians more definite operational diagnostic criteria, data regarding the prevalence of psychiatric disorders in cancer patients were rapidly collected. In the first multicenter study in the US, the PSYCOG study, Derogatis et al. (1983) showed that almost 50 % of cancer patients met the criteria for a DSM-III psychiatric diagnosis, mainly in the area of adjustment. PSYCOG results were confirmed by a number of other investigations in several countries, such as the United Kingdom (Hardman et al. 1989), Belgium (Razavi et al. 1990), Italy (Grassi et al. 1993, 2000), Australia (Kissane et al. 1998, 2004), Spain (Prieto et al. 2002), and Germany (Singer et al. 2013) All these studies, both using the DSM or the World Health Organization (WHO) International Classification of Disease (ICD), indicated that at least one-third of cancer patients present symptoms indicative of a psychiatric disorder, with changes in the prevalence according to the cancer site (e.g., pancreatic cancer is at risk for a higher prevalence of depressive disorders), stage (advanced stages are at risk for a higher prevalence of delirium), and clinical settings (inpatient and palliative care settings are at higher risk than outpatient settings). Recent meta-analyses have also confirmed that 25–30 % of cancer patients in oncology and hematology meet the criteria for a psychiatric diagnosis, mainly depressive disorders, anxiety, and adjustment and stress-related disorders, across the trajectory of their disease (Singer et al. 2010; Mitchell et al. 2011), with higher prevalence in the advanced phases of illness (Miovic and Block 2007; LeGrand 2012).

1.2 The Role of Psychotropic Drugs in Oncology and Palliative Care

From these studies, it derives that the treatment of psychiatric disorders has been part, from the beginning of psycho-oncology, of daily clinical practice. Helping cancer patients to deal with the many challenges they have to face, relieving them from unnecessary distress and psychiatric symptoms, and improving their quality of life are mandatory components of psycho-oncology. With regard to this, evidence regarding the pattern and rationale of use of psychotropic drugs has in fact accumulated over the last 35 years. In one of the first reports on this topic, Derogatis et al. (1979) indicated that 51 % of 1,579 cancer patients were prescribed psychotropic drugs, especially hypnotics (48 % of total prescriptions), antipsychotics (26 %), antianxiety agents (25 %), while a low percentage of patients were prescribe antidepressants (1 %). Similar data were reported in a further study of patients in advanced stages of cancer (Jaeger et al. 1985), which found that among 840 patients, antipsychotic agents were prescribed for 61.3 %, hypnotics for 55.8 %, and antidepressants for 10 %, with the most common reasons for these medications being psychological distress, sleep disorders, and nausea and vomiting. A slight change was observed in a subsequent study (Stiefel et al. 1990) that showed that, although prescription rates for different drug classes remained relatively stable, psychotropic drugs were used for a greater range of reasons and that the introduction of new agents, at that time, had altered the physician's attitudes and choices in treating cancer patients.

More recently, new data have emerged in terms of the increased use of psychopharmacologic treatment of psychiatric disorders and of cancer-related symptoms, such as hot flashes, neuropathic pain, nausea and vomiting, fatigue, and pruritus (Thekdi et al. 2012; Caruso et al. 2013). Farriols et al. (2012), for example, showed that, among 840 advanced cancer patients treated over a 7-year period (2002–2009), the use of antipsychotics increased from 26.1 % to 40 % (particularly haloperidol and risperidone), antidepressants from 17.8 % to 27.1 % (especially mirtazapine, citalopram, escitalopram, and duloxetine), benzo-diazepines from 72.6 % to 84 % (especially lorazepam and midazolam). In another recent study of 7,298 cancer patients and 14,596 matched controls, it has been found that the prevalence of emotional distress was higher among cancer patients (15.6 % versus 1.4 %) and that the volume and duration of psychotropic drugs prescriptions (i.e., anxiolytics and antipsychotics) was correspondingly higher among cases than controls (Desplenter et al. 2012). These data have been confirmed by De Bock et al. (2012) who studied more than 2,000 breast cancer patients receiving endocrine therapy and found that the prescription of anxiolytics, hypnotics, sedatives, and antidepressants was higher as compared to a group of age- and family physician-matched group of 8,129 women without cancer. Regard-ing antidepressants, a study of 2,389 survivors of childhood, adolescent, and young adult cancer showed an increased likelihood of using all categories of anti-depressants (ADs), and of using drugs from two or more antidepressant categories, compared to birth-cohort and gender-matched randomly selected population of 23,890 subjects (Deyell et al. 2013). The tendency to prescribe psychotropic medications in the advanced phase of cancer and particularly before death has been also pointed out in a retrospective case–control study including a total of 113,887 patients (Ng et al. 2013).

For these reasons and in order to provide indications about the use of psychotro-pic drugs in cancer care, guidelines have been developed for the most effective treatment of several psychiatric disorders. Regarding depression, for example, several algorithms are available both in cancer (Rodin et al. 2007; Okamura et al. 2008) and in palliative care (Rayner et al. 2011a, b), with a number of reviews indicating the efficacy of ADs in cancer (Li et al. 2012; Laoutidis and Mathiak 2013). Algorithms are also available for the treatment of delirium for which several studies have shown the most effective and safest drugs to be used in different settings, especially palliative care (Breitbart and Alici 2012). In a recent Delphi survey among 135 palliative care clinicians in nine countries, the antipsychotic, haloperidol, and the benzodiazepine, midazolam, are considered two of the four essential drugs that should be made available in all settings caring for dying patients with cancer (Lindqvist et al. 2013), within palliative sedation protocols (Cowan and Palmer 2002; Kehl 2004; Maltoni et al. 2012) for their efficacy in contrasting the severe symptoms of suffering (e.g., extreme anxiety, pain, dyspnea, nausea, rest-lessness, and agitated delirium) at the end of life.

A new series of data have also accumulated regarding the use of psychotropic drugs for nonpsychiatric symptoms. The clinical use of antidepressants (ADs) has extended to the treatment of pain, hot flashes, loss of appetite, and fatigue. With regards to pain, ADs, especially those acting on both the noradrenergic and seroto- nergic systems, have been used for a long time as a supplementation of the primary analgesics (Bennett 2011) with the European Society for Medical Oncology (ESMO) Guidelines for cancer pain management have more recently underlined ADs as a co-adjuvant treatment (Ripamonti et al. 2012). A vast literature exists on the use of a number of ADs in treating secondary hot flashes, especially in breast cancer patients, to the use of selective estrogen receptor modulators (SERMs), such as tamoxifen, or more recently aromatase inhibitors (AI) (e.g., letrozole, anastrozole, exemestane) (Bordeleau et al. 2007; Morrow et al. 2011; Fisher et al. 2013), with guidelines and treatment algorithms available for this specific field (Kligman and Younus 2010). The anti-histaminergic properties of some ADs have been capitalized in counteracting nausea and chemotherapy-induced anorexia/ cachexia in cancer patients (Kast and Foley 2007; Riechelmann et al. 2010), whereas cancer-related fatigue seems to benefit from the use of other ADs (e.g., bupropion) and psychostimulants (Breitbart and Alici-Evcimen 2007; Minton et al. 2008). The latter class of drugs because of their activating properties, improving alertness, attention, and wakefulness, has also shown a role in oncology and palliative care (Breitbart and Alici 2010; Minton et al. 2011). Regarding both the old and new generation of antipsychotics, an extensive literature exists showing their efficacy as adjunctive drugs in combination with antiemetic drugs, in the treatment of chemotherapy-induced nausea and vomiting. Similar data have been documented by the use of benzodiazepines (BDZ) that, for their amnesic properties, may favor the reduction of the conditioning mechanisms underlying chemotherapy-induced nausea and vomiting. Finally, the use of first and second generation anticonvulsants that also are employed as mood stabilizers (e.g., carbamazepine, topiramate, gabapentin) has shown to be helpful in the treatment of pain and chemotherapy-induced neuropathy (Wolf et al. 2008; Bennett et al. 2013).

1.3   Psychopharmoncology as an Integrated Approach for the Treatment of Psychiatric Disorders

It is clear, on the basis of what has been mentioned, that the progress of research and clinical application of psychopharmacology has been extremely significant in the last years and that a comprehensive review of psychotropic drugs use in oncology and palliative care settings is an urgent need (Grassi et al. 2014). However, the possibility to prescribe psychotropic drugs to control symptoms and to treat psychi- atric syndromes or disorders has to consider the complexity of the needs of the cancer patient and the dimensions we have summarized above. From this point of view, the concept of *psychopharmoncology* may help in representing the integrative way in which psychopharmacological and psychosocial intervention in cancer and palliative care settings can be provided by taking into account the multiple needs that cancer patients have and that only a multidimensional approach can address. This approach may seem quite obvious, since data regarding integration of psychotherapy and psychopharmacotherapy, especially sequential integration, have existed for a long time and, as far as depression is concerned, have shown that it is a viable strategy for the treatment and the prevention of relapse and recurrence (Guidi et al. 2011). Only recently, however, both evidence-based psychotherapy and evidence-based psychopharmacology have met in a more structured way and, although problems of communication still exist between psychotherapists and psychopharmacologists (Kalman and Kalman 2012), integrating the two is more frequent in clinical practice (De Oliveira et al. 2014). In general, psychotropic drug and psychotherapy in combination are better than mono-therapy and are more effective that the sum of the single components in terms of therapeutic synergism; furthermore, for almost all psychiatric disorders, an integrative approach has been shown to favor the outcome of the disorders themselves in a significant way, with psychotherapy acting in a manner similar or complementary to drugs (Stahl 2012).

For these reasons, a close interaction between psychiatrists with expertise in oncology and palliative care and other health professionals (e.g., clinical psychologists, nurses, social workers, rehabilitation professionals) involved in the care of cancer patients and their families is extremely important for the development of integrated treatment (see also Kogon and Spiegel 2014). According to this, there is strong evidence that services providing integrated intervention to patients and their families as part of standard regular care reduce the distress and psychiatric morbidity associated with cancer and foster a better quality of life during and after cancer treatment. Guidelines with respect to the role of integrated management of the most common psychiatric disorders, such as adjustment, anxiety, and depressive disorders, have been developed in several countries and are available (Turner et al. 2005; Adler and Page 2008; Howell et al. 2010; Holland et al. 2013). From a different perspective, the quality of death is also an extremely important area in which psychiatry and mental health, when integrated in oncology and palliative care, play an important role in alleviating the symptoms of suffering for the individual at the end of their life (Raijmakers et al. 2012) (see also Caraceni and Ferrari 2014).

Conclusions

Psychiatric disorders are common in patients with cancer and strongly influence, in a negative way, their quality of life. Thus, complete information about the most important psychotropic drugs and their correct use in clinical practice is essential for healthcare professionals working in cancer and palliative care settings. A proper knowledge of the characteristics of the several medications, their interactions, efficacy, and safety for a rational administration and treatment of the several psychiatric consequences secondary to cancer is urgently needed. Furthermore, when discussing the treatment of both psychiatric disorders and other symptoms in cancer patients, it is necessary to have information about the multifunctional pharmacologic profile of the drugs, that is the different therapeutic mechanisms and different functions at different doses that a molecule may have, depending upon the potency of its multiple pharmacologic actions (Stahl 2009, 2013), diurnal variation, interactions, etc.

Findings from research and clinical experience over the last twenty years have clearly demonstrated the need for integrated intervention, including psychosocial/psychotherapeutic, psychopharmacologic, and complementary therapies (Ouwens et al. 2009; Chandwani et al. 2012) in oncology. The improvement of the collaboration between oncologists, surgeons, radiation oncologists, physiatrists, anesthesiologists and other clinicians, and mental health professionals, the implementation of research protocols regarding pharmacological and psychosocial approaches to psychiatric disorders across the trajectory of the disease, the attention to the cultural aspects of cancer, including the different expression of psychological distress, and the possible different biological responses to psychotropic drugs represent some of the challenges for the clinician when setting up multicomponent and multidisciplinary intervention programs in psycho-oncology.

References

Adler NE, Page EK, editors. Cancer care for the whole patient: meeting psychosocial health needs. Washington, DC: The National Academies Press; 2008.

Bennett MI. Effectiveness of antiepileptic or antidepressant drugs when added to opioids for cancer pain: systematic review. Palliat Med. 2011;25:553–39.

Bennett MI, Laird B, Van Litsenburg C, Nimour M. Pregabalin for the management of neuropathic pain in adults with cancer: a systematic review of the literature. Pain Med. 2013;5.

Bordeleau L, Pritchard K, Goodwin P, Loprinzi C. Therapeutic options for the management of hot flashes in breast cancer survivors: an evidence-based review. Clin Therapeut J. 2007;29(2): 230–41.

Breitbart W, Alici Y. Evidence-based treatment of delirium in patients with cancer. J Clin Oncol. 2012;30:1206–14.

Breitbart W, Alici-Evcimen Y. Update on psychotropic medications for cancer-related fatigue. J Natl Compr Canc Netw. 2007;5:1081–91.

Breitbart W, Alici Y. Psychostimulants for cancer-related fatigue. J Natl Compr Canc Netw. 2010; 8:933–42.

Caruso R, Grassi L, Nanni MG, Riba M. Psychopharmacology in psycho-oncology. Curr Psychiatry Rep. 2013;15(9):393.

Chandwani KD, Ryan JL, Peppone LJ, Janelsins MM, Sprod LK, Devine K, Trevino L, Gewandter J, Morrow GR, Mustian KM. Cancer-related stress and complementary and alternative medicine: a review. Evid Base Compl Alternative Med. 2012;2012:979213.

Cowan JD, Palmer TW. Practical guide to palliative sedation. Curr Oncol Rep. 2002;4(3):242–9.

De Bock GH, Musters RF, Bos HJ, Schröder CP, Mourits MJ, de Jong-van den Berg LT. Psychotropic medication during endocrine treatment for breast cancer. Support Care Cancer. 2012;20:1533–40.

Derogatis LR, Morrow GR, Fetting J, Penman D, Piasetsky S, Schmale AM, Henrichs M, Carnicke Jr CL. The prevalence of psychiatric disorders among cancer patients. JAMA. 1983;249(6): 751–7.

Derogatis LR, Feldstein M, Morrow G, Schmale A, Schmitt M, Gates C, Murawski B, Holland J, Penman D, Melisaratos N, Enelow AJ, Adler LM. A survey of psychotropic drug prescriptions in an oncology population. Cancer. 1979;44:1919–29.

Desplenter F, Bond C, Watson M, Burton C, Murchie P, Lee AJ, Lefevre K, Simoens S, Laekeman G. Incidence and drug treatment of emotional distress after cancer diagnosis: a matched primary care case–control study. Br J Cancer. 2012;107:1644–51.

Deyell RJ, Lorenzi M, Ma S, Rassekh SR, Collet JP, Spinelli JJ, McBride ML. Antidepressant use among survivors of childhood, adolescent and young adult cancer: a report of the Childhood, Adolescent and Young Adult Cancer Survivor (CAYACS) Research Program. Pediatr Blood Canc. 2013;60:816–22.

Farriols C, Ferrández O, Planas J, Ortiz P, Mojal S, Ruiz AI. Changes in the prescription of psychotropic drugs in the palliative care of advanced cancer patients over a seven-year period. J Pain Symptom Manage. 2012;43:945–52.

Fisher WI, Johnson AK, Elkins GR, Otte JL, Burns DS, Yu M, Carpenter JS. Risk factors, pathophysiology, and treatment of hot flashes in cancer. CA Cancer J Clin. 2013;63(3):167–92.

Gorgias: Encomium of Helena (edited with Introduction, note and translation by M.C. MacDowell). London: Bristol Classical Press; 1982

Grassi L, Rosti G, Lasalvia A, Marangolo M. Psychosocial variables associated with mental adjustment to cancer. Psycho-Oncology. 1993;2:11–20.

Grassi L, Gritti P, Rigatelli M, Gala C, Italian Consultation-Liaison Group. Psychosocial problems secondary to cancer: an Italian multicentre survey of consultation-liaison psychiatry in oncology. Eur J Cancer. 2000;36:579–85.

Grassi L, Caruso R, Hammelef K, Nanni MG, Riba M. Efficacy and safety of pharmacotherapy in cancer-related psychiatric disorders across the trajectory of cancer care: a review. Int Rev Psychiatry. 2014;26(1):44–62.

Grassi L, Riba M. Clinical psycho-oncology: an international perspective. Chichester: Wiley; 2012.

Guidi J, Fava GA, Fava M, Papakostas GI. Efficacy of the sequential integration of psychotherapy and pharmacotherapy in major depressive disorder: a preliminary meta-analysis. Psychol Med. 2011;41:321–31.

Hardman A, Maguire P, Crowther D. The recognition of psychiatric morbidity on a medical oncology ward. J Psychosom Res. 1989;33:235–9.

Holland JC, Andersen B, Breitbart WS, Buchmann LO, Compas B, Deshields TL, Dudley MM, Fleishman S, Fulcher CD, Greenberg DB, Greiner CB, Handzo GF, Hoofring L, Hoover C, Jacobsen PB, Kvale E, Levy MH, Loscalzo MJ, McAllister-Black R, Mechanic KY, Palesh O, Pazar JP, Riba MB, Roper K, Valentine AD, Wagner LI, Zevon MA, McMillian NR, Freedman-Cass DA. Distress management. J Natl Compr Canc Netw. 2013;11(2):190–209.

Howell D, Keller-Olaman S, Oliver T, Hack T, Broadfield L, Biggs K, Chung J, Esplen M-J, Gravelle D, Green E, Gerin-Lajoie C, Hamel M, Harth T, Johnston P, Swinton N, Syme A. A Pan-Canadian practice guideline: screening, assessment and care of psychosocial distress (depression, anxiety) in adults with cancer. Toronto: Canadian Partnership Against Cancer (Cancer Journey Action Group) and the Canadian Association of Psychosocial Oncology; 2010.

Jaeger H, Morrow GR, Carpenter PJ, Brescia F. A survey of psychotropic drug utilization by patients with advanced neoplastic disease. Gen Hosp Psychiatry. 1985;7:353–60.

Kalman TP, Kalman VN. Granet RmDo psychopharmacologists speak to psychotherapists? A survey of practicing clinicians. Psychodyn Psychiatry. 2012;40(2):275–85.

Kast RE, Foley K. Cancer chemotherapy and cachexia: mirtazapine and olanzapine are 5-HT3 antagonists with good anti nausea effects. F Eur J Cancer Care (Engl). 2007;16:351–4.

Kehl KA. Treatment of terminal restlessness: a review of the evidence. J Pain Palliative Care Pharmacother. 2004;18(1):5–30.

Kissane DW, Clarke DM, Ikin J, Bloch S, Smith GC, Vitetta L, McKenzie DP. Psychological morbidity and quality of life in Australian women with early-stage breast cancer: a cross-sectional survey. Med J Aust. 1998;169:192–6.

Kissane DW, Grabsch B, Love A, Clarke DM, Bloch S, Smith GC. Psychiatric disorder in women with early stage and advanced breast cancer: a comparative analysis. Aust N Z J Psychiatry. 2004;38:320–6.

Kligman L, Younus J. Management of hot flashes in women with breast cancer. Curr Oncol. 2010;17:81–6.

Laoutidis ZG, Mathiak K. Antidepressants in the treatment of depression/depressive symptoms in cancer patients: a systematic review and meta-analysis. BMC Psychiatry. 2013;13:140. doi:10. 1186/1471-244X-13-140.

LeGrand SB. Delirium in palliative medicine: a review. J Pain Symptom Manage. 2012;44:583–94.

Li M, Fitzgerald P, Rodin G. Evidence-based treatment of depression in patients with cancer. J Clin Oncol. 2012;30(11):1187–96.

Lindqvist O, Lundquist G, Dickman A, Bükki J, Lunder U, Hagelin CL, Rasmussen BH, Sauter S, Tishelman C, Fürst CJ. OPCARE9. Four essential drugs needed for quality care of the dying: a Delphi-study based international expert consensus opinion. J Palliative Med. 2013;16:38–43.

Maguire GP, Lee EG, Bevington DJ, Küchemann CS, Crabtree RJ, Cornell CE. Psychiatric problems in the first year after mastectomy. Br Med J. 1978;15(1):963–5.

Maltoni M, Scarpi E, Rosati M, Derni S, Fabbri L, Martini F, Amadori D, Nanni O. Palliative sedation in end-of-life care and survival: a systematic review. J Clin Oncol. 2012;30:1378–83.

Minton O, Richardson A, Sharpe M, Hotopf M, Stone P. A systematic review and meta-analysis of the pharmacological treatment of cancer-related fatigue. J Natl Cancer Inst. 2008;100: 1155–66.

Minton O, Richardson A, Sharpe M, Hotopf M, Stone PC. Psychostimulants for the management of cancer-related fatigue: a systematic review and meta-analysis. J Pain Symptom Manage. 2011;41:761–7.

Miovic M, Block S. Psychiatric disorders in advanced cancer. Cancer. 2007;110:1665–76.

Mitchell AJ, Chan M, Bhatti H, Halton M, Grassi L, Johansen C, Meader N. Prevalence of depression, anxiety, and adjustment disorder in oncological, haematological, and palliative-care settings: a meta-analysis of 94 interview-based studies. Lancet Oncol. 2011;12:160–74.

Morrow PK, Mattair DN, Hortobagyi GN. Hot flashes: a review of pathophysiology and treatment modalities. Oncologist. 2011;16:1658–64.

Ng CG, Boks MP, Smeets HM, Zainal NZ, de Wit NJ. Prescription patterns for psychotropic drugs in cancer patients; a large population study in the Netherlands. Psychooncology. 2013;22: 762–7.

Okamura M, Akizuki N, Nakano T, Shimizu K, Ito T, Akechi T, Uchitomi Y. Clinical experience of the use of a pharmacological treatment algorithm for major depressive disorder in patients with advanced cancer. Psychooncology. 2008;17(2):154–60.

Ouwens M, Hulscher M, Hermens R, Faber M, Marres H, Wollersheim H, Grol R. Implementation of integrated care for patients with cancer: a systematic review of interventions and effects. Int J Qual Health Care. 2009;21:137–44.

Plumb M, Holland J. Comparative studies of psychological function in patients with advanced cancer–I. Self-reported depressive symptoms. Psychosom Med. 1977;39:264–76.

Plumb M, Holland J. Comparative studies of psychological function in patients with advanced cancer. II. Interviewer-rated current and past psychological symptoms. Psychosom Med. 1981; 43:243–54.

Prieto JM, Blanch J, Atala J, Carreras E, Rovira M, Cirera E, Gasto C. Psychiatric morbidity and impact on hospital length of stay among hematologic cancer patients receiving stem-cell transplantation. J Clin Oncol. 2002;20:1907–17.

Raijmakers NJ, van Zuylen L, Costantini M, Caraceni A, Clark JB, De Simone G, Lundquist G, Voltz R, Ellershaw JE, van der Heide A. OPCARE9: Issues and needs in end-of-life decision making: an international modified Delphi study. Palliat Med. 2012;26:947–53.

Rayner L, Price A, Evans A, Valsraj K, Hotopf M, Higginson IJ. Antidepressants for the treatment of depression in palliative care: systematic review and meta-analysis. Palliat Med. 2011a; 25(1):36–51.

Rayner L, Price A, Hotopf M, Higginson IJ. The development of evidence-based European guidelines on the management of depression in palliative cancer care. Eur J Cancer. 2011b;47(5):702–12.

Razavi D, Delvaux N, Farvacques C, Robaye E. Screening for adjustment disorders and major depressive disorders in cancer in-patients. Br J Psychiatry. 1990;156:79–83.

Reis de Oliveira I, Schwartz T, Stahl SM. Integrating psychotherapy and psychopharmacology: a handbook for clinicians. London: Routledge; 2014.

Riechelmann RP, Burman D, Tannock IF, Rodin G, Zimmermann C. Phase II trial of mirtazapine for cancer-related cachexia and anorexia. Am J Hosp Palliat Care. 2010;27:106–10.

Ripamonti C, Santini D, Maranzano E, Berti M, Roila F. on behalf of the ESMO Guidelines Working Group. Management of cancer pain: ESMO clinical practice guidelines. Ann Oncol. 2012; 23(Supplement 7): 139–54

Rodin G, Lloyd N, Katz M, Green E, Mackay JA, Wong RK. Supportive care guidelines group of cancer care Ontario Program in evidence-based care. The treatment of depression in cancer patients: a systematic review. Support Care Cancer. 2007;15(2):123–36.

Singer S, Szalai C, Briest S, Brown A, Dietz A, Einenkel J, Jonas S, Konnopka A, Papsdorf K, Langanke D, Löbner M, Schiefke F, Stolzenburg JU, Weimann A, Wirtz H, König HH, Riedel-Heller S. Co-morbid mental health conditions in cancer patients at working age - prevalence, risk profiles, and care uptake. Psychooncology. 2013. doi:10.1002/pon.3282.

Singer S, Das-Munshi J, Brähler E. Prevalence of mental health conditions in cancer patients in acute care–a meta-analysis. Ann Oncol. 2010;21:925–30.

Stahl SM. Multifunctional drugs: a novel concept for psychopharmacology. CNS Spectr. 2009; 14(2):71–3.

Stahl SM. Psychotherapy as an epigenetic 'drug': psychiatric therapeutics target symptoms linked to malfunctioning brain circuits with psychotherapy as well as with drugs. J Clin Pharm Ther. 2012;37:249–53.

Stahl SM. Stahl's essential psychopharmacology. Neuroscientific basis and practical applications. 4th ed. New York: Cambridge University Press; 2013.

Stiefel FC, Kornblith AB, Holland JC. Changes in the prescription patterns of psychotropic drugs for cancer patients during a 10-year period. Cancer. 1990;65:1048–53.

Sutherland AM. Psychological impact of cancer and its therapy. Med Clin North Am. 1956; 40:705–20.

Sutherland AM. Psychological impact of postoperative cancer. Bull N Y Acad Med. 1957;33: 428–45.

Thekdi SM, Irarrazaval ME, Dunn L. Psychopharmacological interventions. In: Grassi L, Riba M, editors. Clinical psycho-oncology: an international perspective. Chichester: Wiley; 2012. p. 109–26.

Turner J, Zapart S, Pedersen K, Rankin N, Luxford K, Fletcher J, National Breast Cancer Centre, Sydney, Australia, National Cancer Control Initiative, Melbourne. Clinical practice guidelines for the psychosocial care of adults with cancer. Psychooncology. 2005;14:159–73.

Wolf S, Barton D, Kottschade L, Grothey A, Loprinzi C. Chemotherapy-induced peripheral neuropathy: prevention and treatment strategies. Eur J Cancer. 2008;44(11):1507–15.

Kogon MK, Spiegel D. Integration of psychopharmacology with psychotherapy and other psycho-social treatment. In: Grassi L, Riba M, editors. Psychopharmacology in oncology and palliative care: a practical manual. Heidelberg: Springer; 2014.

Caraceni A, Ferrari L. Sedation for psychological distress at the end-of-life. In: Grassi L, Riba M, editors. Psychopharmacology in oncology and palliative care: a practical manual. Heidelberg: Springer; 2014.

General Principles of Psychopharmacological Treatment in Psycho-Oncology

2

Andrew J. Roth and Yesne Alici

Abstract

Understanding the principles of Pharmacokinetics and Pharmacodynamics is extremely important in the psychiatric care of cancer patients. Otherwise the medical milieu can lead to intolerance or ineffectiveness of psychotropic medications. This chapter provides an overview of important basic principles to be aware of when considering the use of psychotropic medications, in terms of how a person absorbs, distributes, metabolizes, and excretes medications, and the effects that medications can have on a patient's body. It is important to also be aware of the effects of drug concentrations and responses on both intended beneficial effects as well as adverse reactions. Awareness of drug–drug interactions, CYP450 interactions, and the effects of compromised body systems will also be discussed in order to help psycho-oncologists understand, prevent, and treat subtherapeutic and toxic dosing of the major psychotropic medications including antidepressants, neuroleptics, anxiolytics and hypnotics, mood stabilizers, and psychostimulants in cancer patients.

A.J. Roth (✉) • Y. Alici
Weill Cornell Medical College, New York, NY, USA

Department of Psychiatry and Behavioral Sciences, Memorial Sloan Kettering Cancer Center, New York, NY, USA
e-mail: rotha@mskcc.org; Aliciy@mskcc.org

L. Grassi and M. Riba (eds.), *Psychopharmacology in Oncology and Palliative Care*,
DOI 10.1007/978-3-642-40134-3_2, © Springer-Verlag Berlin Heidelberg 2014

2.1   Introduction

The eyes of clinically oriented psychiatrists' sometimes glaze over during discussions of pharmacokinetics and pharmacodynamics. The importance of these areas is not often evident in the everyday clinical care of patients with psychiatric syndromes, until a patient has an adverse reaction that may have been prevented if thought through more thoroughly. Understanding these principles is extremely important when taking care of medically ill patients in general, and cancer patients in particular. It is not unusual for a patient's medical milieu to lead to intolerance or ineffectiveness of psychotropic medications. This may be prevented or more easily dealt with, given a better understanding and practice of proper pharmacokinetics and pharmacodynamics. This chapter will provide an overview of the principles of pharmacokinetics and pharmacodynamics with a focus on psychotropic medications commonly used in patients with cancer and in palliative care settings.

2.2   Pharmacokinetics

Pharmacokinetics is simply described as "what the body does to the drug." (Ferrando 2010) See Fig. 2.1.

Bioavailability is the rate and extent of drug delivery to the systemic circulation from the point of administration and depends largely on the route of administration. Intravenous route ensures 100 % bioavailability. See Fig. 2.2.

Most drugs pass through the stomach and are then absorbed in the small intestine. Acid labile drugs may degrade in the stomach before reaching the small intestine. Rates of gastric emptying may slow absorption (such as in diabetes patients with gastroparesis). Gut flora may metabolize drugs, and the gut flora can be altered in various medical settings. See Fig. 2.3.

After medications are absorbed through the small intestine, the process known as the "first pass metabolism" may play a significant role in drug bioavailability to the systemic circulation. First pass metabolism is the transport and metabolism of drugs from the gut lumen to the systemic circulation with the portal vein and liver.

Hepatic first pass metabolism of drugs from the gut to the portal system is limited by:
• P-glycoprotein transport pump that decreases absorption
• Cytochrome P450 3A4 enzymes' metabolism of drugs within the gut wall

---

Bioavailability may be further decreased by hepatic extraction of drugs as they pass through the liver before gaining access to the systemic circulation. Intravenous, sublingual, and topical routes of administration bypass the first pass metabolism and therefore may be preferred in certain patients. Although the rate and extent of rectal absorption is erratic, the first pass metabolism effect could be reduced by about 50 % via this route of drug delivery.

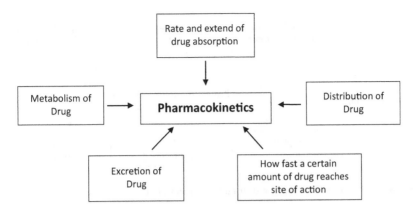

Fig. 2.1 Pharmacokinetics: physiological mechanisms of action on medications

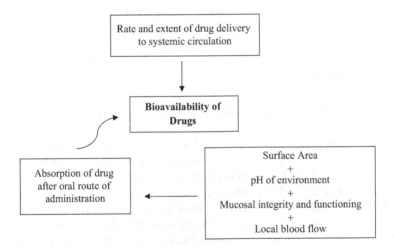

Fig. 2.2 Factors related to the bioavailability of medications

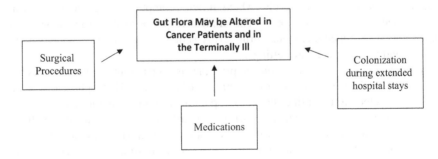

Fig. 2.3 Factors that impact gut metabolism of medications

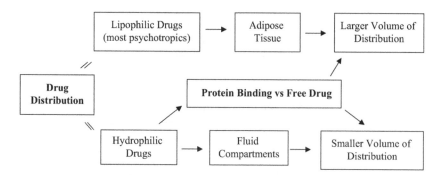

Fig. 2.4 Determinants of volume of distribution of medication

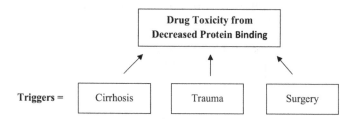

Fig. 2.5 Factors determining impact of protein binding on drug toxicity

Following bioavailability, the second element of pharmacokinetics is *drug distribution*. Volume of distribution (Vd) describes the relationship between the bioavailable dose of the drug and the plasma concentration of the drug. See Fig. 2.4.

Drug distribution is additionally affected by protein binding. Free, or unbound, drug is the pharmacologically active form of the drug. Decreased protein binding can be caused by multiple triggers and lead to drug toxicity. See Fig. 2.5.

An important consideration in treating patients with decreased protein binding is the interpretation of therapeutic drug monitoring. Therapeutic drug monitoring procedures mostly measure total drug levels that could mislead the clinician by suggesting subtherapeutic levels, which might prompt a dosage increase with unintended possible toxic effects. The clinical response to the drug, rather than laboratory determined therapeutic drug levels, should guide dosage in patients with cancer and in palliative care settings.

Drug metabolism and excretion comprise the last step before the drug reaches the site of action. Kidneys are the primary organs of excretion. Hydrophilic drugs are readily excreted through urine and feces. Lipophilic drugs require biotransformation to more hydrophilic compounds, occurring primarily in liver and intestinal wall.

Clinicians are most familiar with cytochrome P450 enzymes due to drug–drug interactions that can take place when drugs are a substrate, an inducer, or an inhibitor of these enzyme systems. Cytochrome P450 enzymes result in oxidation reactions. A small percentage of the population has one or more cytochrome P450 enzymes with significantly altered activity. For example, polymorphisms of the

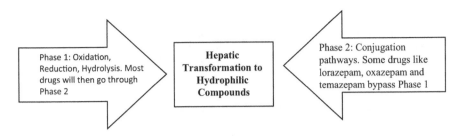

Fig. 2.6 Phase I and phase II effects on liver metabolism of medications

2D6 gene give rise to populations with the capacity to metabolize CYP 2D6 substrates extensively (most commonly), poorly (5–14 % of Caucasians, 1 % of Orientals), or ultra-extensively (1–3 % of the population). These polymorphisms can clearly lead to differences in drug metabolism. The P450 cytochromes CYP1A2, 2C9, 2C19, 2D6, and 3A4 are the most important enzymes for drug metabolism in human beings.

Monoamine oxidases, dehydrogenases, and hydrolysis are the other systems involved in Phase I metabolism. Phase I metabolism may produce active or inactive metabolites. See Fig. 2.6.

Phase II metabolism produces inactive metabolites via conjugation. The only exception to this is morphine-6-glucuronide, an active metabolite of morphine, which is a Phase II metabolite. Lorazepam, oxazepam, and temazepam are the benzodiazepines that primarily go through Phase II metabolism with resultant hydrophilic inactive metabolites and are considered to be safer in patients with hepatic impairment when compared to other benzodiazepines.

Lithium, gabapentin, and pregabalin are essentially excreted unchanged through the kidneys. Dose adjustments are required in patients with renal impairment. Although measurement of the creatinine clearance from serum creatinine is important in the assessment of renal excretion capacity, there may be reduced creatinine production in older patients due to decreased muscle mass resulting in erroneous calculations of the actual glomerular filtration rate. Twenty-four hour urine creatinine measurement is a more reliable indicator of renal function than is serum creatinine in the elderly.

2.3   Pharmacodynamics

The previous section on Pharmacokinetics described how a person absorbs, distributes, metabolizes, and excretes medications. This section on Pharmacodynamics discusses variables leading to both intended beneficial effects as well as undesirable adverse reactions and consequences of medications on the body (Ferrando 2010). See Fig. 2.7.

Some medications produce side effects even at low or subtherapeutic levels, often related to drug–receptor interactions. Some medications will only produce

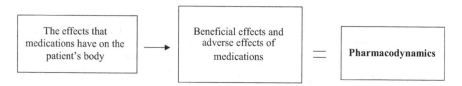

Fig. 2.7 Pharmacodynamics: how medications effect the body's physiology

side effects at higher than therapeutic blood levels, while others produce side effects even at therapeutic levels.

The rule of thumb in the medically ill is to "start low and go slow" with gradual titration of doses, especially with older or debilitated patients; to have as a goal the minimal effective dose of a medication; and to consider giving activating medications in the morning and sedating medication in the evening.

Before starting a psychotropic medication, educate patients about:
• The duration of onset of action and extent of common adverse and therapeutic effects (i.e., gastrointestinal symptoms anxiety, fatigue) and the likelihood of uncommon though popular side effects (i.e., suicidal ideation)
• What to do about missed doses
• The importance of complying with dosage and titration recommendations

We will discuss the effects of serotonin, norepinephrine, and dopamine reuptake blockade of antidepressants; the effects of dopamine 2 blockade of antipsychotics; the antihistaminic effects of antidepressants and antipsychotics; and what the psycho-oncologist should be aware of in terms of how these effects as well as drug interactions and liver function play a role in the cancer setting.

2.3.1 Antidepressants

Reuptake Inhibitors: Selective Serotonin Reuptake Inhibitors
Most of the new generation of antidepressants, both Selective Serotonin Reuptake Inhibitors (SSRIs) and Serotonin Norepinephrine Reuptake Inhibitors (SNRIs), function through serotonergic (5HT) reuptake blockade—SSRIs working primarily on the serotonergic system and SNRIs as well as some of the older tricyclic and MAOI antidepressants working incrementally on the serotonin system with additional norepinephrine reuptake blockade. TCAs are rarely used to treat depression because of their problematic side effect profile (i.e., anticholinergic side effects, cardiac conduction delays, and sedation). MAOIs too are rarely used today because of strict dietary restrictions that may already be burdensome in cancer patients for fear of drug–diet interactions that can cause life-threatening hypertensive crises. There are multiple serotonin receptors in the brain and in the body's periphery responsible for side effects, namely gastric disturbances, anxiety, and in particular sexual dysfunction, which is one of the most common reasons people stop using

antidepressants. Serotonin receptors have also been implicated in extrapyramidal side effects, in particular akathisia, which leads to significant subjective distress. Additionally an overabundance of serotonin either from overdosages or combinations of serotonergic medications and/or Monoamine Oxidase Inhibitors (MAOIs) can cause a serotonin syndrome, a life-threatening disorder (Sternbach 1991).

Serotonin syndrome is Herald by:
• Agitation
• Mental Status Changes
• Myoclonus
• Hyperreflexia
• Diaphoresis
• Fever

Medications and substances that can cause serotonin syndrome

SSRIs
Meperidine
SNRIs
Sumatriptan
MAOIs, including procarbazine
Lithium
TCAs
Buspirone
Linezolid
Lysergic acid diethylamide (LSD)
Fentanyl
MDMA (3,4-methylenedioxy-N-methylamphetamine) Ecstasy
Tramadol

Reuptake Inhibitors: Serotonin Norepinephrine Reuptake Inhibitors

Medications like SNRIs and tricyclic antidepressants (TCAs) which block reuptake of norepinephrine are often used to treat neuropathic pain syndromes, often showing more efficacy with more balanced serotonin: norepinephrine ratios. For instance, the S:N ratio for duloxetine is about 10:1 and considered a better SNRI analgesic medication, than venlafaxine whose S:N is about 30:1. Side effects may include tremors, tachycardia, erectile and ejaculatory dysfunction, and augmentation of pressor effects of sympathomimetic amines.

Norepinephrine reuptake blockade pros and cons

Pros	Cons
Improves mood	Tremors
Treats neuropathic pain	Tachycardia, hypertension
	Erectile and ejaculatory dysfunction

Reuptake Inhibitors: Dopamine

Bupropion is the only antidepressant that works primarily as a dopamine reuptake blocker. Its side effect profile can be helpful in people with slowed down depressions as dopamine blockade offers a stimulating, or activating, effect. However this can overshoot into uncomfortable side effects. Bupropion is the only antidepressant that does not cause any sexual side effects (Mirtazapine causes fewer sexual side effects than SSRIs and SNRIs but still more than bupropion).

Bupropion (dopamine reuptake inhibitor) pros and cons

Pros	Cons
Improves mood	May cause uncomfortable anxiety, agitation, and insomnia
Smoking cessation	May aggravate psychotic symptoms
Stimulating or activating effect (counter fatigue)	May lower seizure threshold
Does NOT cause any sexual side effects	

Other important receptor interactions of antidepressants include antihistaminic effects often seen with the tricyclic antidepressants, MAOIs, and some of the SSRIs. This problematic and uncomfortable side effect profile includes sedation, hypotension, and weight gain and has led to the disuse of many of these antidepressants. Dosing at night may prevent daytime sleepiness, however with nighttime awakenings, falls can occur. The newer antidepressants most likely to cause weight gain are mirtazapine and paroxetine. It was originally thought that medications like mirtazapine that caused increased appetite and secondary weight gain would be ideal for a cancer population. Though it is often used when patients have decreased appetite and weight loss, anecdotally it does not appear to consistently stimulate appetite and weight gain for all patients. Most of the SSRI's and SNRI's are weight neutral.

The TCAs, MAOIs, and some SSRIs like paroxetine have anticholinergic effects, which can be uncomfortable and can be a primary reason for patient noncompliance. Anticholinergic side effects are caused by blockage of muscarinic or nicotinic acetylcholine receptors. These complications are particularly unpleasant for cancer patients who may already have a significant burden from other medications.

The problems with anticholinergic side effects:
• Cognitive impairment or delirium
• Increased body temperature
• Blurred Vision; dilated pupils
• Dry mouth, eyes, decreased sweating
• Flushed face
• Increased heart rate
• Constipation
• Urinary retention

An occasional upside of the anticholinergic effects of antidepressants such as amitriptyline, imipramine, and clomipramine is their use in patients with irritable bowel syndrome or in patients whose gastric side effects make other antidepressants prohibitive. Antihistamines like diphenhydramine and hydroxyzine may have uncomfortable anticholinergic effects as well, making concomitant use with similarly acting antidepressants prohibitive.

Medications that have anti-α1 adrenergic effects can prevent smooth muscle contraction, leading to orthostatic hypotension when patients move from reclining to sitting or sitting to standing positions. These side effects can also lead to dizziness and a compensatory tachycardia. Like anticholinergic side effects, these anti-α1 adrenergic effects were a major problem with the older, less used TCAs and MAOIs. It is good for younger generation psychiatrists to know why the current collection of common antidepressants is so much more patient friendly, given their more expensive prices even for generic usage in poorer countries.

Drug Interactions can lead to problematic effects for cancer patients. Drug interactions are caused by the combined adverse effects of medications taken together; impaired or enhanced drug metabolism; net therapeutic indices of combined medications; alterations in protein binding due to liver disease or cachexia; half-lives of combined medications; and concomitant organ system disease.

As noted earlier, most psychotropic drugs are highly protein bound. This means that they may displace other protein bound drugs, e.g., warfarin, and they are not dialyzable in overdose. Half-life significance may vary greatly with various antidepressants. Four to five half-lives are required to reach steady state, and a similar amount of time is required for the drug to clear the circulation. Fluoxetine has the longest half-life of the newer antidepressants, because it is broken down into its active metabolite norfluoxetine, whose half-life is 7–10 days. On the one hand it allows forgiveness if a patient does not take the medication daily. On the other hand if there is a reason to stop the medication because of a problem like SIADH or akathisia, it will take a while for the medication to be cleared. Drugs with shorter half-lives include venlafaxine, bupropion, sertraline, paroxetine and mirtazapine. These medications will disappear from the circulation faster if they need to be stopped due to an adverse drug interaction. Unfortunately, this attribute also predisposes to drug discontinuation syndrome or withdrawal symptoms if the medication is stopped abruptly; this syndrome may be quite uncomfortable, though it is not dangerous, as is withdrawal from benzodiazepines. The syndrome often consists of a flu-like syndrome (lethargy, dysphoria, anxiety and restlessness, insomnia, dizziness, and nausea).

There are many clinical examples of problematic drug–drug interactions in the cancer setting. Interactions that raise the dose of either the psychotropic or chemotherapeutic agent require us to be aware of possible toxicity and side effects even at usual doses; lower than usual starting doses and slower than usual titration periods would be prudent. For instance, the use of the chemotherapy agent procarbazine, an MAOI, has often been avoided with antidepressants because of concern of serotonin syndrome or hypertensive reaction; a recent retrospective review counters such caution (Kraft et al. 2014).

Cytochrome P450 System Interactions

The number of potential interactions between medications metabolized by the CYP P450 system, where most psychotropic medications are metabolized, is vast. Using reference charts regularly that can easily be found online is a good practice. Experience with potentially clinically important interactions is invaluable. Drugs may be substrates, inhibitors, or inducers of the cytochrome p450 enzymes. Sometimes, medications can be both substrates and inhibitors. It is important to remember that all patients are not the same and there can be clinically important genetic differences. The most important p450 cytochromes for psychotropic medications are: 2D6, 3A4, 1A2, 2C9, 2C19.

Useful Rules of Thumb

Clinicians working with cancer patients need to have a high degree of vigilance when prescribing psychotropic medications. The more medications a patient is on, the more awareness is suggested. Many drug–drug interaction tables and computer programs are available at the bedside today on smart phones. Get your thumbs moving and use them! Be aware that some medications may have more than one metabolic pathway or interact differently with different competing medications. High-risk situations include older patients with multiple medical comorbidities who are on multiple medications; low therapeutic indices of some of the medications on board; and patients who are not compliant with their drug regimens, either because of cognitive deficits or substance abuse.

The 3A3,4 cytochrome P450 isoenzymes are the most abundant of these liver enzymes. They can be associated with fatal arrhythmias in some cases (e.g., terfenadine, astemizole, cisapride). Fluoxetine and fluvoxamine are the most likely antidepressants to interact with these CYPs. 3A3,4 substrates include the antidepressants sertraline, citalopram, escitalopram, and mirtazapine. Other 3A4 substrate medications often used in the cancer setting are methadone, morphine, and some steroids. The wakefulness agent modafinil can interact with ketoconazole, used as an antiandrogen in men with prostate cancer. This can cause anxiety and other side effects. A new medication that inhibits biosynthesis of testosterone in the testes, adrenal glands, and prostate tumor tissues, abiraterone, can interact at the 2D6 and C3A4 isoenzymes, as an inhibitor and as a substrate, respectively. Some antidepressant levels may subsequently increase, causing toxicity.

The most common CYP enzyme for psychotropics is the CYP 2D6, where there is critical genetic polymorphism. Enzyme inhibitors will lead to "Poor metabolizers," and inducers will lead to "rapid metabolizers." Polymorphism can be found in 5–14 % of Caucasians and African Americans and 1 % of Asians. CYP 2D6 antidepressant substrates include SSRIs fluoxetine, paroxetine, and the SNRI venlafaxine as well as the TCAs (amitriptyline, imipramine, nortriptyline, and desipramine). In the last few years there has been controversial yet inconsistent interpretation of findings that antidepressants with Cyp 450 2D6 inhibition can block the metabolism of the breast cancer hormonal agent, tamoxifen, to its active metabolite endoxifen, decreasing its effectiveness to prevent recurrence of the cancer (Henry et al. 2008).

Body Systems

Another way to look at pharmacodynamics is to consider which psychotropics will lead to a higher effective dose in a particular body system, thus increasing susceptibility to complications, either because of their inherent ability to affect that system or because of a drug interaction.

The cardiovascular system is vulnerable to TCAs because of the combination of receptor system interactions including anticholinergic-induced tachycardia, antiadrenergic-induced orthostatic hypotension, quinidine-like anti-arrhythmias, as well as intraventricular conduction delays. Thus with patients who have prolonged QRS, QTc, or bundle branch blocks, extreme caution should be maintained if using TCAs. There has been recent concern about using higher doses of citalopram because of QTc prolongation. SSRI's are otherwise safe cardiologically as is bupropion. Venlafaxine can cause dose-dependent hypertension, especially in its immediate release formulation.

SSRIs have been found to cause decreased *platelet aggregation* and may lead to aberrant prothrombin (PT), INR, and bleeding times. The risk for patients already vulnerable to bleeding (i.e., those already being treated with medications that have anticoagulant properties or those with low platelets) may be more at risk. More frequent monitoring of PT and bleeding times may be needed when starting SSRIs or changing doses. Discontinuing an SSRI prior to surgery may be beneficial if there is an increased bleeding time or PT.

More often SSRIs and SNRIs have *intestinal* mucosal 5-HT3 receptor binding with increases in GI motility causing gastric upset with diarrhea and abdominal pain. Some patients will become constipated with these medications.

For the most part, antidepressants do not have significant *renal* clearance, so dose adjustments are not needed. Patients with *hepatic* disease may be prone to subclinical encephalopathy. Those sedating medications that can affect cognition such as the TCAs should be monitored carefully. Medications that are highly protein bound will be more displaced. This is less likely with venlafaxine which is less protein bound. Sertraline, citalopram, and escitalopram may be SSRIs of choice in patients with hepatic dysfunction because of their minimal CYP interactive profiles. The 5HT3 blocking effects of mirtazapine make it a strong antiemetic and is useful for patients experiencing nausea from chemotherapy regimens or directly from the cancer. Mirtazapine's antihistaminic effect helps make it a good sedating and sleeping agent to assist people who have insomnia. It may cause fewer sexual side effects than other SSRI's and SNRIs.

2.3.2   Antipsychotics

Antipsychotics treat psychotic symptoms such as hallucinations and delusions by blocking mesolimbic dopamine pathways. They are used most often in the cancer setting to treat patients with delirium. Through dopamine deprivation antipsychotics may cause parkinsonian symptoms such as extrapyramidal side effects,

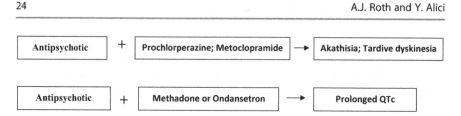

Fig. 2.8 Drug interactions to be watchful for with antipsychotic medications

including cogwheeling, masked facies, shuffling gait, and akathisia. They may also cause hyperprolactinemia and sexual dysfunction.

Antihistaminic effects, anticholinergic effects, and anti-α1 adrenergic effects may be seen with lower potency neuroleptics used in the cancer setting for delirium as we saw with the TCAs. Many of the atypical and lower potency antipsychotics are prone to causing unwanted weight gain in people without medical illnesses with longer-term use. Higher potency antipsychotics may cause parkinsonian symptoms because of their impact on dopamine receptors particularly in the basal ganglia. Most typical antipsychotics can cause dystonia, tardive dyskinesia, and neuroleptic malignant syndrome. The atypical antipsychotics are less likely to cause tardive dyskinesia and dystonias; however, they can cause metabolic syndromes and weight gain over time, causing concern about development of diabetes. Anecdotal experience of using atypical antipsychotics, such as olanzapine in cancer patients for short-term treatment of delirium, has found no significant changes in fasting blood sugar or body weight. Long-term use of neuroleptics is not common in the cancer population, unless a patient has an underlying primary psychiatric disorder such as schizophrenia or bipolar disorder.

Drug Interactions with antipsychotics often lead to exacerbation of common side effect of sedation, Parkinsonism, and akathisia. See Fig. 2.8.

Cytochrome P450 In general, neuroleptics are not involved meaningfully in P450 interactions. Haloperidol and risperidone are 2D6 substrates, so their concentrations may be increased or decreased by inhibitors or inducers.

Cardiovascular In recent years, all antipsychotics have received warnings for potential cardiovascular effects. It has long been known that haloperidol could cause a Torsades de Pointes arrhythmia. Concern for prolonged QTc intervals and life-threatening arrhythmias has increased, though there are still no clear guidelines other than to monitor for QTc prolongation regularly. Concern arises when the QTc interval exceeds 450 ms. Discontinuation of antipsychotics should be considered if the QTc exceeds 500 ms.

Another cardiovascular warning for neuroleptics involves their use with older people who have dementia. There is concern for an increased risk of cardio-vascular-related death. A retrospective, exploratory, secondary analysis of the association between antipsychotic use and mortality in elderly patients with delirium found that administration of antipsychotics was not associated with a statistically significant increased risk of mortality (Elie et al. 2009). Attention to other medications in the cancer setting that can also prolong QTc intervals, such as methadone, olanzapine, and tricyclics, is suggested, while monitoring EKG QTc regularly.

A Cochrane review (Lonergan et al. 2007) found that despite the risks associated with antipsychotic drugs, there is insufficient evidence to suggest that psychotropics other than antipsychotics represent an effective, safer, or better treatment choice for psychosis or agitation in dementia (or delirium).

Hepatic Phenothiazine neuroleptics have been known to cause hepatic toxicity; liver functions should be monitored accordingly. Though other neuroleptics are not known to cause significant hepatic problems, liver functions should be monitored periodically and lower doses considered with compromised liver function. *Renal* toxicity from neuroleptics is rare.

Neuroleptic Malignant Syndrome is a rare complication of neuroleptic use marked by a sudden decrease in dopamine activity.

Signs of neuroleptic malignant syndrome:
• A sudden decrease in dopamine activity
• Fever
• Muscle rigidity
• Autonomic instability
• Confusion
• Increase Creatine Phosphokinase
• Increase white blood cell count
• Myoglobinuria

A rapid increase in dosage and longer acting formulations of medication may increase risk. This is a life-threatening entity and should be treated as a medical emergency. Neuroleptics should be discontinued with the consideration of intensive medical support and the use of dopaminergic agents.

2.3.3 Sedative Hypnotics

The sedative hypnotic medications are used to decrease anxiety and improve sleep. Benzodiazepines are the most common type of drug in this class. They increase the efficiency of synaptic transmission of the neurotransmitter GABA. The resulting increase in the concentration of Cl- ions in the postsynaptic neuron immediately hyperpolarizes this neuron, thus making it less excitable. There is a relatively rapid onset of effectiveness. The lipophilic nature of benzodiazepines allows for quick entry into the brain. Benzodiazepines give relatively fast relief of anxiety and periodic panic attacks. These medications also help improve insomnia, control seizures, act as muscle relaxants, relieve akathisia, and treat alcohol withdrawal.

These medications are best used in acute crisis situations rather than for long-term treatment.

The pros of benzodiazepines:
• Fast acting anxiolytics for many anxiety syndromes
• Relieves panic attacks
• Treats phobic symptoms (i.e., MRI scans, awaiting test results)
• Relieves akathisia caused by other medications such as antiemetics
• Controls agitation during acute manic and psychotic episodes in medical settings
• Treats alcohol withdrawal

Just as with alcohol, benzodiazepines can lead to excess drowsiness; impaired coordination; impaired concentration; toxicity in vulnerable, frail patients like the elderly, which can lead to falls; paradoxical anxiety and agitation; and amnesia which may be welcome during chemotherapy sessions. Medications with longer half-lives (i.e., clonazepam) decrease the potential for end-of-dose rebound anxiety, but they may lead to accumulation and potential for confusion and falls. The likelihood of withdrawal from longer acting medications is less than with shorter acting drugs. The shorter acting medications like alprazolam on the other hand will not accumulate over time, causing less daytime sedation and cognitive impairment, but they often cause interdose rebound of anxiety symptoms and may require more frequent dosing, potentially leading to medication abuse.

Lorazepam has been found to help with chemotherapy-related nausea and is thus frequently used as an adjunct antiemetic in the cancer setting. Benzodiazepines may also induce amnesia and sometimes make a difficult experience like chemotherapy easier to deal with.

Long-term use of benzodiazepines can lead to physical dependence and dangerous withdrawal syndrome when discontinued abruptly, whether they are used for anxiety or chemotherapy-related nausea. The importance of tapering the medication should be explained to patients. Benzodiazepines can also cause physical tolerance, leading to a patient requiring higher doses over time. They rarely cause psychological addiction in the cancer setting. Older patients and those with impaired cognition may experience confusion. These medications can also cause respiratory compromise and should therefore be used with caution in those already having respiratory difficulties. Some patients complain of headaches. Clinicians should be aware of the interactions with alcohol and other CNS depressants, which can cause cognitive problems and sedation.

CYP P450

Some benzodiazepines may have a reduced half-life with hepatic inducers such as phenytoin and barbiturates. Benzodiazepines that rely on glucuronidation (e.g., lorazepam, oxazepam, and temazepam) are less vulnerable to drug–drug interactions with hepatic failure or metabolic inhibition of Cytochrome p450 enzymes; however, caution should be used with these drugs in patients with renal compromise.

Non-benzodiazepines used for insomnia include zolpidem, zaleplon, and eszopiclone, which work via the GABA system, and ramelteon which works on the melatonin system. The biggest pharmacodynamic concern for these medications is interactions with other sedating medications that can cause cognitive dysfunction if awakened, and falls. Hallucinations and sleepwalking have been reported.

2.3.4 Psychostimulants

Psychostimulants are useful medications in cancer patients. They work on the dopaminergic system and are relatively fast acting, compared with the antidepressants.

Psychostimulants in the cancer setting are useful for:
• Treating opioid related fatigue or cognitive slowing
• Fatigue related to chemotherapy or hormonal therapy
• Fast relief of depressive symptoms for those near the end of life
• Combining with an antidepressant to speed mood improvement

They can relieve depressive symptoms in people nearing the end of life who cannot wait an extended time for mood elevation. They can be used either alone or in combination with an SSRI or an SNRI while the antidepressant begins to work. Side effects at low doses include anxiety, insomnia, tachycardia, euphoria, and mood lability, especially when used in combination with other medications that can cause similar effects. High doses and long-term use may produce nightmares, insomnia, tics, and paranoia. Patients should be cardiologically and neurologically stable without a history of arrhythmias or seizures before starting on a stimulant, as these disorders can be exacerbated by these stimulants.

Modafinil and armodafinil are gentler wakefulness agents, are usually good drugs for frail, debilitated patients. Many patients who cannot tolerate the potentially harsher side effects of the more traditional psychostimulants such as methylphenidate and amphetamine, or who may not be able to take them because of a history of cardiac arrhythmia or seizures, may benefit from these gentler stimulants. Modafinil can have p450 3A4 interactions with medications like ketoconazole and abiraterone.

2.3.5 Mood Stabilizers

In the cancer setting, acute mood stabilization is attained with the newer atypical antipsychotic medications such as olanzapine or quetiapine or with a combination of haloperidol and a benzodiazepine like lorazepam. These medications can bring rapid relief to agitation and high energy states caused by manic exacerbations of bipolar disorder or by medications like the corticosteroids. Patients who have been receiving lithium carbonate for bipolar affective disorder prior to developing cancer should be maintained on the agent throughout cancer treatment, although close monitoring is necessary when the intake of fluids and electrolytes is restricted, such as during preoperative, postoperative, and bone marrow or stem cell transplant periods. The maintenance dose of lithium may have to be reduced in seriously ill patients. Lithium should be prescribed with caution in patients receiving cisplatin or other potentially nephrotoxic drugs. Thyroid function tests should be monitored regularly. Impaired renal function will reduce lithium clearance, increasing toxicity. Caution should be taken with patients who have cognitive deficits as chronic lithium administration can cause impaired concentration capacity (nephrogenic diabetes insipidus). If needed, hemodialysis will remove lithium rapidly.

Use of carbamazepine as a mood stabilizer can be problematic in cancer patients because of its bone marrow-suppressing properties. As with physically healthy people, valproic acid in cancer patients may cause gastric distress, liver function problems, and sedation. These medications can have a synergistic sedating effect when used with other potentially sedating medications such as central nervous system depressants.

Conclusion

Psycho-oncologists have a unique role to play in providing psychopharmacologic interventions for the distressing psychiatric syndromes or disorders experienced by cancer patients that are not amenable or fully treated by psychotherapy. Psychotropic medications are selected based on the specific symptom clusters (if not the full disorder), the side effect profile of the medication, drug–drug interactions, and the pharmacokinetic factors (including the changes in lean body mass, total body fat, hepatic functioning, and creatinine clearance) that dictate the body's response to the drug. Psycho-oncology clinicians should therefore be familiar with the basic principles of psychopharmacology that includes familiarity with the basics of pharmacokinetics and pharmacodynamics. As reviewed in this chapter, it is of utmost importance for psycho-oncology clinicians to vigilantly take into consideration the fine balance between "creative psychopharmacology" and "primum non nocere," the "do no harm" principal in treating cancer patients.

Clinical Case

A 78-year-old man with primary central nervous lymphoma presents to the psychiatry outpatient clinic, referred by his oncologist, for assessment and management of depression. The patient completed chemotherapy and whole brain radiation about 6 months prior and has been in remission since. He also has benign prostate hypertrophy (BPH), chronic hepatitis C, chronic renal insufficiency with a creatinine of 1.6 to 1.8, atrial fibrillation, and orthostatic hypotension. His presentation is consistent with mood disorder due to general medical condition with depressive features. The primary sources of distress are fatigue, anhedonia, depressed mood, poor concentration, and apathy.

The psycho-oncology clinician should take into consideration at the very least the following before initiating treatment for depressive symptoms with antidepressants or psychostimulants:

1. Attention to pharmacokinetics:
   (a) Calculate the creatinine clearance for dose adjustments
   (b) Dose adjustments may be required based on patient's lean body mass.
   (c) Evaluate liver functioning for dose adjustments and to avoid medications that undergo significant hepatic metabolism in the presence of hepatic impairment.
2. Attention to pharmacodynamics:
   (a) Review the medication list for drug–drug interactions (warfarin and SSRIs.
   (b) Stay away from medications that lower seizure threshold or may exacerbate arrhythmias.
   (c) Stay away from medications with anticholinergic side effects due to risk of urinary retention (BPH) and due to risk of worsening cognitive symptoms.
   (d) Stay away from medications that might exacerbate orthostatic hypotension.

▶ **Key Points**

Pharmacokinetics is simply described as "what the body does to the drug," or how a person absorbs, distributes, metabolizes, and excretes medications.

Pharmacodynamics are the effects that medications can have on the patient's body and the effects of drug concentrations and responses on both intended beneficial effects as well as adverse reactions.

Understanding pharmacodynamics of drug–drug interactions, CYP450 interactions, and the effects of compromised body systems such as hepatic, renal, and cardiovascular systems will help psycho-oncologists understand, prevent, and treat subtherapeutic and toxic dosing of the major psychotropic medications including antidepressants, neuroleptics, anxiolytics and hypnotics, mood stabilizers, and psychostimulants in cancer patients.

Understand pharmacokinetics and pharmacodynamics and improve your ability to "primum non nocere," "do no harm."

Suggested Further Reading

- Braun I, Pirl W. Psychotropic medications in cancer care. In: Holland et al. (eds.), Psycho-Oncology. 2nd ed. Oxford University Press; 2010. p. 378–85.
- Breitbart W, Alici Y. Evidence-based treatment of delirium in patients with cancer. J Clin Oncol. 2012;30(11):1206–14.
- Breitbart W, Alici Y. Psychostimulants for cancer-related fatigue. J Natl Compr Canc Netw. 2010;8(8):933–42.
- Ferrando SJ, Levenson JL, Owen JA. Clinical manual of psychopharmacology in the medically Ill. Washington, DC: APPI; 2010.
- Brunton LL, Chabner BA, Knollmann BC. Goodman & Gilman's, The pharmacological basis of therapeutics. 12th ed. New York: Mc Graw Hill Education; 2011.

References

Elie M, Boss K, Cole MG, McCusker J, Belzile E, Ciampi A. A retrospective, exploratory, secondary analysis of the association between antipsychotic use and mortality in elderly patients with delirium. Int Psychogeriatr. 2009;21(3):588–92.

Ferrando SJ, Levenson JL, Owen JA. Clinical manual of psychopharmacology in 582 the medically ill. Washington, DC: APPI; 2010.

Henry NL, Stearns V, Flockhart DA, Hayes DF, Riba M. Drug interactions and pharmacogenomics in the treatment of breast cancer and depression. Am J Psychiatry. 2008;165(10):1251–5.

Kraft SL, Baker NM, Carpenter J, Bostwick JR. Procarbazine and antidepressants: a retrospective review of the risk of serotonin toxicity. Psychooncology. 2014;23(1):108–13.

Lonergan E, Britton AM, Luxenberg J, Wyller T. Antipsychotics for delirium. Cochrane Database Syst Rev. 2007;2, CD005594.

Sternbach H. The serotonin syndrome. Am J Psychiatry. 1991;148:705–13.

Diagnostic Issues

3

Luigi Grassi, Maria Giulia Nanni, and Michelle Riba

Abstract

The chapter provides a summary of the main issues related to the assessment of the psychological reactions and/or psychopathological disorders in oncology and palliative care. A careful psychiatric interview and a proper mental status examination (MSE) are the means by which a psychiatric diagnosis is made, as a mandatory step when prescribing psychotropic drugs. During the assessment, a detailed description and evaluation of the emotional and behavioral signs and symptoms indicative of a psychiatric disturbance should be carried out. Several other variables need also to be considered (e.g., attachment styles, coping, defense mechanisms, stressful life events, social support) in order to fully understand the patient's status. Furthermore, a definite assessment of the patient's physical functioning and the general medical condition, in liaison with the healthcare professionals, is a necessary component of the psychiatric diagnostic process. The Diagnostic and Statistical Manual for Mental Disorders (DSM-5) and the International Classification of Diseases (ICD-10) are the most common taxonomic systems to classify psychiatric disorders. Changes in the diagnostic criteria, especially with regard to the rubrics of adjustment disorders, depressive disorders, somatic symptom disorders, and psychological factors affecting a medical condition, have however been proposed when the DSM or the ICD are applied in oncology and palliative care settings. The

L. Grassi (✉) • M.G. Nanni
Institute of Psychiatry, Department of Biomedical and Specialty Surgical Sciences, University of Ferrara, Ferrara, Italy
e-mail: luigi.grassi@unife.it; mariagiulia.nanni@unife.it

M. Riba
Department of Psychiatry, University of Michigan, Ann Arbor, MI, USA

Director, Psycho-Onclology Program, University of Michigan Comprehensive Cancer Center, Ann Arbor, MI, USA
e-mail: mriba@med.umich.edu

Diagnostic Criteria for Psychosomatic Research (DCPR) are useful for a more precise identification of psychosocial conditions affecting cancer patients, including health anxiety, demoralization, and somatic symptom presentation of distress. A psychosomatic integrative approach is thus necessary in the psychiatric diagnostic process.

3.1   Introduction

The evaluation of the psychological reactions and/or psychopathological disorders in response to cancer and related treatment is a main aim of clinical work in psycho-oncology.

As in general psychiatry, in psycho-oncology the distinction between symptoms (the subjective complain of the patient) and signs (the indicator of a specific disease observed during the examination) is not easy, since both are elicited during the encounter and the conversation with the patient and are contained in what the patient expresses to the examiner (descriptive evaluation) (Sims 2012). Furthermore, the issues related to the medical condition are always to be determined as possible concomitant causes of the patient's disorder (explanatory evaluation).

Also, the distinction between acceptable and normal (healthy, physiological) experiences and abnormal (unhealthy, pathological) experiences may be complicated in the psycho-oncology diagnostic process. Both the Diagnostic and Statistical Manual for Mental Disorders (DSM) (2013) and the International Classification of Diseases (ICD) (2010), which are the most common taxonomic systems of psychiatric classification, use a broad definition of a mental disorder: "a clinically recognizable set of symptoms or behavior associated in most cases with distress and with interference with personal function" (ICD-10) or "a syndrome characterized by clinically significant disturbance in an individual's cognition, emotion regulation or behavior" reflecting a psychobiological dysfunction and causing "significant distress or disability in social, occupational, or other important activities" (DSM-5). Examining these aspects in patients that are facing serious life challenges and conditions threatening their lives and affecting their future in profound ways is a special challenge in psychiatry in medicine and it needs possible reformulation of diagnostic approaches (McHugh and Clark 2006). As indicated elsewhere (Grassi 2013; Grassi and Nanni 2013) and in Chap. 1 of this book, a diagnostic process in oncology and palliative care cannot be complete if all the several dimensions of the cancer patient (physical or *ümwelt*; the individual psychological or *eigenwelt*; the interpersonal or *mitwelt*; and spiritual dimensions or *überwelt*) are not taken into account. The aim of this chapter is to summarize some of the most significant issues in the psychiatric diagnostic process of cancer patients when psychopharmacological treatment is indicated.

3.2   Psychiatric Interview and Examination

In the encounter with the cancer patient, setting a proper framework for conducting the psychiatric evaluation of the patient's mental state is the most important part of the diagnostic process.

The psychiatric evaluation has several aims (APA 2006), such as establishing whether a psychiatric disorder or other condition requiring clinical psychiatric/psychosocial attention is present; collecting data to support the differential diagnosis and a comprehensive clinical formulation; collaborating with the patient to develop an initial treatment plan and fostering treatment adherence; and to evaluate the change of symptoms and mental state across time, according to the intervention prescribed. In the specific setting of psycho-oncology, however, as well as of consultation-liaison psychiatry (Smith et al. 2011), the process of the assessment should also consider other issues. First, the liaison with referring physicians and the multidisciplinary team is extremely important. Information of all the possible aspects of the medical disease and its treatment, review of the patient's chart and medical document, and information from the staff and healthcare providers should be gathered. Secondly, when proposing a psychopharmacological intervention for established psychiatric disorders (e.g., delirium), the engagement of the patient and the family, as well as the oncology or palliative care staff, is usually the rule both for the immediate treatment and for further assessment in follow-up care. Psycho-pharmacological intervention for other disorders (e.g., depression, stress-related disorders) and integrated care (i.e., psychological intervention and rehabilitation, referred in this book as *psychopharmoncology*) may be provided by other multi-disciplinary teams as part of the hospital care, or from the community health care or the palliative care systems (Grassi et al. 2013b; Turner 2010; Loscalzo and von Gunten 2009).

3.2.1   Psychiatric Interview and Mental State Examination

Establishing a rapport and creating a good atmosphere in the relationship with the patient (and the family) are the cornerstones of the examination and the framework in which the interview should be conducted. The main aspects of communication, exploration, validation, and empathic understanding are provided in another chapter in this book (Baile et al. 2014, Chap. 5).

The steps and the areas to be covered by the psychiatric interview are summarized in Table 3.1. Likewise psychosomatic medicine (Groves and Muskin 2011), psychiatric interview, and mental state examination in psycho-oncology must consider a series of variables that should be evaluated in order to differentiate possible abnormal and maladaptive from normal and adaptive aspects of the psychological and behavioral response of the patient affected by cancer (Spencer et al. 1998) (Fig. 3.1).

Attachment style is an example of a significant area to be explored in consultation settings in oncology and palliative care, since the way in which the patient

Table 3.1 Psychiatric interview in oncology settings

Medical area

- Cancer history: Diagnosis, phase, stage, type of past and current treatment, side effects
- Other medical disorders other than cancer
- Physical status: Current physical symptoms (e.g., pain, sleep, appetite and eating problems, fatigue, vegetative symptoms); performance status and functioning

Psychiatric area

- Present psychiatric condition
  - Patient chief complaint and its duration; reason for seeking evaluation by the patient and other involved (e.g., family, healthcare professionals)
  - Symptoms experienced by the patient (e.g., anxiety, worries; depression, suspicions; delusions, hallucinatory experiences; changes in sleep, concentration, memory; suicidal or aggressive behaviors); severity and duration of the symptoms)
- Past psychiatric history
  - Previous episodes of psychopathology or psychiatric disorder; nature and diagnosis; duration; precipitating or aggravating factors; treatment received (psychopharmacology: dose of drugs, efficacy, side effects, treatment duration, adherence; psychotherapy: type, duration, adherence)
  - History of suicide attempts or aggressive behaviors
  - History of alcohol and other substance use (type, quantity, frequency of use, pattern and route of use, tolerance or withdrawal symptoms)
  - Previous psychiatric hospitalization
- Personal and interpersonal history
  - Individual psychological development
  - Functioning (family, sexuality, work, interpersonal relationships)
  - Cultural, religious, and spiritual beliefs
  - Life events (most important events in the patient's life; traumatic experiences or adversities)
  - Coping styles (i.e., individual styles in dealing with life events, with particular emphasis to the stress of cancer
  - Social support (i.e., support from close and diffuse interpersonal bonds; nature, quantity, density, and quality of the available support)
- Family history
  - History of psychiatric disorders in the family members
  - History of alcohol or drug abuse
  - History of suicide or violent behavior

has experienced early relations with caregiving figures in the past relates to her view of herself and to the expectation she has from the healthcare provider (or healthcare system). In medically ill patients, Maunder and Hunter (2009, 2012) have described four possible patterns of attachment, namely secure, preoccupied, dismissing, and fearful, which are related to illness behavior, healthcare relationships, and health outcomes (Hunter and Maunder 2001). In the setting of palliative care, Tan et al. (2005) have described the importance of attachment processes as critically important determinants of therapeutic relationships, particularly when the aims of clinicians are to improve the quality of life of patients and to address the suffering that encompasses the physical, psychosocial, and spiritual realms of individuals' and families' experiences with terminal illness. Coping, as

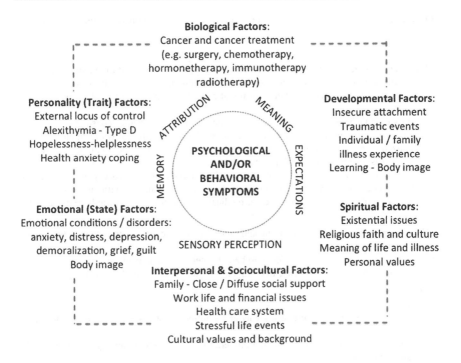

Personality (Trait) Factors:
External locus of control
Alexithymia - Type D
Hopelessness-helplessness
Health anxiety coping

Biological Factors:
Cancer and cancer treatment
(e.g. surgery, chemotherapy,
hormonetherapy, immunotherapy
radiotherapy)

Developmental Factors:
Insecure attachment
Traumatic events
Individual / family
illness experience
Learning - Body image

ATTRIBUTION   MEANING

MEMORY   PSYCHOLOGICAL
AND/OR
BEHAVIORAL
SYMPTOMS   EXPECTATIONS

SENSORY PERCEPTION

Emotional (State) Factors:
Emotional conditions / disorders:
anxiety, distress, depression,
demoralization, grief, guilt
Body image

Spiritual Factors:
Existential issues
Religious faith and culture
Meaning of life and illness
Personal values

Interpersonal & Sociocultural Factors:
Family - Close / Diffuse social support
Work life and financial issues
Health care system
Stressful life events
Cultural values and background

Fig. 3.1 Possible variables involved in determining psychological and behavioral symptoms and needing to be examined

the pattern of thoughts, beliefs, and behaviors in response to stressful events, should also be always examined in cancer patients in a longitudinal manner (Greer and Watson 1987). In the psycho-oncology literature, the relationship of coping styles with psychological disorders has been studied in detail, with data showing that certain styles of coping are maladaptive and are associated with maladjustment to illness and are intrinsically related to psychopathology. Defense mechanisms, as automatic, intrapsychic psychological processes by which the mind deals with psychological threats or conflicts between wishes and the reality, can also inform the physician about that particular patient, explaining his/her emotional and behavioral response to cancer. A summary of the attachment styles, coping, and defense mechanisms associated with dysfunctional adjustment to illness is presented in Table 3.2.

The evaluation of personality traits—in part derivable by attachment and coping styles—also provides important information about the way in which the patient experiences cancer and consequently behaves towards the disease and the staff. Without going into the details of personality assessment and the huge literature related to the association between personality and adaptation to illness, some personality traits can cause difficult problems within the patient–family/physician–staff. Some constructs, which are in part overlapping, such as type D (distressed) and Type C personality, and alexithymia have been particularly studied in medical

Table 3.2 Attachment styles, coping, defense mechanisms favoring psychological morbidity in cancer

Attachment styles
• Preoccupied attachment: Dependency, amplified expressiveness, need to maintain emotional and physical closeness to attachment figures (e.g., family members, healthcare staff); sense of personal fragility and hypervigilance for threat caused by cancer; high levels of perceived stress
• Dismissing attachment: Proximity seeking reduced, attachment figures considered unimportant and signs of personal vulnerability or distress suppressed with symptoms minimized or reported too late; possible interference with collaboration with healthcare staff (e.g., mistrust or impatience with professionals)
• Fearful attachment: High attachment anxiety (characteristic of the preoccupied pattern) and high attachment avoidance (characteristic of the dismissing pattern), with untenable combination of distress and avoidance of medical help, ambivalence towards healthcare staff
Coping
• Hopelessness: The tendency to give up and to feel at a loss about cancer, with inability to react and to return to life
• Anxious preoccupation: The tendency to be extremely worried about cancer and its implications, allowing the disease to dominate life; attention-focused on the body
Defense mechanisms
• Neurotic defenses
– Conversion: expression of unacknowledged emotional distress in the guise of a physical symptom
– Control: tendency to control the environment to avoid or reduce anxiety; loss of control causes anxiety
• Immature defenses
– Passive aggression: Indirect and passive expression of anger
– Acting out: Direct expression of impulse or wish
– Projection: Attribution of unacceptable impulse or ideas to others
– Devaluation: depreciation of others
– Denial: refusal to acknowledge painful realities
• Psychotic defenses
– (pathological) denial: Refuse to confront with the reality (e.g., cancer) that is completely obliterated
– (delusional) projection: Externalization of conflicts and distress in the reality (reality testing is minimal or absent)

settings (Lumley et al. 2007; Mols and Denollet 2010a, b; Zozulya et al. 2008) and in psycho-oncology (De Vries et al. 2012; Mols et al. 2012). The main characteristics of these constructs are the following:

Type D (distressed): Negative affectivity and social inhibition, consisting in a general propensity to distress (feelings of negativity, anxiety, depression, loneliness), tendency to overreact to stressful situations, to conceal one's own feelings from others; fear of disapproval and rejection; lack self-assurance.

Type C: Denial or repression of one's own feelings (especially anger) and/or inability to ventilate them; tendency to conform to social standards; patience, unassertiveness, cooperativeness and appeasing with work, social, and family relationships, and compliance with external authority; concern with meeting

Table 3.3 Risk factors for psychiatric disorders in cancer and palliative care

• Biological factors
– Type of cancer and site (e.g., lung, pancreas, head-neck, central nervous system)
– Stage (metastatic vs. local/loco-regional)
– Phase (secondary/recurrence vs. primary)
– Physical symptoms (e.g., uncontrolled pain, nausea, vomiting, fatigue)
– Low performance status and disability
– Treatment (e.g., chemo-radio-hormone; other medications)
– Other possible concomitant physical problems or medical conditions
• Individual factors
– History of psychological or psychiatric disorders
– Previous experiences of physical illness or cancer in the family
– Poor defense/coping mechanisms (e.g., giving-up; hopelessness; pathological denial)
– Personality traits (e.g., tendency not to express emotions, tendency to consider life events as uncontrollable and unavoidable)
• Interpersonal factors
– History of stressful events in the past
– Current stress and problems (both cancer- or non/cancer-related) (e.g., economical problems, conflicts at work, in the family, losses)
– Lack of resources in the interpersonal context
Poor support from the family and close friends
Poor support from other sources (e.g., colleagues at work, neighbors, associations, community and health services)

others' needs and insufficiently engagement in meeting one's own needs; tendency to self-sacrificing.

Alexithymia: Difficulty identifying feelings and distinguishing between feelings and the bodily sensations of emotional arousal; difficulty describing feelings to other people; difficulty in distinguishing and appreciating the emotions of others, with unempathic and ineffective emotional responding; constricted imaginal processes, as evidenced by a scarcity of fantasies; a stimulus-bound, externally oriented cognitive style.

The assessment of other risk factors is also important during the interview since psycho-oncology literature has clearly shown the role of several variables in favoring the onset of psychiatric disorders across the many phases of cancer trajectory (Table 3.3). The National Comprehensive Cancer Network (NCCN) has summarized risk factors for psychopathology in the distress management guideline (NCCN 2013), in order to alert and guide physicians taking care of cancer patients.

During the interview the mental status examination (MSE) is also performed, as an essential component of the psychiatric diagnostic assessment. The MSE is characterized by a systematic collection of data based by observing and inquiring the patient's psychological and behavioral conditions, in terms of signs and symptoms gathered during the encounter with (and interview of) the patient

Table 3.4 Areas of mental functioning in the Mental Status Examination (MSE)

1. General description
   (a) Appearance: apparent age, height, weight, position, manner of dress, cleanliness and grooming, eye contact, physical abnormalities (related to cancer or other causes)
   (b) Attitude: patient's approach to the interview process and the interaction with the examiner
2. Sensorium and cognition
   (a) Level of consciousness (alert, drowsy, somnolent, stuporous, fluctuating)
   (b) Vigilance, orientation (person, place, time, situation), ability to focus, attention and concentration, memory (e.g., registration, short-term, long-term)
3. Motor Behavior: Level of activity and arousal, motor activity (abnormal movements, tics, posturing
4. Language and speech: Rate, rhythm, volume, amount, accent, inflection, fluency, and articulation
5. Affect and mood: Current subjective sustained emotional state as described by the patient (mood), and examiner's inferences of the quality of the patient's emotional state based on objective observation (affect)
6. Thought
   (a) Process: Patient's associations and flow of ideas (e.g., vagueness, incoherence, circumstantiality, tangentiality, neologisms, perseveration, flight of ideas, loose or idiosyncratic associations, and self-contradictory statements)
   (b) Content: Patient's spontaneously expressed worries, concerns, thoughts, and impulses (e.g., ruminations, obsessions, compulsions, phobias, ideas of reference, delusions, suicidal or self-injurious thoughts)
7. Perception: Possible perceptual disturbances (e.g., depersonalization and derealization, illusions and hallucinations)
8. Insight: Patient's awareness of internal (one's mind) and external realities (environment, other people), of his/her problems and their implications
9. Judgment: Capacity to consider and formulate opinions, by weighing and comparing the relative values of different issues, understanding if the illness and the treatment offered

(Trzepacz and Baker 1993). In psycho-oncology, the MSE is not different from what is carried out when assessing patients in the psychiatric or psychosomatic medicine fields. The different components and domains of the mental status examination (MSE) are reported in Table 3.4.

The psychiatric interview and the MSE may also be completed by a number of tests that have been developed in psycho-oncology. Their use can also help confirm the diagnosis by assessing the several domains for which psychological tools are routinely employed in oncology and palliative care, including those assessing psychiatric symptoms, psychosocial functioning and quality of life, neuropsychological and cognitive issues, as well as attachment styles and coping mechanisms. More details about screening for psychological well-being and distress, clinical assessment (case finding) of psychosocial well-being and rating psychological health, and the challenges and benefits of screening for psychological comorbidity are provided by Mitchell and Bultz (2014) in this book.

3.2.2 Medical and Psychosocial Assessment

When assessing cancer patients, evaluation of the patient's physical status and the general medical condition is always necessary to understand the many different variables possibly implicated in the current psychiatric symptoms or disorder. Psycho-oncology is by definition part of a multidisciplinary team, which usually includes different healthcare professionals who, by working together, provide their expertise derived by their own specialty (e.g., geneticists, radiologists, surgeons, medical oncologists, nurses, palliative care physicians) (Grassi et al. 2013b). Thus, laboratory tests (e.g., examination of basic blood conditions, endocrine and metabolic functions), radiological tests, neuroimaging studies (e.g., computed tomography, magnetic resonance imaging, electroencephalogram), and liaison with other medical staff (e.g., examination of the patient's chart, list of medications and type of treatment) are part of the patient's assessment. Screening for general medical conditions and drugs may clarify which other factors are involved in etiology (e.g., delirium) or may give the clinician information to be used in choosing psychopharmacological treatment (e.g., side effects of psychotropic drugs, drug–drug interaction) (Grassi et al. 2014).

According to the results of the interview, the MSE, and the psychological and diagnostic tools, it is usually possible to make a working diagnosis and, consequently, to decide a possible psychopharmacology treatment strategy.

3.3   Diagnostic Issues

As Wise (1986) indicated, there are different levels of psychiatric diagnosis that should be considered as not mutually exclusive but integrated in psychopharmacology and, in general, in consultation psychiatry and psychosomatic medicine: the clinical diagnosis, which is a nosologically oriented diagnosis and allows clinicians to communicate with one another about the signs and symptoms the patient is presenting (e.g., DSM, ICD); the dynamic-interpersonal diagnosis, which is an interpersonally oriented diagnosis and includes the psychological and social variables (or forces) involved in the presentation of symptoms and description of the patient's vulnerabilities and strengths; and the genetic diagnosis, which is historically oriented and it is based on the history of the patient in terms of early experiences and life events (e.g., attachment early experiences).

For the aims of deciding what psychopharmacological intervention is necessary for a specific patient's psychiatric condition, and for the purpose of having a common ground for communication within the multidisciplinary team, the clinical diagnosis is usually what clinicians use in the different settings (e.g., emergency vs. general settings; inpatient vs. outpatient; hospital vs. community), although both interpersonal and genetic diagnosis are provided when discussing a case in multidisciplinary teams.

Table 3.5 The most common disorders (and relative codes) observable in cancer patients according to the DSM-5 and ICD-10

DSM-5	ICD-10
Anxiety disorders • 300.29: Specific phobia (e.g., blood, injection, injury; situational)	Neurotic, stress-related and somatoform disorders • F40: Phobic anxiety disorder • F41: Other anxiety disorders • F43: Reaction to severe stress (including PTSD) and adjustment disorders • F45: Hypochondriacal disorder (including nosophobia)
Depressive disorders • 296: Major depressive disorder (single episode; recurrent) • 293: Depressive disorders due to another medical condition • Substance-medication induced depressive disorder	Mood (affective) disorders • F32: Depressive episode • F33: Recurrent depressive disorder
Trauma- and stressor-related disorder • 309: Adjustment disorders (with depressed mood; with anxiety; with mixed anxiety and depression, with disturbance of conduct; with mixed disturbance of emotions and conduct) • 309.81: Post-traumatic stress disorder	See above neurotic, stress-related, and somatoform disorders
Somatic symptom and related disorders • 300.7: Illness anxiety disorder • 316: Psychological factors affecting other medical conditions	Behavioral syndromes associated with physiological disturbances and physical factors • F54: Psychological and behavioral factors associated with disorders or diseases classified elsewhere
Neurocognitive disorders • 293: Delirium (due to another medical condition; due to multiple etiologies)	Organic, including symptomatic, mental disorders • F05: Delirium not induced by alcohol and other psychoactive drugs • F06: Other mental disorders due to brain damage and dysfunction and to physical disease (e.g., organic affective disorder)

3.3.1 ICD and DSM Diagnosis

It s not the aim of this chapter to describe the development of DSM and ICD, their specific characteristics, and their applications in consultation-liaison psychiatry, psychosomatic medicine, or psycho-oncology. Since the beginning of psychosocial research in oncology settings, both ICD and DSM have been the most common taxonomy instruments used to classify psychopathological signs and symptoms and to formulate a psychiatric diagnosis in cancer settings. The most common disorders that psycho-oncology literature has pointed out can be subsumed under certain categories as indicated in Table 3.5, while the diagnostic criteria for these disorders are summarized in the relevant chapters of this book.

A series of questions and unanswered problems persist, however, in assessing psychosocial disorders in psycho-oncology clinical practice. In particular, the specificity of the criteria of some psychiatric disorders (see below) has been questioned: the risk that a pure psychiatric approach may reduce instead of enlarging the vision of the multiform phenomenology of psychosocial suffering in cancer patients has also been raised as a problem. With respect to the previous editions of the DSM, the most recent DSM-5 has tried to overcome some of the problems of categorical diagnoses by introducing a more dimensionally oriented approach, but data about possible changes in terms of psycho-oncology diagnostic approach are not yet available.

Adjustment Disorders

The problem of making a diagnosis of adjustment disorders in medical settings has been repeatedly pointed out, since psychiatric nosological systems seem to fail to provide specific diagnostic criteria and to clearly guide clinicians on distinguishing them from normal adaptive reactions to stress, on the one side, and from recognized mental disorders (e.g., depressive episode, post-traumatic stress disorder), on the other (Casey 2009; Casey and Bailey 2011). The ICD-10 and DSM-5 criteria underline that, in order to make a diagnosis of adjustment disorder, the distress should be marked and out of proportion to the severity and intensity of the stressor and that by definition it should begin within 3 months of onset of a stressor and last no longer than 6 months after the stressors (or its consequences) have terminated. These criteria are difficult to apply to a chronic situation such as cancer. In a study of 800 medically ill patients, including cancer patients, those receiving a diagnosis of adjustment disorder were actually characterized by many different psychosocial dimensions, only partially belonging to anxiety, depression, and disturbance of conduct, as indicated in DSM-5 or ICD-10 (Grassi et al. 2007).

Depressive Disorders

For the last 30 years, psycho-oncology clinicians struggled with some significant diagnostic problems within the category of mood or depressive disorders. To make a diagnosis of major depression, any physiological effect of a substance or of a medical disease needed to be excluded. Thus, if this criterion was scrupulously followed and met, all depressive disorders in cancer could be diagnosed as depressive disorders substance/medication induced or secondary to the medical condition, and none as a "pure" major depressive episode. It is in fact not easy, given the number of drugs and interactions between drugs used to treat cancer or the role of inflammation due to cancer (e.g., interleukins and cytokines), to exclude their role in causing depression.

A second problem regarded the need to modify the DSM criteria of major depression when applied to cancer, or medical illness in general, since many symptoms, such as loss of appetite, loss of weight, insomnia, loss of interest and cognitive impairment, fatigue, and loss of energy may be a consequence of cancer or cancer treatment rather than depression. Different opinions and conceptualizations and several proposals have been suggested over the years (Endicott 1984;

Von Ammon Cavanaugh 1995; Akechi et al. 2009): to include all the symptoms irrespective of the fact that these symptoms may or may not be attributable to cancer (inclusive approach); to replace somatic symptoms with cognitive-affective items (substitute approach); to add some new affective symptoms to the original criteria (alternative approach); and to exclude somatic symptoms and use only affective symptoms to make the diagnosis (exclusive approach). An agreement on which method is the most specific has not been reached.

A third complex problem is related to the diagnosis of depression in patients with advanced stages of cancer, where the need to have a clear-cut framework is particularly important. The European Palliative Care Collaborative (EPCRC) (http://www.epcrc.org/) has developed a set of guidelines to better assess depression in patients with advanced stages of illness (Rayner et al. 2009; Wasteson et al. 2009), but the difficulty in the area of palliative care is quite evident, given the poor physical condition of the patients, the number of somatic symptoms caused by cancer and treatment, and the number and variety of interactions between the several drugs administered.

A fourth problem is that, in oncology, some taxonomic distinctions (e.g., DSM-5 between depressive episode with insufficient symptoms, recurrent brief depression, short duration depressive episodes) seem not useful in cancer and palliative care settings.

Somatic Symptom Disorder (Somatization)

Somatization and somatic symptom presentation in oncology is a complex area due to the presumption that if somatic symptoms occur in a patient with cancer, these are caused by the disease itself and/or its progression. Complaints of feeling tired, sensory symptoms, fatigue, and poor concentration likely related to psychological factors and interpretable as expression of abnormal illness behavior are frequently reported by cancer patients (Chaturvedi et al. 2006). The complexity, yet the importance of this clinical and research area has been underlined by Grassi et al. (2013a) who indicated that somatic symptoms may magnify disability resulting from cancer, interfere with treatment adherence and decisions, cause delay in recovery, result in poor outcome and recurrence, and reduce overall well-being and quality of life. Secondly, somatic symptoms in cancer may complicate the diagnosis of major depression due to the overlap of symptoms occurring as a result of the underlying disease, depression, or somatoform disorder. Lastly, somatic symptoms in cancer are unique in being often interrelated with each other, with one somatic symptom possibly causing other somatic symptoms (e.g., pain causing fatigue).

Psychological Factors Influencing a Medical Condition

A large area of emotional reactions and other psychosocial factors or dimensions seem to be neglected or oversimplified by both the ICD-10 and the DSM-5. The former summarizes this area in Chap. 21 under the rubric "Factors influencing health status and contact with health system" (code Z00-Z99); the latter has recently given more dignity to this section by integrating it (code 316;

corresponding to F54 code in the ICD-10) within the chapter "Somatic symptom and related disorders," in the rubric "Psychological factors affecting a medical condition." According to the criteria, psychological or behavioral factors should be not better explained by another mental disorder, but may affect cancer (i) by influencing its course as shown by a close temporal association between the psychological factors and the development or exacerbation of, or delayed recovery from, the cancer; (ii) by interfering with the treatment (e.g., poor adherence); (iii) by representing additional well-established health risks for the individual; (iv) by influencing the underlying pathophysiology, precipitating or exacerbating symptoms, or necessitating medical attention.

Some problems arise in this classification, however. No specific explanation is in fact given about how to assess the psychological and behavioral factors, indicating that more detailed examination of the different psychosocial dimensions involved in medically ill patient is needed (Fava and Sonino 2005).

3.3.2 Diagnostic Criteria for Psychosomatic Research

A more recent approach that tries to solve some of the above-mentioned difficulties when using the DSM-5 and the ICD-10 systems in medical settings is the Diagnostic Criteria for Psychosomatic Research (DCPR) (Fava et al. 1995). The DCPR has been specifically developed and proposed with the aim of translating psychosocial variables that were derived from psychosomatic research into operational tools for psychosocial variables, with prognostic and therapeutic implications in clinical settings whereby medically ill patients can be identified. The DCPR consists of 12 clinical categories (or clusters) which, through a semi-structured interview, explore a variety of possible psychological conditions and emotional responses to medical illness. Four clusters are related to patients' ways of perceiving, experiencing, evaluating, and responding to their health status that are subsumed into the construct of abnormal illness behavior (AIB) (disease phobia, thanatophobia, health anxiety, and illness denial), four clusters related to the concept of somatization (functional somatic symptoms secondary to psychiatric disorders, persistent somatization, conversion symptoms, and anniversary reaction), and four related to psychological dimensions that have been frequently and consistently found in medical patients (alexithymia, type A behavior, irritable mood, and demoralization). These dimensions, which were proposed to be integrated in the DSM-5 (Fava et al. 2007), have been found clinically significant in medically ill patients (Porcelli and Rafanelli 2010).

The DCPR have been proven to have an adjunctive role in increasing the understanding of psychosocial dimensions in comparison with DSM or ICD approaches in oncology settings (Grassi et al. 2007). The dimension of demoralization, as a syndrome that the DCPR is able to assess in medically ill patients (Mangelli et al. 2005), has been shown to be extremely important in oncology. Loss of meaning and hope can determine a sense of worthlessness on one's own life and in the future and impair the sense of mastery and competence which according to several authors (Angelino and Treisman 2001; Kissane et al. 2001; Cockram et al. 2009) is the hallmark of demoralization, as a clinical syndrome separated from major depression. Furthermore, the DCPR, with its specific rubric dedicated to somatization and somatic symptom presentation (Fava and Wise 2007; Sirri and Fava 2013), can also help in answering some of the questions related to the problem of somatic symptom presentation in cancer patients, mainly those with early stage of cancer, after completion of treatment and long-term survivors.

3.3.3   Other Conditions That May Be a Focus of Clinical Attention

By using the taxonomy system such as the DSM-5 or the ICD-10, it is common that in oncology many situations observed in clinical practice may be classified as part of the rubric "Other conditions that may be a focus of clinical attention" (code V in the DSM-5 and code Z in the ICD-10). These conditions can be elicited during the interview or through the adjunctive use of problem checklists (e.g., the National Comprehensive Cancer Network—NCCN Distress Thermometer and Problem List) (see Mitchell and Bultz 2014 in this book). The most common conditions mentioned are summarized in Table 3.6. Relational problems and sexuality issues are extremely significant in oncology and palliative care. When one member of the family has cancer, children may be at risk for suffering. The occupational and economical problems determined by having cancer (loss of work, cost of medication and treatment, insurance issues) should be also regularly assessed in the diagnostic phase. In palliative care, the problem of anticipatory grief and bereavement are a mandatory part of the assessment of the family, since it is by definition a condition needing clinical attention and, in about 20% of the cases, a condition that may complicate a psychopathological disorder (e.g., persistent complex bereavement disorder and other forms of complicated grief) (Shear et al. 2013). In DSM-5, frank disturbances of grief and mourning reaction are described in the chapter "Other specified trauma- and stressor-related disorder (code 309.89), specifically as Persistent complex bereavement disorder.

Conclusions

A careful examination of the psychological and behavioral signs and symptoms is extremely important in cancer care settings to make a diagnosis and to set up the most proper treatment, including psychopharmacological intervention. Both oncologists and palliative care physicians should be informed of the several clinical disorders observable in cancer patients and the characteristics of the diagnostic process as performed by psychiatrists and psycho-oncologists.

It is clear that using a system, such as the ICD-10 or the DSM-5, is mandatory to have a common language for the description and the classification of psychiatric disorders in cancer and palliative care settings. A broader multidimensional diagnostic process however helps clinicians in integrating information deriving from classical psychiatric nosology with that coming from psychosocially and psychosomatically oriented approaches. The specific problems arising from

Table 3.6 Possible cancer-related problems as classified in the DSM-5 (or ICD-10) under the rubric "Other conditions that may be a focus of clinical attention"

Problems related to family upbringing
• Parent–child relational problem (code V61.20; Z62.820)
• Child affected by parental relationship distress (code V61.29; Z62898)
Problems related to primary support group
• Relationship distress with spouse or intimate partner (code V61.10; Z63.0)
• Uncomplicated bereavement (code V68.82; Z63.4)
Occupational problems
• Other problems related to employment (code V62.29; Z56.9)
Economic problems
• Low income (code V60.2; Z59.6)
• Insufficient social insurance or welfare support (code V60.2; Z59.7)
Other problems related to the social environment
• Phase of life problems (code V62.89; Z60.0)
• Acculturation difficulty (code V60.3; Z60.2)
Other health service encounters for counseling and medical advice
• Sex counseling (code V65.49; Z70.9)
• Other counseling or consultation (code V65.40; Z71.9)
Problems related to other psychosocial, personal, and environment circumstances
• Religious or spiritual problems (code V62.89; Z65.8)
• Other problems related to psychosocial circumstances (code V62.9; Z65.9)
Problems related to access to medical and other health care
• Unavailability or inaccessibility of healthcare facilities (code V63.9; Z75.3)
Non adherence to medical treatment (code V15.81; Z91.19)

cancer and cancer treatments (e.g., depression in pancreatic cancer), the multiple expression of emotional suffering among cancer patients (e.g., demoralization, health anxiety, alexithymia), and the role of psychosocial dimensions, other than psychiatric categories, in negatively influencing the patients' quality of life and behavior (e.g., illness behavior, maladaptive coping) should be carefully taken into account during the diagnostic process. Thus, the application of the criteria that are useful to make a psychiatric diagnosis should be partnered with the assessment of psychosocial factors affecting individual vulnerability (e.g., attachment and coping styles, life events and acute and chronic stress, family functioning).

References

Akechi T, Ietsugu T, Sukigara M, Okamura H, Nakano T, Akizuki N, Okamura M, Shimizu K, Okuyama T, Furukawa TA, Uchitomi Y. Symptom indicator of severity of depression in cancer patients: a comparison of the DSM-IV criteria with alternative diagnostic criteria. Gen Hosp Psychiatry. 2009;31:225–32.

American Psychiatric Association: Diagnostic and Statistical Manual for Mental Disorders – Fith edition (DSM5). American Psychiatric Publishing, Washington, DC. 2013.

American Psychiatric Association (APA). Practice guideline for the psychiatric evaluation of adults. 2nd ed. Washington, DC: American Psychiatric Press; 2006.

Angelino AF, Treisman GJ. Major depression and demoralization in cancer patients: diagnostic and treatment considerations. Support Care Cancer. 2001;9:344–9.

Casey P. Adjustment disorder: epidemiology, diagnosis and treatment. CNS Drugs. 2009;23: 927–38.

Casey P, Bailey S. Adjustment disorders: the state of the art. World Psychiatry. 2011;10:11–8.

Chaturvedi SK, Maguire P, Somashekar BS. Somatization in cancer. Int Rev Psychiatry. 2006;18: 49–54.

Cockram CA, Doros G, de Figueiredo JM. Diagnosis and measurement of subjective incompetence: the clinical hallmark of demoralization. Psychother Psychosom. 2009;78:342–5.

De Vries AM, Forni V, Voellinger R, Stiefel F. Alexithymia in cancer patients: review of the literature. Psychother Psychosom. 2012;81:79–86.

Endicott J. Measurement of depression in patients with cancer. Cancer. 1984;53 (10 Suppl):2243–9.

Fava GA, Sonino N. The clinical domains of psychosomatic medicine. J Clin Psychiatry. 2005;66:849–58.

Fava GA, Wise TN. Issues for DSM-V: psychological factors affecting either identified or feared medical conditions: a solution for somatoform disorders. Am J Psychiatry. 2007;164:1002–3.

Fava GA, Freyberger HJ, Bech P, Christodoulou G, Sensky T, Theorell T, Wise TN. Diagnostic criteria for use in psychosomatic research. Psychother Psychosom. 1995;63:1–8.

Fava GA, Fabbri S, Sirri L, Wise TN. Psychological factors affecting medical condition: a new proposal for DSM-V. Psychosomatics. 2007;48:103–11.

Grassi L. Quam bene vivas referre: curing and caring in psycho-oncology. Psycho-Oncology. 2013;22:1679–87.

Grassi L, Nanni MG. Beyond psychiatric classification in oncology: psychosocial dimensions in cancer and implications for care. Psycho-Oncologie. 2013;7:235–242.

Grassi L, Biancosino B, Marmai L, Rossi E, Sabato S. Psychological factors affecting oncology conditions. In: Sononi N, Porcelli P, editors. Psychological factors affecting medical conditions. A new classification for DSM-V, vol. 28. Basel: Karger; 2007. p. 57–71.

Grassi L, Caruso R, Nanni MG. Somatization and somatic symptom presentation in cancer: a neglected area. Int Rev Psychiatry. 2013a;25:41–51.

Grassi L, Caruso R, Nanni MG. Psycho-oncology and optimal standards of cancer care: developments, multidisciplinary team approach and international guidelines. In: Wise TN, Biondi M, Costantini A, editors. Psycho-Oncology. Arlington, VA: American Psychiatric Publishing Press; 2013b. p. 315–39.

Grassi L, Caruso R, Hammelef K, Nanni MG, Riba M. Efficacy and safety of pharmacotherapy in cancer-related psychiatric disorders across the trajectory of cancer care: a review. Int Rev Psychiatry. 2014;26(1):44–62.

Greer S, Watson M. Mental adjustment to cancer: its measurement and prognostic importance. Cancer Surv. 1987;6(3):439–53.

Groves MS, Muskin PR. Psychological responses to illness. In: Levenson JL, editor. The American Psychiatric Publishing textbook of psychosomatic medicine: psychiatric care of the medically III. 2 revisedth ed. Washington, DC: American Psychiatric Press; 2011. p. 45–67.

Hunter JJ, Maunder RG. Using attachment theory to understand illness behavior. Gen Hosp Psychiatry. 2001;23:177–82.

Kissane DW, Clarke DM, Street AF. Demoralization syndrome. A relevant psychiatric diagnosis for palliative care. J Palliat Care. 2001;17:12–21.

Loscalzo MJ, von Gunten CF. Interdisciplinary team work in palliative care: compassionate expertise for serious complex illness. In: Chochinov HM, Breitbart W, editors. Handbook of psychiatry in palliative medicine. 2nd ed. New York, NY: Oxford University Press; 2009. p. 172–85.

Lumley MA, Neely LC, Burger AJ. The assessment of alexithymia in medical settings: implications for understanding and treating health problem. J Pers Assess. 2007;89(3):230–46.

Mangelli L, Fava GA, Grandi S, Grassi L, Ottolini F, Porcelli P, Rafanelli C, Rigatelli M, Sonino N. Assessing demoralization and depression in the setting of medical disease. J Clin Psychiatry. 2005;66:391–4.

Maunder RG, Hunter JJ. Assessing patterns of adult attachment in medical patients. Gen Hosp Psychiatry. 2009;31:123–30.

Maunder RG, Hunter JJ. A prototype-based model of adult attachment for clinicians. Psychodyn Psychiatry. 2012;40:549–73.

McHugh PR, Clark MR. Diagnostic and classificatory dilemmas. In: Blumenfield M, Strain JJ, editors. Psychosomatic medicine. Philadelphia, PA: Lippincott Williams & Wilkins; 2006. p. 40–5.

Mitchell A, Bultz B. Psychological assessment in psychopharmoncology. In: Grassi L, Riba MB, editors. Psychopharmacology in oncology and palliative care: a practical manual. Heidelberg: Springer; 2014.

Mols F, Denollet J. Type D personality in the general population: a systematic review of health status, mechanisms of disease, and work-related problems. Health Qual Life Outcomes. 2010a; 8:9.

Mols F, Denollet J. Type D personality among noncardiovascular patient populations: a systematic review. Gen Hosp Psychiatry. 2010b;32(1):66–72.

Mols F, Thong MS, van de Poll-Franse LV, Roukema JA, Denollet J. Type D (distressed) personality is associated with poor quality of life and mental health among 3080 cancer survivors. J Affect Disord. 2012;136:26–34.

Porcelli P, Rafanelli C. Criteria for psychosomatic research (DCPR) in the medical setting. Curr Psychiatry Rep. 2010;12:246–54.

Rayner L, Loge JH, Wasteson E, Higginson IJ, EPCRC, European Palliative Care Research Collaborative. The detection of depression in palliative care. Curr Opin Support Palliat Care. 2009;3:55–60.

Shear MK, Ghesquiere A, Glickman K. Bereavement and complicated grief. Curr Psychiatry Rep. 2013;15(11):406.

Sims A. Descriptive phenomenology. In: Gelder M, Andreasen N, Lopez-Ibor J, Geddes J, editors. New Oxford textbook of psychiatry. 2nd ed. Oxford: Oxford University Press; 2012. p. 47–61.

Sirri L, Fava GA. Diagnostic criteria for psychosomatic research and somatic symptom disorders. Int Rev Psychiatry. 2013;25:19–30.

Smith FA, Levenson JL, Stern TA. Psychiatric assessment and consultation. In: Levenson JL, editor. The American Psychiatric Publishing Textbook of Psychosomatic Medicine Psychiatric Care of the Medically Ill. 2 revisedth ed. Washington, DC: American Psychiatric Press; 2011. p. 3–17.

Spencer SM, Carver CS, Price AA. Psychological and social factors in adaptation. In: Holland JC, editor. Psycho-oncology. New York: Oxford University Press; 1998. p. 211–54.

Tan A, Zimmermann C, Rodin G. Interpersonal processes in palliative care: an attachment perspective on the patient_/clinician relationship. Palliat Med. 2005;19:143–50.

Trzepacz PT, Baker RW. The psychiatric mental status examination. New York: Oxford University Press; 1993.

Turner J. Working as a multidisciplinary team. In: Kissane DW, Bultz BD, Butow PM, Finlay IG, editors. Handbook of communication in oncology and palliative care. New York: Oxford University Press; 2010. p. 245–57.

Von Ammon Cavanaugh S. Depression in the medically ill. Critical issues in diagnostic assessment. Psychosomatics. 1995;36:48–59.

Wasteson E, Brenne E, Higginson IJ, Hotopf M, Lloyd-Williams M, Kaasa S, Loge JH, European Palliative Care Research Collaborative (EPCRC). Depression assessment and classification in palliative cancer patients: a systematic literature review. Palliat Med. 2009;23:739–53.

Wise T. Clinical strategies for evaluating the medical patient. In: Derogatis LR, editor. Clinical psychopharmacology. Menlo Park: Addison-Wesely Publishing Company; 1986. p. 1–16.

World Health Organization: International Statistical Classification of Diseases and Related Health Problems 10th Revision. Version 2010. WHO, Geneve. 2010.

Zozulya AA, Gabaeva MV, Sokolov OY, Surkina ID, Kost NV. Personality, coping style, and constitutional neuroimmunology. J Immunotoxicol. 2008;5(2):221–5.

Psychological Assessment in Psychopharmacology

4

Alex J. Mitchell and Barry D. Bultz

Abstract

A key element of supportive care is the reliable measurement of psychological health and psychosocial problems. This may include detection and measurement of frank psychiatric disorders as well as broader psychological symptoms and generalised distress. Many organisations have made recommendations for assessment of distress but despite the potential benefits uptake has been slow and evidence mixed. There is however momentum building for multi-domain screening for distress as the 6th vital sign. Psychosocial assessment can be pragmatically divided into screening, clinical assessment (case-finding) and assessment of adaptation and daily function. Screening for distress is designed to quickly ascertain which individuals in a large population need further assessment followed by specific additional care and intervention; however, the evidence base for screening needs to be improved. The target of screening may be mood disorders, distress, cognitive decline, unmet needs or a multi-domain approach. A multidimensional approach may be preferable and a multidimensional tool can be valuable as it can serve as a roadmap to a more effective way of addressing patient concerns in a timely way with appropriate referral to the right professional. Most forms of screening are seen as at least a slight burden to patients and clinicians. In some circumstances this burden can be significant and rate-limiting. Therefore screening implementation can be limited as much by acceptability as by accuracy. Screening for distress and/or psychological assessment should not be considered a one-off exercise but part of routine high quality

A.J. Mitchell (✉)
Department of Psycho-oncology, Cancer Studies & Molecular Medicine, University of Leicester, Leicester, UK
e-mail: ajm80@le.ac.uk

B.D. Bultz
Department of Psychosocial Oncology, Tom Baker Cancer Centre, University of Calgary, Calgary, AB, Canada
e-mail: bdbultz@ucalgary.ca

L. Grassi and M. Riba (eds.), *Psychopharmacology in Oncology and Palliative Care*,   49
DOI 10.1007/978-3-642-40134-3_4, © Springer-Verlag Berlin Heidelberg 2014

of care that involves all healthcare professionals. Thorough and timely psychological assessment will enhance trust and therapeutic alliance. Psychosocial needs are the most overlooked of all cancer complications. Psychological assessment together with appropriate follow-up and tailored acceptable interventions will help reduce this gap in unmet psychosocial needs.

4.1   Introduction

Supportive care in oncology is not the responsibility of any one professional group but shared across many professions. An important element of supportive care is the reliable measurement of psychological health and psychosocial problems. Sharing a common professional language and agreeing on how to assess and diagnose cancer patients' psychological health will strengthen the science and practice of psychosocial oncology. There have always been challenges in the assessment of psychological complications of cancer because many reactions to life-threatening conditions do not fit the common psychiatric diagnostic criteria. Only a minority have frank psychiatric disorders whereas the majority of patients have psychological symptoms and generalised distress. It is therefore important not to reply only on measures developed for diagnosis of mental illness but to consider measures which broadly defined emotional issues, unmet needs and poor adjustment resulting from cancer and its treatment. A great deal of progress has been made over the past three decades in the development of measures that are appropriate for cancer patients, and it is timely to review and describe what is now accepted as good clinical practice in the assessment of psychosocial needs and outcomes.

Psychological health covers a wide area including broad concepts of quality of life (QoL) and distress, as well as traditional mental health diagnoses, such as depression and anxiety. Based on robust evidence from interview-based studies, the prevalence of interview-defined major depression and anxiety is approximately twice that of healthy controls (Mitchell et al. 2011a, 2013). Adjustment disorder with broadly defined distress is present in between 30 % and 50 % early in the course of cancer. Unfortunately, many cancer patients report that their psychological concerns are not addressed and that they continue to experience unmet psychosocial needs (Harrison et al. 2009; Puts et al. 2012). Although distress tends to diminish with time in long-term cancer survivors, longitudinal studies have also reported that anxiety is often elevated in the five years or more after a diagnosis (Mitchell et al. 2013). In addition, in patients with advanced cancer, anxiety and depression are also elevated compared with healthy controls but perhaps not significantly great than in early stages of cancer (Mitchell et al. 2011a; Lo et al. 2010). Concerning, less than a third of patients recall being asked about emotions or mood, about half of medical notes show no evidence of any assessment for psychosocial symptoms or well-being and in observed clinical interviews emotional issues are often not emphasised during medical consultations (Jacobsen et al. 2011; Rodriguez et al. 2010; Bonito et al. 2013). Yet untreated physical or psychological or social problems may reduce quality of life and adversely reduce or delay receipt of medical treatment for cancer (Waller et al. 2012; Baillargeon et al. 2011).

As a result, many organisations have made recommendations: distress be assessed routinely and considered as the 6th vital sign (Bultz and Carlson 2005; Bultz et al. 2011). Most consider screening for distress to be part of high quality guideline concordant supportive care (Howell et al. 2012). This includes necessity to undertake a thorough and timely screen for distress followed by appropriate follow-up such as clinical assessment of symptom severity for every patient. Although it is important to recognise that frontline cancer clinicians may have only limited time or expertise to assess psychosocial concerns, it is imperative that psychosocial care should not be overlooked during routine care. Indeed, even in the absence of a local system of implementation, recognition of distress is the responsibility of all cancer professionals. Distress is too common to be managed by one profession alone.

Psychosocial assessment can be pragmatically divided into screening, clinical assessment (case-finding) and assessment of adaptation and daily function (see also Bultz, Loscalzo, Clark (2012) in Chap. 7). Clinical assessment includes fostering trust and therapeutic alliance, screening and case-finding. On the other hand screening for distress is a method widely used in oncology to quickly ascertain which individuals in a large population need further assessment followed by specific additional care and intervention. Within systems with limited resources, it is important to match specialist services to those who need and want them. Screening for distress initiatives include the application of validated tools to improve the recognition of frequently reported biopsychchosocial concerns over and above the accuracy clinician judgement alone. Assessment of adaptation and daily function includes the process of quantifying severity of physical, social, practical and psychological complications, clarifying coping styles and measuring function. In this chapter we will not consider structured/semi-structured psychiatric interviews often designed for research to establish a criterion reference (for further information, see Chap. 3).

4.2 Clinical Psychological Assessment

4.2.1 Clinical Approach

Evidence indicates that a sensitive, collaborative and confidential approach to patients fosters a trusting therapeutic relationship (Heyland et al. 2006). Trust between clinician and patient is in itself influential in determining clinical outcomes (Hillen et al. 2011; Underhill and Kiviniemi 2012). Clinicians who have a professional but approachable style are honest but flexible in their discussion of sensitive information and offer helpful but realistic therapeutic goals that are more likely to be trusted and by developing a strong alliance enhance psychosocial well-being and increase treatment adherence in patients with cancer (Trevino et al. 2013).

4.2.2 Improving Communication

A number of authors have commented on suboptimal communication strategies by clinicians. For example, clinicians appear to miss most cues and concerns and adopt behaviors that discourage disclosure (Deveugele et al. 2004). Tai-Seale et al. (2007) observed that a typical mental health discussion lasted approximately 2 min in routine practice. Difficult topics are often infrequently raised by clinicians and perceived as a communication gap by patients. Examples include discussion of emotional symptoms, practical needs, spiritual concerns, proxy appointment/ advocates, living will, resuscitation and life support preferences, hospice options and discussions of prognsosis (Nelson et al. 2011). This has led to communication skills training both in oncology and in other settings. In oncology results suggest a modest effect on communication behaviour, but effects on patient outcomes have been harder to demonstrate (Uitterhoeve et al. 2010; Barth and Lannen 2011). Nevertheless, good communication skills improve patient disclosure of problems during clinical interviews and hence aid detection as well as psychological intervention.

4.2.3 Operational Criteria for Mental Disorder

The criteria for major depression, minor depression, dysthymia, adjustment disorder and anxiety disorders (including PTSD) are listed in ICD10 and DSM5. Ideally, clinicians should make reference to the official criteria when making a diagnosis but in reality this rarely happens (Mitchell et al. 2008). A complication is that ICD10 and DSMIV differ. For example, the DSMIV criteria for GAD are excessive, difficult to control anxiety for at least 6 months and at least three of the following symptoms: restlessness or feeling keyed up or on edge, easily fatigued, difficulty concentrating or mind going blank, irritability, muscle tension and sleep disturbance. ICD10, on the other hand, requires 4 out of 22 possible symptoms. Similarly in DSM5, Major Depressive Disorder (MDD) is defined by depressed mood or loss of interest for at least 2 weeks, accompanied by an additional three (for a total of five) symptoms, but in ICD10 the core symptoms of depression include decreased energy or increased fatigability, in addition to low mood and loss of interest. Further, only four symptoms are required for a mild episode and six symptoms qualify as moderate depressive episode. An important qualifier is that all of the above disorders should cause significant distress or impairment in social, occupational or other important areas of functioning. Clinicians should therefore ask patients routinely about distress and impaired daily function with a question such as 'How difficult is it to do your work, take care of things at home or get along with people?' Several authors have suggested possible contamination of criteria for depression (and perhaps anxiety) due to physical symptoms of cancer itself. Yet recent studies suggest that somatic symptoms of depression (e.g. fatigue, insomnia, anorexia) appear to remain valid determinants of major depression even in the context of cancer (Mitchell et al. 2012b).

4.2.4 Clinicians Accuracy Using Clinical Assessment

There have been many studies examining the unassisted ability of cancer clinicians to identify depression and cognitive impairment, but fewer regarding distress and almost no studies concerning anxiety or other emotional domains such as anger. Sollner et al (2001) examined the accuracy of oncologists' evaluations of 298 cancer patients. Against moderate or severe distress on the HADS (using a 12v13 cut-off), oncologists' clinical sensitivity was 80 % but their specificity was only 33 %. Using a HADS cut-off of 18 representing severe distress, sensitivity dropped to 37 % and specificity increased to 88 %. Mitchell and colleagues (2011e) looked at identification of distress by chemotherapy cancer nurses using distress defined by the DT in 400 patients (Mitchell and colleagues 2011d). Nurse practitioners had a detection sensitivity of 50 % and specificity 80 %. Interestingly, there was higher sensitivity but lower specificity in those clinicians with high self-rated confidence. It is rarely appreciated that modest specificity can translate into a significant number of false positive errors. Assuming distress is present in 40 % of cancer patients, clinicians would miss 20 patients (false negatives) and misidentify 12 patients (false positives) for every 100 people seen in routine cancer care. Thus the decision and action that follow initial judgement is a critical step in clinical diagnoses as well as in screening. The rate of false positives increases further when clinicians are under study (Hawthorne effect) and indeed in any situation where the prevalence of depression is low. There are many possible reasons for diagnostic error, including both patient and provider factors. For example, not all patients want to talk about their emotional problems and many may not mention key psychological terms early in the consultation. Clinician related factors linked with low detection include the willingness to look for emotional problems, clinical confidence, clinical communication skills and duration of the clinical consultation. Detection is generally easier in high prevalence settings where mental health problems are common. Here the challenge may be to allocate sufficient time to deal with regular mental health issues. In a low prevalence setting, it may be useful to watch out for 'red flags' that is, symptoms such as tearfulness, isolation, trouble sleeping, irritability, agitation which may reveal a more serious disorder. In all patients, it is reasonable to ask generic questions such as 'how are you feeling?' or 'how are you coping at the moment?' If there is a positive response, or if the patient has persistent concerns or where there is clear distress, clinicians should move on to ask about symptoms of clinical disorder such as depression. Even in the absence of a formal scale, a positive answer to either persistent low mood or loss of interest is enough to suspect clinical depression and would warrant further questions. It may also be useful to ask 'is this out of the ordinary for you' and 'are things generally getting better or worse at the current time'. Lastly, clinicians should not be afraid to see the patient again in order to clarify a diagnosis. When compared to a single assessment, a repeat assessment was projected to increase unassisted accuracy from 79 % to 93 % in one study (Mitchell et al. 2009).

4.3   Psychological Assessment Using Screening

Screening can be considered the pro-active rapid initial identification of commonly experienced key indicators that allow for further assessment, diagnosis, treatment and referral. It is the application of a diagnostic test or clinical assessment in order to optimally rule out those *without* the disorder in question with minimal false negatives (missed cases) (Mitchell et al. 2010a, b). Screening is often applied to a large population who may or may not have an identified concern. Case-finding is often performed as a second step in a selected population at high risk for the condition following initial screening. Thus false negatives are the currency of screening and false positives the currency of case-finding. Screening is rarely perfect and is likely to lead to some false positives (misidentifications) and some false negatives (missed cases). Effects that minimise the effects of screening errors should be a priority. Misidentifications can be reduced by a second step assessment. False negatives can be reduced by applying screening to a high-risk population or by following up screen-negative cases (particularly those where there is a clinical concern). Initial screening can be broad and multidimensional. When symptoms and unmet needs have been identified, second stage assessment (such as of anxiety/depression) can be organised.

4.3.1   Screening for Depression/Anxiety

Early research focussed on screening for depression, a valid target but only one from a range of complex emotional responses to cancer. The best-known conventional self-report mood scale is probably the Hospital Anxiety and Depression Scale (HADS) (Zigmond and Snaith 1983). Two recent reviews found that the HADS could not be recommended as a case-finding (diagnostic) instrument, but it may be suitable as an initial screening tool for anxiety and depression (Luckett et al. 2010; Mitchell et al. 2010a). However, the 14-item HADS is probably too long for routine use, at least in paper and pencil format, although it has appeared to have been successfully implemented by touch screen in some well-resourced areas (Strong et al. 2008). Screening tools for depression have been comprehensively reviewed. According to the Depression in Cancer Consensus Group, as of 2012, there were 63 diagnostic validity studies involving 19 tools designed to help clinicians identify depression in cancer settings (Mitchell et al. 2012c). However, only eight tools had reasonable independent replication and, of these, best evidence supported the two stem questions (PHQ2) if acceptability was a key consideration and the Beck Depression Inventory (BDI-II) where a longer scale was acceptable. For every 100 people screened in a cancer setting, where 20 were depressed, the BDI-II would likely accurately detect 17 cases, missing 2 and correctly re-assure 70, with 11 falsely identified as cases.

In contrast to screening for depression, screening for anxiety has been overlooked but anxiety is no less important in cancer settings. Clinicians rarely use formal instruments when assessing anxiety but typically rely on verbal and nonverbal cues (Fröjd et al. 2007). Anxiety scales include the anxiety subscale of the HADS, the State-Trait Anxiety Inventory (STAI), the Generalised Anxiety Disorder scale (GAD7), the GAD for DSM and Fear of Disease Progression Scale (FoP) (Herschbach et al. 2005). These tools all have only modest acceptability and shorted single item, and brief multi-domain tools are under development (see Sect. 4.3.4).

4.3.2   Screening for Distress in Cancer Care

Given the limitations of focussing on specific psychiatric disorders, an alternative approach is to look for broadly multidimensionally defined distress. In a cancer context, distress has been defined by National Comprehensive Cancer Network (NCCN) as 'A multifactorial unpleasant emotional experience of a psychological (cognitive, behavioural, emotional), social and/or spiritual nature that may interfere with the ability to cope effectively with cancer, its physical symptoms and its treatment'. Distress should be considered a treatable complication of cancer that can present at any stage in the cancer pathway. Distress is not a specific category in DSM-IV or ICD10 but appears as a qualifier (also known as clinical significance criteria) to notate a disorder as clinically important. Details of how and how often to screen are subject to much local variation. According to the National Comprehensive Cancer Network (NCCN), distress should be recognised and monitored through regular and repeated screening and treated promptly at all stages of disease (Bultz and Holland 2006). In 1998 the NCCN released a one-item, visual-analogue scale (VAS) known as the Distress Thermometer (DT) (Roth et al. 1998; NCCN 2008). Subsequently validation studies suggest modest to good sensitivity and specificity and high acceptability. (Mitchell 2007, 2010). Alternatives to the DT include the Psychological Distress Inventory (Morasso et al. 1996), Brief Symptom Inventory (BSI), General Health Questionnaire (GHQ), Symptom Checklist 90-R (SCL-90), the Edmonton Symptom Assessment System (ESAS) and Canadian Problem Checklist (Bultz et al. 2011). Validation attempts against interview-defined distress are sparse and acceptability of longer tools is a limitation.

4.3.3   Screening for Cognitive Decline

Dementia and milder forms of cognitive impairment are import complications of various cancers particularly brain tumours and brain metastases. Cognitive impairment impairs function, quality of life and independence. Yet cognitive impairment, particularly in milder forms, is often ignored in clinical practice until family member raise concern (Mitchell et al. 2011). Yet many tools have been developed to help clinicians assess cognition, and these have often been extensively validated in other settings, usually involving older people. Extensive cognitive testing can be conducted by trained staff such as neuropsychologists or occupational therapists. Brief testing (often called bedside cognitive testing) can often be conducted in less than 10 min. The most well-known tool is the Mini-Mental State Examination or MMSE (Folstein et al. 1975), but this is often used out of habit or convention as its accuracy for delirium, mild cognitive impairment and dementia is modest. More accurate tools are available such as the Addenbrooke's Cognitive Assessment—Revised (ACE-R), and briefer tools are also available such as the Abbreviated mental test score (AMTS) and 6-Item cognitive impairment test (6CIT). Accuracy of these tools is promising for dementia but less robust in the case of mild cognitive impairment. In addition, validation research and implementation research are urgently needed in oncology settings.

4.3.4 Screening for Well-being

Well-being is the overall sense of satisfaction with self, not a specific mental health complication. Some clinicians prefer to concentrate on health rather than ill health and hence may prefer to screening for well-being rather than distress. This can be achieved using QoL assessment. Generic QoL instruments have been used in cancer settings. These include the mental health inventory short form (MHI-5), the short form health survey 36 (SF36) and the Nottingham Health Profile (NHP). Generic QoL instruments may omit important cancer related complications and therefore several cancer-specific QoL instruments have been developed and validated. The most extensive studied include the EORTC QLQ-C30 (European Organization for Research and Treatment of Cancer Quality of Life Core Questionnaire) (Aaronson et al. 1993) and the FACT-G (Functional Assessment of Cancer Therapy-General) (Cella et al. 1993) and its various modules. The EORTC QLQ-C30 was originally validated in multiple European countries and published in 1993 and since used in almost 10,000 clinical studies. Specific QoL instruments have been used in trials comparing different oncologic treatment regimens, but such instruments have rarely made the transition into clinical practice (Bezjak et al. 1997, 2001; Morris et al. 1998).

4.3.5 Multi-domain Screening

Several multi-domain tools have been developed which encompass several bio-psychosocial domains.

The well-validated and multilingual Edmonton Symptom Assessment System (ESAS) includes six physical symptoms of cancer (pain, tiredness, nausea, depression, anxiety, drowsiness, appetite, well-being, shortness of breath) and three psychosocial symptoms (well-being, depression, anxiety). The tool originally designed to address common concerns by palliative patients is also being applied as a primary Screening for distress tool for cancer patients, given the multitude of biopsychosocial symptoms experienced by oncology patients. In the original version of the ESAS, patients rated the intensity of symptoms, using visual analogue scales, by placing a mark along a line ranging from 0 (no symptom) to 100 mm (worst possible symptom) although later versions used 11-point numerical rating scales. Evidence suggests appealing psychometric properties (Nekolaichuk et al. 2008; Richardson and Jones 2009). Mitchell and colleagues proposed a multi-domain extension to the distress thermometer called the Emotion thermometers (see http://www.psycho-oncology.info/ET.htm) including distress, depression, anxiety and anger. This also has an 11-point visual-analogue scale. Preliminary validation in early and late stage cancers and also in cardiology and neurology settings suggest the ET improves upon the accuracy of the DT (Mitchell et al. 2010b).

Other multi-domain tools have been developed in mental health and primary care settings that are of interest. Gaynes et al. (2010) tested the My Mood Monitor (M-3) checklist, a patient-rated 27-item tool (Gaynes et al. 2010). Using a sample of 647 consecutive primary care, the M-3 was examined against major depression, bipolar disorder, any anxiety disorder and post-traumatic stress disorder (PTSD) using the MINI. As a screen for any psychiatric disorder, sensitivity was 83 % and specificity was 76 %. Houston and colleagues asked 343 patients to complete a self-reported list of 85 DSM-IV symptom-based candidate questions against the SCID (Houston et al. 2011). The authors reduced the 85 items to a 17-item instrument for provisional differential diagnosis of GAD, MDE, past/present mania and ADHD. Sensitivities and specificities were 83 % and 75 % for GAD, 80 % and 80 % for MDE, 83 % and 82 % for mania and 82%and 73 % for ADHD.

4.3.6 Screening for Unmet Needs

The application of a screening test for emotional complications is unlikely to be diagnostically sufficient to facilitate a change in patient outcomes. Clinicians may require assistance to pinpoint the cause of a physical, psychological or practical distress as well as whether patients wish to receive input from clinical services (only the minority of patients with emotional complications want professional help at any point in time (Baker-Glenn et al. 2011). In an up-to-date review, Carlson and colleagues found 38 studies investigating psychometric qualities of 29 needs assessment tools (Carlson et al. 2012). Evidence of validity and reliability varies considerably between tools. Like distress, there is no accepted gold standard, therefore construct validity is often used. From this review only three tests had inter-rater reliability (3LNQ, NAT:PD-C and PNAT) and nine had test–retest reliability (CaNDI, CARES, CARES-SF, CaSUN, CCM, NA-ACP, NEQ, PCNQ and PNAT). At the current time, unmet needs tools are probably best chosen on the basis of ease of application and interpretation, possibly with consideration of reliability.

4.3.7 Effectiveness of Screening for Emotional Disorders in Clinical Practice

Despite the potential benefits of either selected or routine screening for anxiety, depression uptake has been slow and evidence mixed (Mitchell et al. 2011b; Thombs et al. 2011). Large-scale studies comparing care before and after screening (sequential cohort) or in groups randomised to screening have been uncommon (Luckett et al. 2009; van Scheppingen et al. 2011; Carlson et al. 2012). There is however momentum building for multi-domain Screening for Distress, as the 6th vital sign globally. Twelve randomised trials that have examined screening for psychological problems (or wellbeing) divided in six concerning emotional complications and six involving QL and one that studied both domains (Table 4.1) (Maunsell et al. 1996; Sarna 1998; McLachlan et al. 2001; Detmar et al. 2002; Velikova et al. 2004; Mills et al. 2009; Carlson et al. 2010b, 2012; Braeken et al. 2011; Klinkhammer-Schalke et al. 2012; Hollingworth et al. 2012). For example, in one British study, 28 oncologists treating 286 cancer patients were randomly assigned to an intervention group who underwent screening along with feedback of results to physicians, a screen-only group who completed questionnaires without feedback and a control group with no screening at all (Velikova et al. 2004, 2010). The questionnaires used were the EORTC QLQ-C30 and a touch screen version of HADS. A positive effect on emotional well-being was seen in the intervention compared with the control group, but there is no detectable effect on patient management. More recently, Carlson et al. (2010a, b) examined the effect of screening for distress on the level of distress in lung and breast cancer patients randomised to minimal screening (no feedback), full screening (with feedback) or screening with optional triage and referral (enhanced screening) (Carlson et al. 2010a, b). This was one of the largest studies to date with over 1,000 patients, 365 in minimal screen, 391 in full screen and 378 in screening with triage. In lung cancer patients receiving enhanced screening distress at follow-up was reduced by 20 % compared to other groups. In breast cancer, the full screening and enhanced screening, both had lower distress at follow-up than minimal screening. These results suggest a modest but potentially significant beneficial effect of Screening for distress in oncology clinical practice, provided follow-up care is provided to those who screen positive.

There is much interest in what determines whether screening leads to an effective psychological assessment. Evidence suggests screening can benefit communication and clinician referral patterns, but it has a weaker effect on the ability of clinicians to correctly identify cases. When mandated screening can be widely disseminated and therefore acceptability to both clinicians and patients is key. Acceptability to frontline clinicians, who are busy with other responsibilities, cannot be assumed (Mitchell et al. 2012a). Acceptability can be enhanced by using a brief tool that is multidimensional, with simple scoring, one that generates meaningful results and does not duplicate work. Staff who are involved in tool development and dissemination tend to be more invested in the screening programme itself. To be effective screening must be allied with appropriate

Table 4.1 Summary of common tools for psychological assessment in cancer settings

Distress/multi-domain	Depression	Anxiety	Unmet needs	Adaptation/function	QoL	Adjustment/coping	Cognition
Brief Symptom Inventory (BSI)	Beck Depression Inventory (BDI-II)	Fear of Progression Scale (FoP12)	Cancer Rehabilitation Evaluation System (CARES)	ECOG-PSR	Functional Assessment of Cancer Therapy (FACT)	Brief Cope	Addenbrooke's Cognitive Examination (ACE-R)
Distress Thermometer (DT)	Centers for Epidemiological Studies Depression Scale (CES-D)	Generalised Anxiety Scale (GAD9)	Cancer Survivors Unmet Needs measure (CaSun)	Functional Independence Measure (FIM)	European Organization for the Research and Treatment of Cancer Quality-of-Life Questionnaire (EORTC QLQ)	Cancer Coping Questionnaire	The Montreal Cognitive Assessment (MoCA)
Edmonton Symptoms Assessment Scale (ESAS)	Geriatric Depression Scale (GDS)	Generalised Anxiety Scale for DSM5 (GAD-DSM)	Needs Assessment Tool (NAT: PD-C)	Katz Activities of Daily Living	Medical Outcome Study-Short Form-36 (MOS SF-36)	COPE	Mini-COG
Emotion Thermometer (ET)	Hamilton Depression Rating Scale (HDRS)	Generalised Anxiety Disorder QQ (GAD7)	Cancer Care Monitor (CCM)	Lawton Instrumental Activities of Daily Living	Cancer Rehabilitation Evaluation System (CARES)	Dealing with Illness Inventory	Abbreviated Mental test score (AMTS)
General Health Questionnaire (GHQ)	Hospital Anxiety and Depression Scale-Depression (HADS)	Hospital Anxiety and Depression Scale-Anxiety (HADS-A)	Three-Levels-of-Needs Questionnaire (3LNQ)	Karnofsky Performance Scale (KPS)	Functional Living Index-Cancer (FLIC)	Mental Adjustment to Cancer (MAC)	Mini-Mental State Examination (MMSE)
General Health Questionnaire (GHQ28)	Montgomery Asperg Depression Scale (MARDS)	Impact of Events Scale (IES)	Needs Evaluation Questionnaire (NEQ)	IFS-CA, Inventory of Functional Status Cancer	Sickness Impact Profile (SIP)	Mini-MAC	cognitive impairment test (6-CIT)

(continued)

Table 4.1 (continued)

Distress/multi-domain	Depression	Anxiety	Unmet needs	Adaptation/function	QoL	Adjustment/coping	Cognition
Kessler-10 (K10)	Patient Health Questionnaire (PHQ9)	MHI-38 (Anxiety)	Needs Assessment of Advanced Cancer Patients (NA-AC)	Global Assessment of Functioning (GAF	Quality of Life Index (QLI)	Perceived Control of Life Questionnaire	CAMCOG
Symptom Checklist 90-R (SCL-90)	Zung Depression Scale (ZSDS)	State-Trait Anxiety Inventory (STAI)	Patient Needs Assessment Tool (PNAT)	Barthel Index (Loewen and Anderson)		Ways of Coping Questionnaire (WCQ)	GPCog

follow-up and effective treatment. Screening should work in combination with good quality of care because good quality screening cannot compensate for poor quality care in other areas.

4.4   Assessment of Coping and Adaptation to Disease

4.4.1   Measuring Adaptation to Disease

Living with cancer can be demanding if not challenging to the patient and their family. There are regular threats from physical complications, adverse treatment effects and the prospect of relapse, deterioration or death. People living with all stages of cancer are faced with considerable uncertainty and unpredictability as well as multiple biopsychosocial symptoms. Individuals may have multiple losses, an unexpected sick role and low sense of control. Several scales have been used to assess successful and unsuccessful adaptation to these challenges. For example health-related quality of life, distress, depression and anxiety are all markers of the degree to which an individual is coping emotionally. Global adaptation may be measured with measured of daily function. Coping with cancer can be defined as the perception of being able to maintain integrity, autonomy and function in the face of a diagnosis of cancer. The transactional theory of stress and coping, developed by Lazarus and Folkman, is the most widely used framework for evaluating the processes of coping with stressful events (Endler and Parker 1990). According to this theory, the stressor is initially appraised in terms of personal relevance to the individual and, subsequently, the resources available to deal with the stressor are evaluated. Several generic self-report measures of coping now exist—for example, the Ways of Coping Questionnaire (WCQ) (Folkman 1988) and the Coping Inventory (Carver et al. 1989). In cancer, the Mental adjustment to cancer (MAC) is the best known (Watson et al. 1989). Watson and colleagues (1988) developed the Mental Adjustment to Cancer (MAC) scale which identifies five styles of coping: denial/avoidance, fighting spirit, fatalism, helplessness/hopelessness and anxious preoccupation. They found that the last three coping styles were significantly associated with depression as measured by the HAD scale which was simultaneously administered. They also reported that helplessness/hopelessness but not 'fighting spirit' was significantly associated with survival. A criticism of these coping scales is their length. The mini-MAC is a 29-item scale focusing on five coping responses: helplessness-hopelessness (e.g. 'I feel like giving up'), anxious preoccupation (e.g. 'I am apprehensive'), cognitive avoidance (e.g. 'Not thinking about it helps me cope'), fatalism (e.g. 'At the moment I take one day at a time') and fighting spirit (e.g. 'I see my illness as a challenge'). A number of studies examining the psychometric properties of the mini-MAC have supported the reliability of all five subscales (Watson et al. 1994).

4.5   Discussion

Screening for distress, the 6th vital sign (Bultz and Carlson 2005) and psychological assessment is an integral part of high quality whole person cancer care. A large body of work has attempted to develop and validate tools for screening for distress and psychological assessment, but comparatively little work has tested the implementation of these tools in clinical practice. Routine psychological assessment by clinicians is subject to large individual differences. Significant influences include clinicians' skills, experience and past training, availability of audit and work pressures. Studies suggest that clinicians own routine ability to detection psychological symptoms, and psychiatric diagnoses is often poor with about 50 % sensitivity and 80 % specificity. However, the routine clinical method often fosters trust and therapeutic alliance and may actually be the method most preferred by patients. Most forms of screening are seen as a slight burden to patients and clinicians. In some circumstances this burden can be significant and rate-limiting. Therefore screening implementation can be limited as much by acceptability as by accuracy. Relatively little attention has been paid to the acceptability and comparative formats of screening tools. Previously most screening focussed on one narrow domain, such as depression. A multidimensional approach may be preferable but it is more difficult to validate. A multidimensional tool can be valuable as it can serve as a roadmap to a more effective way of addressing patient concerns in a timely way with appropriate referral to the right professional. A number of new application strategies are being explored including: screening online, at home or in the waiting room and kiosk screening, screening using smart phones and tables. Ideally each method should be tested for effects on acceptability and accuracy. Screening for distress is an attractive first cut at a board-based multidimensional assessment method that aims to improve upon usual care. Well-designed studies have compared screening with 'diagnosis as usual' demonstrate small but potentially important gains, notably in communication and referral. However, screening is insufficient in isolation and must be followed up by appropriate treatment and aftercare. In a national survey of US oncologists, 65.0 % reported screening patients for distress routinely, but only 14.3 % used a screening instrument (Pirl et al. 2007). In a survey of 84 Canadian cancer institutions, only 36.5 % routinely screened patients for emotional distress at the time of admission (Moller 2000). In short, there is no country that has yet mandated routine screening, and this may be because the evidence base for distress screening has been limited by methodological considerations or because individual institutions have yet to invest in worthwhile programmes.

In the past, much clinical and training focussed on rather narrow construct of 'breaking bad news'. Similarly screening tended to focus only on clinical depression. Thus, both clinical assessment and screening have overlooked other valuable physical, social, practical and psychological domains. Screening for depression, although important, cannot encompass the whole patient experience. Similarly communicating a diagnosis is only one aspect of the patient journey with cancer. Assessment may be enhanced by consideration of evaluation of unmet needs, clarification of any desire for help and questions about the acceptability of the treatment offered. These may be essential rate-limiting steps in determining the effectiveness of psychological assessment in the real world. For example less than half of patients are ready to accept psychological help when it is offered in the clinic.

Screening for distress and/or psychological assessment should not be considered a one-off exercise but part of routine high quality of care that involves all healthcare professionals. Thorough and timely psychological assessment will enhance trust and therapeutic alliance particularly when it involves the clinician directly. Psychosocial needs are the most overlooked of all cancer complications. Psychological assessment, together with appropriate follow-up and tailored acceptable interventions, will help reduce this gap in unmet psychosocial needs.

References

Aaronson NK, Ahmedzai S, Bergman B, Bullinger M, Cull A, Duez NJ, Filiberti A, Flechtner H, Fleishman SB, de Haes JC. The European Organization for Research and Treatment of Cancer QLQ-C30: a quality-of-life instrument for use in international clinical trials in oncology. J Natl Cancer Inst. 1993;85:365–76.

Baillargeon J, Kuo YF, Lin YL, Raji MA, Singh A, Goodwin JS. Effect of mental disorders on diagnosis, treatment, and survival of older adults with colon cancer. J Am Geriatr Soc. 2011; 59(7):1268–73. doi:10.1111/j.1532-5415.2011.03481.x. Epub 2011.

Baker-Glenn EA, Park B, Granger L, Symonds P, Mitchell AJ. Desire for psychological support in cancer patients with depression or distress: validation of a simple help question. Psychooncology. 2011;20(5):525–31. doi:10.1002/pon.1759.

Barth J, Lannen P. Efficacy of communication skills training courses in oncology: a systematic review and meta-analysis. Ann Oncol. 2011;22(5):1030–40. doi:10.1093/annonc/mdq441. Epub 2010 Oct 25.

Bezjak A, Ng P, Taylor K, et al. A preliminary survey of oncologists' perceptions of quality of life information. Psychooncology. 1997;6:107–13.

Bezjak A, Ng P, Skeel R, et al. Oncologists' use of quality of life information: results of a survey of Eastern Cooperative Oncology Group physicians. Qual Life Res. 2001;10:1–13.

Bonito A, Horowitz N, McCorkle R, Chagpar AB. Do healthcare professionals discuss the emotional impact of cancer with patients? Psychooncology. 2013;22(9):2046–50. doi:10.1002/pon.3258.

Braeken AP, Kempen GI, Eekers D, et al. The usefulness and feasibility of a screening instrument to identify psychosocial problems in patients receiving curative radiotherapy: a process evaluation. BMC Cancer. 2011;11:479.

Bultz BD, Holland JC. Emotional distress in patients with cancer: the sixth vital sign. Commun Oncol. 2006;3(5):311–4.

Bultz BD, Carlson LE. Emotional distress: the sixth vital sign in cancer care. J Clin Oncol. 2005;23 (26):6440–1.

Bultz BD, Groff SL, Fitch M, Claude-Blais M, Howes J, Levy K. Implementing screening for distress, the 6th vital sign: a Canadian strategy for changing practice. Psychooncology. 2011;20:463–9.

Bultz BD, Loscalzo MJ, Clark KL. Screening for distress, the 6th vital sign, as the connective tissue of health care systems: a roadmap to integrated interdisciplinary person-centred care. In: Grassi L, Riba M, editors. Clinical psycho-oncology: an international perspective. New York: Wiley; 2012. p. 83–96.

Carlson LE, Clifford SK, Groff SL, Maciejewski O, Bultz B. Screening for depression in cancer care. In: Mitchell AJ, Coyne JC, editors. Screening for depression in clinical practice. New York: Oxford University Press; 2010a. p. 265–98.

Carlson LE, Groff SL, Maciejewski O, Bultz BD. Screening for distress in lung and breast cancer outpatients: a randomized controlled trial. J Clin Oncol. 2010b;28(33):4884–91. Epub 2010 Oct 12.

Carlson LE, Waller A, Mitchell AJ. Screening for distress and unmet needs in patients with cancer: review and recommendations. J Clin Oncol. 2012;30(11):1160–77. doi:10.1200/JCO.2011.39. 5509. Epub 2012 Mar 12.

Carver CS, Scheier MF, Weintraub JK. Assessing coping strategies: a theoretically based approach. J Person Soc Psychol. 1989;56:267–83.

Cella DF, Tulsky DS, Gray G, Sarafian B, Linn E, Bonomi A, Silberman M, Yellen SB, Winicour P, Brannon J. The functional assessment of cancer therapy scale: development and validation of the general measure. J Clin Oncol. 1993;11:570–9.

Detmar SB, Muller MJ, Schornagel JH, Wever LD, Aaronson NK. Health-related quality-of-life assessments and patient-physician communication: a randomized controlled trial. JAMA. 2002;288:3027–34.

Deveugele M, Derese A, De Bacquer D, van den Brink-Muinen A, Bensing J, De Maeseneer J. Is the communicative behavior of GPs during the consultation related to the diagnosis? A cross-sectional study in six European countries. Patient Educ Couns. 2004;54(3):283–9.

Endler NS, Parker JD. Multidimensional assessment of coping: a critical evaluation. J Pers Soc Psychol. 1990;58:844–54.

Folkman S, Lazarus RS. Manual for the ways of coping questionnaire. Palo Alto, CA: Consulting Psychologists Press; 1988.

Folstein MF, Folstein SE, McHugh PR. 'Mini-mental state'. A practical method for grading the cognitive state of patients for the physician. J Psychiatr Res. 1975;12:189–98.

Fröjd C, Lampic C, Larsson G, Birgegård G, von Essen L. Patient attitudes, behaviours, and other factors considered by doctors when estimating cancer patients' anxiety and desire for information. Scand J Caring Sci. 2007;21:523–9.

Gaynes BN, DeVeaugh-Geiss J, Weir S, Gu H, MacPherson C, Schulberg HC, Culpepper L, Rubinow DR. Feasibility and diagnostic validity of the M-3 checklist: a brief, self-rated screen for depressive, bipolar, anxiety, and post-traumatic stress disorders in primary care. Ann Fam Med. 2010;8(2):160–9.

Harrison JD, Young JM, Price MA, Butow PN, Solomon MJ. What are the unmet supportive care needs of people with cancer? A systematic review. Support Care Cancer. 2009;17(8):1117–28. doi:10.1007/s00520-009-0615-5. Epub 2009 Mar 25.

Herschbach P, Berg P, Dankert A, Duran G, Engst-Hastreiter U, Waadt S, Keller M, Ukat R, Henrich G. Fear of progression in chronic diseases: psychometric properties of the Fear of Progression Questionnaire. J Psychosom Res. 2005;58(6):505–11.

Heyland DK, Dodek P, Rocker G, Groll D, Gafni A, Pichora D, Shortt S, Tranmer J, Lazar N, Kutsogiannis J, Lam M, Canadian Researchers End-of-Life Network (CARENET). What matters most in end-of-life care: perceptions of seriously ill patients and their family members. CMAJ. 2006;174(5):627–33.

Hillen MA, de Haes HC, Smets EM. Cancer patients' trust in their physician-a review. Psychooncology. 2011;20(3):227–41. doi:10.1002/pon.1745.

Hollingworth W, Harris S, Metcalfe C, Mancero S, Biddle L, Campbell R, Brennan J. Evaluating the effect of using a distress thermometer and problem list to monitor psychosocial concerns among patients receiving treatment for cancer: preliminary results of a randomised controlled trial. Psychooncology. 2012; 21(s2)

Houston JP, Kroenke K, Faries DE, Doebbeling CC, Adler LA, Ahl J, Swindle R, Trzepacz PT. A provisional screening instrument for four common mental disorders in adult primary care patients. Psychosomatics. 2011;52(1):48–55.

Howell D, Mayo S, Currie S, Jones G, Boyle M, Hack T, Green E, Hoffman L, Collacutt V, McLeod D, Simpson J. Psychosocial health care needs assessment of adult cancer patients: a consensus-based guideline. Support Care Cancer. 2012;20(12):3343–54. Epub ahead of print.

Jacobsen PB, Shibata D, Siegel EM, Lee JH, Fulp WJ, Alemany C, Abesada-Terk Jr G, Brown R, Cartwright T, Faig D, Kim G, Levine R, Markham MJ, Schreiber F, Sharp P, Malafa M. Evaluating the quality of psychosocial care in outpatient medical oncology settings using performance indicators. Psychooncology. 2011;20(11):1221–7.

Klinkhammer-Schalke M, Koller M, Steinger B, Ehret C, Ernst B, Wyatt JC, Hofstädter F, Lorenz W, Regensburg QoL Study Group. Direct improvement of quality of life using a tailored quality of life diagnosis and therapy pathway: randomised trial in 200 women with breast cancer. Br J Cancer. 2012;106(5):826–38.

Lo C, Zimmermann C, Rydall A, Walsh A, Jones JM, Moore MJ, Shepherd FA, Gagliese L, Rodin G. Longitudinal study of depressive symptoms in patients with metastatic gastrointestinal and lung cancer. J Clin Oncol. 2010;28(18):3084–9. doi:10.1200/JCO.2009.26.9712. Epub 2010 May 17.

Luckett T, Butow PN, King MT. Improving patient outcomes through the routine use of patient-reported data in cancer clinics: future directions. Psychooncology. 2009;18:1129–38.

Luckett T, Butow PN, King MT, Oguchi M, Heading G, Hackl NA, Rankin N, Price MA. A review and recommendations for optimal outcome measures of anxiety, depression and general distress in studies evaluating psychosocial interventions for English-speaking adults with heterogeneous cancer diagnoses. Support Care Cancer. 2010;18(10):1241–62. Epub 2010 Jul 2.

Maunsell E, Brisson J, Deschenes L, Frasure-Smith N. Randomized trial of a psychologic distress screening program after breast cancer: effects on quality of life. J Clin Oncol. 1996;14: 2747–55.

McLachlan SA, Allenby A, Matthews J, Wirth A, Kissane D, Bishop M, et al. Randomized trial of coordinated psychosocial interventions based on patient self-assessments versus standard care to improve the psychosocial functioning of patients with cancer. J Clin Oncol. 2001;19: 4117–25.

Mills ME, Murray LJ, Johnston BT, Cardwell C, Donnelly M. Does a patient-held quality-of-life diary benefit patients with inoperable lung cancer? J Clin Oncol. 2009;27(1):70–7. Epub 2008 Nov 24.

Mitchell AJ. Pooled results from 38 analyses of the accuracy of distress thermometer and other ultrashort methods of detecting cancer-related mood disorders. J Clin Oncol. 2007;25: 4670–81.

Mitchell AJ. Short screening tools for cancer-related distress: a review and diagnostic validity meta-analysis. J Natl Compr Canc Netw. 2010;8(4):487–94.

Mitchell AJ, Kaar S, Coggan C, Herdman J. Acceptability of common screening methods used to detect distress and related mood disorders-preferences of cancer specialists and non-specialists. Psychooncology. 2008;17(3):226–36.

Mitchell AJ, Vaze A, Rao S. Clinical diagnosis of depression in primary care: a meta-analysis. Lancet. 2009;374(9690):609–19. Epub 2009 Jul 27.

Mitchell AJ, Meader N, Symonds P. Diagnostic validity of the hospital anxiety and depression scale (HADS) in cancer and palliative settings: a meta-analysis. J Affect Disord. 2010a; 126(3):335–48.

Mitchell AJ, Baker-Glenn EA, Symonds P. Can the distress thermometer be improved by additional mood domains? Part I. Initial validation of the emotion thermometers tool. Psychooncology. 2010b;19(2):125–33.

Mitchell AJ, Chan M, Bhatti H, Halton M, Grassi L, Johansen C, Meader N. Prevalence of depression, anxiety, and adjustment disorder in oncological, haematological, and palliative-care settings: a meta-analysis of 94 interview-based studies. Lancet Oncol. 2011a;12(2): 160–74. Epub 2011.

Mitchell AJ, Vahabzadeh A, Magruder K. Screening for distress and depression in cancer settings: 10 lessons from 40 years of primary-care research. Psychooncology. 2011b;20(6):572–84.

Mitchell AJ, Meader N, Pentzek M. Clinical recognition of dementia and cognitive impairment in primary care: a meta-analysis of physician accuracy. Acta Psychiatr Scand. 2011c;124(3): 165–83.

Mitchell AJ, Hussain N, Grainger L, Symonds P. Identification of patient-reported distress by clinical nurse specialists in routine oncology practice: a multicentre UK study. Psychooncology. 2011d;20(10):1076–83. doi:10.1002/pon.1815. Epub 2010 Aug 4.

Mitchell AJ, Lord K, Slattery J, Grainger L, Symonds P. How feasible is implementation of distress screening by cancer clinicians in routine clinical care? Cancer 2012a. Cancer. 2012a; 118(24):6260–9.

Mitchell AJ, Lord K, Symonds P. Which symptoms are indicative of DSMIV depression in cancer settings? An analysis of the diagnostic significance of somatic and non-somatic symptoms. J Affect Disord. 2012b;138(1–2):137–48. doi:10.1016/j.jad.2011.11.009. Epub 2012 Feb 5.

Mitchell AJ, Meader N, Davies E, Clover K, Carter GL, Loscalzo MJ, Linden W, Grassi L, Johansen C, Carlson LE, Zabora J. Meta-analysis of screening and case finding tools for depression in cancer: Evidence based recommendations for clinical practice on behalf of the Depression in Cancer Care consensus group. J Affect Disord. 2012c;140(2):149–60. Epub ahead of print.

Mitchell AJ, Ferguson DW, Gill J, Paul J, Symonds P. Depression and anxiety in long-term cancer survivors compared with spouses and healthy controls: a systematic review and meta-analysis. Lancet Oncol. 2013;14(8):721–32.

Moller HJ. Rating depressed patients: observer- vs self-assessment. Eur Psychiatry. 2000;15: 160–72.

Mor V, Laliberte L, Morris JN, Wiemann M. The Karnofsky performance status scale: an examination of its reliability and validity in a research setting. Cancer. 1984;53:2002–7.

Morasso G, Costantini M, Baracco G, Borreani C, Capelli M. Assessing psychological distress in cancer patients: validation of a self-administered questionnaire. Oncology. 1996;53 (4):295–302.

Morris J, Perez D, McNoe B. The use of quality of life data in clinical practice. Qual Life Res. 1998;7:85–91.

National Comprehensive Cancer Network. Distress management. NCCN clinical practice guidelines in oncology. National Comprehensive Cancer Network; 2008. Available from: http://www.nccn.org/professionals/physician_gls/PDF/distress.pdf.

Nekolaichuk C, Watanabe S, Beaumont C. The Edmonton Symptom Assessment System: a 15-year retrospective review of validation studies (1991–2006). Palliat Med. 2008;22(2): 111–2.

Nelson JE, Gay EB, Berman AR, Powell CA, Salazar-Schicchi J, Wisnivesky JP. Patients rate physician communication about lung cancer. Cancer. 2011;117(22):5212–20. doi:10.1002/ cncr.26152. Epub 2011 Apr 14.

Pirl W, Muriel A, Hwang V, Kornblith A, Greer J, Donelan K. Screening for psychosocial distress: a national survey of oncologists. J Support Oncol. 2007;5(1):499–504.

Puts MT, Papoutsis A, Springall E, Tourangeau AE. A systematic review of unmet needs of newly diagnosed older cancer patients undergoing active cancer treatment. Support Care Cancer. 2012;20(7):1377–94. Epub 2012 Apr 4.

Richardson LA, Jones GW. A review of the reliability and validity of the Edmonton symptom assessment system. Curr Oncol. 2009;16(1):55.

Rodriguez KL, Bayliss N, Alexander SC, et al. How oncologists and their patients with advanced cancer communicate about health-related quality of life. Psychooncology. 2010;19(5):490–9.

Roth AJ, Kornblith AB, Batel-Copel L, et al. Rapid screening for psychologic distress in men with prostate carcinoma: A pilot study. Cancer. 1998;82:1904–8.

Sarna L. Effectiveness of structured nursing assessment of symptom distress in advanced lung cancer. Oncol Nurs Forum. 1998;25(6):1041–8.

Sollner W, DeVries A, Steixner E, et al. How successful are oncologists in identifying patient distress, perceived social support, and need for psychosocial counselling? Br J Cancer. 2001; 84(2):179–85.

Strong V, Waters R, Hibberd C, Murray G, Wall L, Walker J, McHugh G, Walker A, Sharpe M. Management of depression for people with cancer (SMaRT oncology 1): a randomised trial. Lancet. 2008;372(9632):40–8.

Tai-Seale M, McGuire T, Colenda C, et al. Two-minute mental health care for elderly patients: Inside primary care visits. J Am Geriatr Soc. 2007;55(12):1903–11.

Thombs BD, Coyne JC, Cuijpers P, et al. Rethinking recommendations for screening for depression in primary care. CMAJ. 2011;184(4):413–8.

Trevino KM, Fasciano K, Prigerson HG. Patient-oncologist alliance, psychosocial well-being, and treatment adherence among young adults with advanced cancer. J Clin Oncol. 2013;31(13): 1683–9.

Uitterhoeve RJ, Bensing JM, Grol RP, Demulder PH, Van Achterberg T. The effect of communication skills training on patient outcomes in cancer care: a systematic review of the literature. Eur J Cancer Care (Engl). 2010;19(4):442–57.

Underhill ML, Kiviniemi MT. The association of perceived provider-patient communication and relationship quality with colorectal cancer screening. Health Educ Behav. 2012;39:555–63.

van Scheppingen C, Schroevers MJ, Smink A, et al. Does screening for distress efficiently uncover meetable unmet needs in cancer patients? Psychooncology. 2011;20(6):655–63.

Velikova G, Booth L, Smith AB, Brown PM, Lynch P, Brown JM, et al. Measuring quality of life in routine oncology practice improves communication and patient well-being: a randomized controlled trial. J Clin Oncol. 2004;22:714–24.

Velikova G, Keding A, Harley C, Cocks K, Booth L, Smith AB, Wright P, Selby PJ, Brown JM. Patients report improvements in continuity of care when quality of life assessments are used routinely in oncology practice: secondary outcomes of a randomised controlled trial. Eur J Cancer. 2010;46(13):2381–8.

Waller A, Garland SN, Bultz BD. Using screening for distress, the sixth vital sign, to advance patient care with assessment and targeted interventions. Support Care Cancer. 2012;20(9): 2241–6. doi:10.1007/s00520-012-1506-8. Epub 2012 Jun 7.

Watson M, Greer S, Young J, Inayat Q, Burgess C, Robertson B. Development of a questionnaire measure of adjustment to cancer: the MAC scale. Psychol Med. 1988;18(1):203–9.

Watson M, Greer S, Bliss JM. Mental adjustment to cancer (MAC) Scale users' manual. Surrey: CRC Psychological Medicine Research Group; 1989.

Watson M, Law M, dos Santos M, Greer S, Baruch J, Bliss J, The Mini-MAC. Further development of the Mental Adjustment to Cancer scale. J Psychosoc Oncol. 1994;12(3):33–46.

Zigmond AS, Snaith RP. The hospital anxiety and depression scale. Acta Psychiatr Scand. 1983; 67:361–70.

Interpersonal Relationship Issues in Psychopharmacology

5

Luigi Grassi, Rosangela Caruso, and Walter Baile

Abstract

Communication is the essential component for good clinical practice within a patient-centered approach, with guidelines empathizing the role of communication and the mandatory need to train physicians in communication in order to assure optimal psychosocial care of cancer patients, including the psychosocial interview patient assessment, prescription, and follow-up. The aim of this chapter is to briefly summarize some principles of communication when dealing with cancer patients with psychiatric disorders in order to facilitate assessment and promote adherence to treatment and to suggest guidelines which the clinician may use to achieve these goals. For these reasons, the protocol SPIKES-Rx has been specifically developed to guide doctors in the appropriate interactions to promote patient agreement with recommendations for psychopharmacological management when psychotropic drugs are prescribed.

5.1 Introduction

The field of communication and interpersonal relationship skills in oncology and palliative care has been the object of a very large number of empirical studies, randomized clinical trials, and meta-analysis. It is a fact that communication is the essential component for good clinical practice within a patient-centered approach,

L. Grassi (✉) • R. Caruso
Institute of Psychiatry, Department of Biomedical and Specialty Surgical Sciences, University of Ferrara, Ferrara, Italy
e-mail: luigi.grassi@unife.it; rosangela.caruso@unife.it

W. Baile
Program for Interpersonal Communication and Relationship Enhancement (I*CARE), Department of Faculty and Academic Development, University of Texas, M.D. Anderson Cancer Center, Houston, TX, USA
e-mail: wbaile@mdanderson.org

L. Grassi and M. Riba (eds.), *Psychopharmacology in Oncology and Palliative Care*,
DOI 10.1007/978-3-642-40134-3_5, © Springer-Verlag Berlin Heidelberg 2014

with guidelines empathizing the role of communication and the mandatory need to train physicians in communication in order to assure optimal psychosocial care of cancer patients (Butow and Baile 2012). Communication skills training mostly has focused on some specific topics in oncology, such as breaking bad news, preparing patients for aversive procedures, giving clear information, promoting shared decision making, eliciting concerns, and responding to emotion. On the other hand, it is clear that communication is intrinsically part of the doctor–patient relationship and emerges as the cornerstone in any encounter with the patient, including the psychosocial interview, patient assessment, prescription, and follow-up.

While we direct the reader, for more details, to the many books dedicated, in the last 20 years, to the area of communication in cancer and palliative care (Faulkner and Maguire 1994; Stiefel 2006; Back et al. 2009; Kissane et al. 2011; Surbone et al. 2013), the aim of this chapter is to briefly summarize some principles of communication when dealing with cancer patients with psychiatric disorders in order to facilitate assessment and promote adherence to treatment and to suggest guidelines which the clinician may use to achieve these goals.

5.2 Specific Aspects of the Interpersonal Relationship in Cancer Care

5.2.1 Communication Process in the Clinical Encounter

In the encounter with cancer patients showing symptoms of psychological distress or psychiatric disorders, it is extremely important that the basic and advanced skills for good communication and a doctor–patient relationship are employed. A correct evaluation needs a respectful, empathic, and nonjudgmental attitude, with special attention to the patient's modalities of interpersonal communication, both verbal and nonverbal, while investigating the several areas of his/her history (see Grassi et al. 2014, Chap. 3 in this book). The main tasks of communication in this process are the promotion of reciprocal trust, the encouragement of the patient's emotional expression, the fostering of shared decision making, the consolidation of the therapeutic alliance, and the provision of support. These tasks, as indicated by Priebe et al. (2011), are relevant to many objectives of clinical care and may directly or indirectly influence outcomes of treatment. At the end of the communication process, in fact, the clinician should have obtained all necessary information from the patient and family. The patient also should have obtained and understood all information that is relevant to him or her. A positive therapeutic relationship should have been established and/or sustained, and all necessary decisions should have been made or discussed.

From the relational point of view, these goals can be achieved if components of effective communication are present, including the clinician's attention to listening, exploring emotions, identifying psychological problems, and providing empathic responses. With reference to this, Baile and Costantini (2013) have provided a series of valued physician behaviors that represent fundamentals of the clinical encounter. These can be summarized as follows: the capacity to impart confidence (e.g., greeting patient with warmth, making eye contact, encouraging patient queries); being empathetic (e.g., eliciting patient's concerns, acknowledging distress, recognizing and being sensitive to emotions); providing a "human touch" (e.g., using appropriate physical contact, being attentive and present to the patient and the situation, showing interest and compassion); relating on a personal level (e.g., asking patient about his/her life, acknowledging patient's family, remembering details about patient's life from visit to visit); being forthright (e.g., being honest and not withholding information, asking patient to recap conversation to ensure understanding); being respectful (e.g., listening carefully and not interrupting, taking care of the dignity of the patient); being thorough (e.g., providing detailed explanations, giving instructions in writing, following up in a timely manner).

If the skills mentioned above are fundamental attributes of the encounter, a sensitive and skilful assessment of the patient's signs and symptoms is then a crucial point of both the diagnostic phase and the treatment planning and decision making. As for the good communication skills necessary in clinical psychiatry, when assessing psychiatric symptoms and in psychosocial assessment in oncology, some techniques and skills have demonstrated to facilitate the interaction and the conduction of the interview, while others have been shown to inhibit or to block the process of the interaction (Faulkner and Maguire 1994; Maguire and Pitceathly 2002) (Table 5.1).

In summary, communication with cancer patients showing psychosocial disorders needs to be founded on cooperation, and the clinician has to be aware that what originates from the relationship with patient is the result of the co-participation of two active counterparts. Unlike simple information exchange, it has intrinsic therapeutic value but requires from the clinician the ability to reflect on him/herself, about his/her relational style, and one's own emotions. In some cases physicians may find it uncomfortable to delve into patients' feelings, because they are concerned that symptoms, once elicited, would be daunting to manage. Attention to countertransference issues is important here. For example, as a reaction to a depressed cancer patient, physicians may adopt a paternalistic attitude, avoiding discussions with an emotional focus, offering inappropriately, providing reassurance, using ambiguous terms, or giving in to the temptation of communicating false hope. In other cases, patients may evoke in clinicians frustrating emotions, such as sadness, anger, boredom, and sense of failure (Grassi et al. 2013). The involvement of family members and significant others, with the patient's permission, is also important when assessing and planning for treatment. In all the possible psychiatric manifestation of suffering, in fact, the presence of a key family member can be extremely helpful both for a broader vision and comprehension of the patient's symptoms and for the educational role that can be favored by creating an alliance with the family.

Table 5.1 Interview techniques

Facilitative styles promoting disclosure	Obstructive styles inhibiting disclosure
Open-ended questions: "Tell me about. . ."; "Can you describe how you have felt?"	Closed (yes–no) questions, direct questions: "Did you have insomnia?", "Are you anxious?"
Facilitation: "Uh-huh", "Please go on", "I see"	Non facilitating messages: Distraction, not making eye contact, following one's own thoughts
Reflection: "You say you are giving up. . .."; "Give up?"	Premature reassurance: "Before continuing I can already say that your depression is curable"
Clarification: "Can you tell me more about. . .?"; "What do you mean exactly when you say. . ..?"	False reassurance: "You need not to worry about these flashbacks, they will go away soon"
Positive reinforcement: encouraging the patient to continue on a specific theme or topic	Inappropriate reinforcement: "Come on! You owe your daughter a less depressed father"
Respectful silence: judicious use of silence, while maintaining the contact	Premature problem solving: "OK, I understand you are depressed and, to be practical, you need to take this drug and I will see you again in a month"
Summarizing: "So, if I have understood well, after the diagnosis of cancer you started to have nightmares. . ."	Switching the topic: when speaking about a significant topic, moving abruptly to a different unrelated topic

5.2.2 Adherence

A further communication issue when psychopharmacology treatment is proposed, regards the need to reinforce adherence to treatment. The debate on the definition of adherence (i.e., extent to which the patient's behavior matches agreed recommendations from the prescriber), compliance (i.e., extent to which the patient's behavior matches the prescriber's recommendations), concordance (i.e., process by which a patient and clinician make decisions together about treatment), and persistence (i.e., the patient's capacity to continue treatment) is still ongoing (Aaronson 2007). What has emerged over the last several years regarding this topic is that an average of 25 % of patients tend not to follow in a correct way their physician's recommendations (non-adherence) (DiMatteo 2004), with variations according to the type of the disease and its severity (DiMatteo et al. 2007). Also for these reasons, the problem of low adherence in medical practice, with negative consequences for outcome, is a special area of interest taken into account by the World Health Organization (WHO 2003). Many factors are involved in adherence, including sociodemographic characteristics, specific aspects of the treatment regimen (type, complexity, side effects, and duration), features of the illness or potential illness (symptoms, duration, disability, and medically defined seriousness), and doctor–patient communication (Arbuthnott and Sharpe 2009; Martin et al. 2000). With regard to the latter area, the literature is extremely extensive, with data showing the role of poor communication and relational issues in non-adherence and subsequently the outcome of both medical and psychiatric disorders (Zolnierek and DiMatteo 2009; Thompson and McCabe 2012). Thus, the problem of adherence in terms of the capacity to correctly follow a shared decision-making process with the clinicians about medication or drug treatment, self-care, healthy lifestyles, intervention in general (e.g., psychotherapy sessions) is an important issue in psychosocial oncology.

When specifically related to psychopharmacology, data exist about the low tendency of patients with psychiatric disorders to follow what the treatment plan agreed upon with their doctors in terms of medication assumption and continuation of treatment. For example, both among people with depressive disorders (DiMatteo et al. 2000) and cancer patients with depression (DiMatteo and Haskard-Zolnierek 2011), reduced motivation toward self-care, negative health beliefs about treatment, social isolation and avoidance of health promoting behavior, and greater difficulty in tolerating treatment side effects are all possible causes of reduced adherence to psychotropic drugs prescription. In primary care initiatives to improve physicians' communication skills regarding mental health issues, and to improve recognition of psychiatric disorders, have been shown to increase the number of patients receiving treatment (Prins et al. 2010). Furthermore, higher rates of guideline adherence tends to be associated with a stronger confidence in depression identification among physicians confirming the importance of developing communication skills in inter-personal doctor–patient relationship (Smolders et al. 2010).

Summarizing what has emerged from the literature, the factors related to communication and interpersonal issues that have been indicated as important in favoring adherence in psychiatry are mainly represented by clinician–patient alliance and specific task-oriented variables. The clinician–patient alliance is based on a strong bond between patient and therapist and the establishment of patient and therapist agreement on the goals of treatment and on the steps to achieve these goals. The essential issues related to clinician–patient alliance are provided in Table 5.2.

More specific communication styles regard clinical messages related to adherence itself, which are important both in the planning of the treatment and follow-up are: encouragement of expression of concerns or problems with the medication; asking about and listening to concerns about medication; helping in solving the problems related to the patient's use of medication are all elements to be taken into consideration. Thus, not only a good interpersonal rapport is important but also educational, active, and task-oriented elements of the alliance are instrumental for adherence (Sawada et al. 2009; Thompson and McCabe 2012). Some issues to be considered to facilitate adherence in psychopharmacological treatment in cancer care are presented in Table 5.3. However, from a more practical and, at the same time, specific point of view, having a road map regarding how to prescribe and reinforce the use of psychotropic drugs is extremely important in cancer settings, as described in the next paragraph.

Table 5.2 Interpersonal relationship ingredients for psychopharmacological approach in cancer care [from Schnur and Montgomery (2010, mod)]

- Therapeutic alliance: A good agreement between therapist and patient on the goals of treatment, the tasks needed to accomplish those goals, and a sense of a personal bond between therapist and patient
- Empathy: Therapist's sensitive ability and willingness to understand the client's thoughts, feelings, and struggles from the client's point of view based on an accurate recognition of the client's experience, the ability to share the client's feelings, and the capacity to express empathy to the client
- Goal consensus: The patient–therapist agreement on the therapeutic goals and the expectations for therapy
- Collaboration: A mutual involvement by patient and therapist in helping the relationship, including patient cooperation, patient resistance, homework completion, hostility, defensive styles, or involvement in the patient role

Table 5.3 Strategies to facilitate adherence in psychopharmacological treatment in cancer care

Education about the disorder
Symptoms and characteristics of the specific disorder (e.g., major depression, stress-related disorder, anxiety disorder)
Risk of complications if untreated, need for early recognition of symptoms for seeking treatment
Education about treatment
Specify the rationale of the use of the drug, its benefits and side effects, dose, duration of treatment
Correct misperceptions and fears about the use of the drug (e.g., potential to be addictive, sedative effects, tolerance, etc.)
Education about healthy behaviors
Promotion of healthy behaviors (e.g., exercise, good sleep hygiene, good nutrition, avoidance of tobacco, alcohol, and other substances)
Involvement of family members and other key figures of the patient's day-to-day life

5.3 Wedding Communication Skills to Psychotropic Drug Prescribing

Prescribing psychopharmacological agents in the oncology setting is not always straightforward. Many patients are already on multiple other medications and may be reluctant to add to the burden that they impose regarding cost and side effects. Moreover, the purpose and importance of a psychiatric consultation may not be well explained by the referring physician who may themselves feel uncomfortable about patient reactions to a psychiatric referral such as "you don't think I'm crazy do you?." In addition patients may have heard negative reports from family or friends about psychotropic medications, had previous negative experiences of their own, or fear that they will become "addicted" to the prescribed drug.

On the other hand most practicing psychiatrists who deal with cancer patients are well aware that depression and anxiety are common accompaniments of psychiatric disorders and can contribute to significant decreases in quality of life for patients already dealing with disability or debility from their cancer. Many have experienced patients who have significantly benefited from improved sleep and mood, decrease in anxiety and panic attacks, reduction in hot flashes, and a more positive outlook toward their cancer treatment that can come with the use of psychotropics in the oncology setting. Moreover, many patients are naïve to psychotropic medication and often respond quickly to the desired effects whether they be anxiolytic, anti-depressive, or hypnotic. This latter characteristic, although not written about much in the literature, can make a significant difference in patient acceptance due to the fact that they can see a difference in their mood or a decrease in their anxiety in a matter of several days. While some have argued that this may be a placebo effect, it may be that patients who are on medications which alter body chemistry or the blood brain barrier are advantaged compared to other patients who have previously been on antidepressants or who are not receiving systemic chemotherapy.

For these reasons it may be particularly important that patients who seem to be a candidate for psychopharmacotherapy have the opportunity to have a complete trial on them. For this reason we believe that certain elements of the communication process are crucial in patient acceptance of psychopharmacological recommendations. A clinician might consider following an acronym we have developed to guide him or her in the appropriate interactions to promote patient agreement with recommendations for psychopharmacological management. This acronym called SPIKES Rx is borrowed from the SPIKES six-step protocol for giving bad news (Baile et al. 2000) that has been extensively shown to help in communication in cancer settings (Finlay and Casarett 2009; Kaplan 2010) and adapted in different cultural context, such as Japan (Fujimori et al. 2003) and Italy (Costantini et al. 2009; Lenzi et al. 2011). SPIKES Rx has been specifically modified to underscore that communication is an essential component of proposing a therapy that many patients may be skeptical of (Table 5.4).

5.4 The SPIKES Rx Protocol in Cancer Settings

5.4.1 S = Setting up the Discussion

As previously pointed out, a trusting relationship is essential to any conversation about psychopharmacological recommendations. Patients who feel that the prescribing physician has an interest in them as a person and is empathic toward their plight will be more likely to accept recommendations for therapy. So before suggesting medications, a clinician should inquire about the patient's medical illness asking them to relate the history of their disease. Not only does every patient has a unique story to tell but the feeling on the part of the patient that the clinician is taking into account the patient's illness experience will be reassuring to them and enhance their trust in the clinician. The history should also include the traditional questions such as the patient's social and employment background and their understanding of their illness and the goals of care. Opportunities for empathic

Table 5.4 The SPIKES Rx protocol

S = Setting	Setting up the discussion: before suggesting medications clinician should inquire about the patient's medical illness (history of their disease, concerns, illness experience, social and employment background), by using basic communication skills (e.g., listening without interrupting, empathizing, and exploring) Example: "Can you tell me about your disease? How did you react? How are you coping with that?"
P = Perception	Perception about psychotropic drugs and treatment (what the patient knows about drugs, previous treatment and experiences, attitudes of family members' and their perspectives) Example: "Can you tell me what you know on the treatment you received?"
I = Invitation	Setting goals for prescribing a psychotropic indicating transition from history taking to giving information. Additional exploration and further information in case of resistance Example: "I'd like to spend the next few moments explaining a medication that I think will help you feel better"
K = Knowledge	Giving information about the medication to be prescribed and how it works, in a jargon-free manner. Knowledge needs to be tailored to the education level of the patient and family member(s) Example: "The effect of this drug, that is an antidepressant, is to reduce spontaneous crying spells, to help you in being more active and interested in what you previously liked, and to improve the sense of fatigue and irritability you have told me are problems for you"
E = Emotions	Explore and validate the patient's emotions (e.g., anger, fear emerging during the course of discussion about psychotropic drugs) Example: " I can see you have had a bad experience previously" (empathic response); "Tell me more about why you feel that way" (exploration); "Most people it seems would be concerned about that" (validation)
S = Strategy and Summary	Summarize what was discussed with the patient, checking if the patient has understood well. Implement strategic plans for treatment (e.g., writing the main points of the discussion, audio record the conversation). Provide information (e.g., phone number) about when and where to call for a feedback (usually in a week) or in case of emergency, make another appointment

statements will likely come up frequently during the discussion with the patient and/or family member. Listening without interrupting, empathizing, and exploring the patient's story in detail can provide important information about patient coping and the impact of their distress on their quality of life.

5.4.2　P = Perception

Many patients are misinformed about psychotropic drugs, previously had bad experiences with them, or know someone who has or have formed negative attitudes based on other factors. On the other hand some patients have responded well to psychotropic drugs in the past, and this is an important information for the prescribing clinician. Asking the patient "tell me what you know" about such and such a drug or class of drugs will help the clinician understand how much and what kind of information the patient and family members need to provide to the patient and family. Knowing if other family members are on psychotropic medications is also useful information, because patients may have formed either positive or negative impressions of psychopharmacological agents based on family members' experience. They may also be more willing to accept the rationale for a psychotropic drug if they know that depression, for example, "runs in the family." When taking such a history, the clinician may take note with the patient that a family member had responded to reinforce or "normalize" its use. Important to note that is the fact that many patients today come to the oncology setting accompanied by family members who are duly concerned about psychiatric symptoms that the patient is experiencing and may be important allies in reinforcing the recommendations of the clinician regarding the use of psychotropic medications. Therefore it may be important to include them in the patient evaluation. Moreover, it is important to elicit family members' perspectives in case they are themselves bias against or uninformed about psychotropic medications that the clinician is considering as a recommendation for care.

5.4.3 I = Invitation

Setting goals for that part of the patient encounter where you want to talk about prescribing a psychotropic will signpost for the patient that you have transitioned from history taking to giving information. The simple statement "I'd like to spend the next few moments explaining a medication that I think will help you feel better" signals to the patient to transition into "listening mode." At this point one might meet resistance that would divert the conversation to additional exploration such as: "I don't want to take medications" or "I've tried those before." This is an opportunity to explore legitimate concerns or experiences which may not have emerged during the initial history taking.

5.4.4 K = Knowledge

Patients are often leery about adding another medication to their current anti-cancer regimen which may be considerable, so the clinician must be very clear and concrete about how the medication is going to help the patient. For example, if patients are depressed and fatigued about not sleeping or having spontaneous crying spells or their irritability is affecting their relationship with others explaining how antidepressants can make this better. If patients are having panic attacks that are keeping them from leaving the house or cannot make it to their MRI because of phobia of closed spaces, one can tout the significant improvements that might occur when medications are introduced. Explaining to patients about psychotropic medications can be tricky. As mentioned previously patients may fear what they call addiction (but usually mean dependency) and taking a medication which affects "the mind" can make patients feel that they have failed in coping with their problems. Sometimes it may help to have patients talk to other patients who have improved on psychotropic medications but finding such a patient may be problematic. We have found it useful to explain to patients the following (even if our information about the mechanisms of action of medications such as antidepressants is incomplete):

1. Depression, anxiety, bipolar disease are disorders and have a biochemical basis, just like diabetes.
2. Although we do not exactly know how the medications work, it appears that they restore normal function to brain mechanisms that have produced the malady.
3. While some patients may become dependent on medications such as anxiolytics, this is different from addiction where patients abuse the medications to "escape " from reality.
4. In most cases the medications will not interfere with medications they may already be taking for their cancer.
5. In many cases patients can stop the medications after a period of time.
6. Dosages need to be regulated based upon the response (or lack therein).

Knowledge of course needs to be tailored to the education level of the patient and family member, and the clinician should explain things in a jargon-free manner as possible.

5.4.5   E = Emotions

Emotions such as fear or anger may emerge at any time during the course of discussion about psychotropic drugs. They should not be met with defensiveness or argumentation but with empathy. Statements such as " I can see you have had a bad experience previously" go a longer way than "fix it" responses which attempt to reassure the patient such as " that happens to very few people and is unlikely to happen to you" or defensive ones such as " I've been giving these medications for many years and I've seen very few problems." Emotions can also be explored (" tell me more about why you feel that way") or validated (" most people it seems would be concerned about that") which go a long way toward presenting to the patient a compassionate face rather than one who is just trying to convince the patient to do what the clinician wants.

5.4.6   S = Strategy and Summary

The "plan" for treatment should be clear to the patient and written so that the anxiety from the visit does not interfere with comprehension. Many times it helps to start psychotropic medications at low dosages so that patients can gain confidence in it since the likelihood of side effects is usually less (see above discussion on adherence). Allowing patients to audio record conversations or when the clinician writes a summary letter has been proven to facilitate retention of information, albeit both of these techniques are somewhat controversial. Since psychotropic medications in the cancer population often work quickly, having the patient call you in week or so to bring you up to date on how they are doing will allow you to assess early on if you need to increase the dose, change the medications, or give the patient a "pep talk".

Conclusions

In conclusion effective communication and the relationship with the patient and family are key factors influencing whether patients accept our recommendations for treatment. Factors such as achieving a good rapport, listening, and empathizing may be more important with psychotropic medications which often have a stigma attached to their use. Paying attention to relationship factors may also increase compliance when a patient trusts you enough to let you know when there is a problem with the medication instead of stopping it altogether. Moreover, effective communication is a skill set, and mindfulness on the part of the prescribing clinician about his or her communication can help promote the desired goals of patient acceptance, adherence, and ultimately improvement in quality of life.

References

Aaronson JK. Compliance, concordance, adherence. Br J Clin Pharmacol. 2007;63:383–4.

Arbuthnott A, Sharpe D. The effect of physician-patient collaboration on patient adherence in non-psychiatric medicine. Patient Educ Couns. 2009;77(1):60–7.

Back A, Arnold R, Tulsky J. Mastering communication with seriously ill patients: balancing honesty with empathy and hope. Washington, DC: Cambridge University Press; 2009.

Baile W, Costantini A. Communicating with cancer patients and their families. In: Wise T, Biondi M, Costantini A, editors. Psycho-oncology. Arlington: American Psychiatric Publishing; 2013. p. 57–90.

Baile WF, Buckman R, Lenzi R, Glober G, Beale EA, Kudelka AP. SPIKES-A six-step protocol for delivering bad news: application to the patient with cancer. Oncologist. 2000;5(4):302–11.

Butow P, Baile W. Communication in cancer care: a cultural perspective. In: Grassi L, Riba M, editors. Clinical Psycho-oncology: an international perspective. Chichester: Wiley; 2012.

Costantini A, Baile WF, Lenzi R, Costantini M, Ziparo V, Marchetti P, Grassi L. Overcoming cultural barriers to giving bad news: feasibility of training to promote truth-telling to cancer patients. J Cancer Educ. 2009;24(3):180–5.

DiMatteo MR. Variations in patients' adherence to medical recommendations: a quantitative review of 50 years of research. Med Care. 2004;42(3):200–9.

DiMatteo MR, Haskard-Zonierek KB. Impact of depression on treatment adherence and survival form cancer. In: Kissane DW, Maj M, Sartorius N, editors. Depression and cancer. Chichester: Wiley; 2011. p. 101–24.

DiMatteo MR, Lepper HS, Croghan TW. Depression is a risk factor for noncompliance with medical treatment: meta-analysis of the effects of anxiety and depression on patient adherence. Arch Intern Med. 2000;160:2101–7.

DiMatteo MR, Haskard KB, Williams SL. Health beliefs, disease severity, and patient adherence: a meta-analysis. Med Care. 2007;45(6):521–8.

Faulkner A, Maguire P. Talking to cancer patients and their families. Oxford: Oxfird Univeristy Press; 1994.

Finlay E, Casarett D. Making difficult discussions easier: using prognosis to facilitate transitions to hospice. CA Cancer J Clin. 2009;59(4):250–63.

Fujimori M, Oba A, Koike M, Okamura M, Akizuki N, Kamiya M, Akechi T, Sakano Y, Uchitomi Y. Communication skills training for Japanese oncologists on how to break bad news. J Cancer Educ. 2003;18(4):194–201.

Grassi L, Caruso R, Nanni MG. Dealing with depression: communication to depressed cancer patients and grieving families. In: Surbone A, Zwitter M, Rajer M, Stiefel R, editors. New challenges in communication with cancer patients. New York: Springer; 2013. p. 63–76.

Grassi L, Nanni MG, Riba MB. Diagnostic issues. In: Grassi L, Riba MB, editors. Psychopharmacology in oncology and palliative care: a practical manual. Heidelberg: Springer; 2014.

Kaplan M. SPIKES: a framework for breaking bad news to patients with cancer. Clin J Oncol Nurs. 2010;14(4):514–6.

Kissane D, Bultz B, Butow P, Finlay I, editors. Handbook of communication in oncology and palliative care. New York: Oxford University Press; 2011.

Lenzi R, Baile WF, Costantini A, Grassi L, Parker PA. Communication training in oncology: results of intensive communication workshops for Italian oncologists. Eur J Cancer Care (Engl). 2011; 20(2):196–203.

Maguire P, Pitceathly C. Key communication skills and how to acquire them. BMJ. 2002;325: 697–700.

Martin DJ, Garske JP, Davis MK. Relation of the therapeutic alliance with outcome and other variables: a meta-analytic review. J Consult Clin Psychol. 2000;68(3):438–50.

Priebe S, Dimic S, Wildgrube C, Jankovic J, Cushing A, McCabe R. Good communication in psychiatry–a conceptual review. Eur Psychiatry. 2011;26:403–7.

Prins MA, Verhaak PF, Smolders M, Laurant MG, van der Meer K, Spreeuwenberg P, van Marwijk HW, Penninx BW, Bensing JM. Patient factors associated with guideline-concordant treatment of anxiety and depression in primary care. J Gen Intern Med. 2010;25(7):648–55.

Sawada N, Uchida H, Suzuki T, Watanabe K, Kikuchi T, Handa T, Kashima H. Persistence and compliance to antidepressant treatment in patients with depression: a chart review. BMC Psychiatry. 2009;9:38. doi:10.1186/1471-244X-9-38.

Schnur JB, Montgomery GH. A systematic: review of therapeutic alliance, group cohesion, empathy, and goal consensus/collaboration in psychotherapeutic interventions in cancer: Uncommon factors? Clin Psychol Rev. 2010;30:238–47.

Smolders M, Laurant M, Verhaak P, Prins M, van Marwijk H, Penninx B, Wensing M, Grol R. Which physician and practice characteristics are associated with adherence to evidence-based guidelines for depressive and anxiety disorders? Med Care. 2010;48(3):240–8.

Stiefel F. Communication in cancer care. Berlin: Springer; 2006.

Surbone A, Zwitter M, Rajer M, Stiefel R, editors. New challenges in communication with cancer patients. Berlin: Springer; 2013.

Thompson L, McCabe R. The effect of clinician-patient alliance and communication on treatment adherence in mental health care: a systematic review. BMC Psychiatry. 2012;12:87.

World Health Organization. Adherence to long-term therapies: evidence for action (PDF). Geneva: World Health Organisation; 2003. ISBN 92-4-154599-2.

Zolnierek KB, Dimatteo MR. Physician communication and patient adherence to treatment: a meta-analysis. Med Care. 2009;47:826–34.

Integration of Psychopharmacotherapy with Psychotherapy and Other Psychosocial Treatment

6

Manuela Kogon and David Spiegel

> **Abstract**
>
> The effective use of psychotropic medication in cancer care involves attention to both pharmacology and symbolic communication. Prescribing is part of a therapeutic relationship in which meaning as well as medication is dispensed. Numerous factors influence the meaning of medication, including preexisting psychiatric condition, personal history, disease phase, disease stage, ethnic, cultural and individual differences, and cancer-specific symptoms. Cancer patients are understandably sensitive to the implications of what their doctors say and do, so both a prescription and the lack of one are communications about the doctors' perception of the nature and severity of their patients' condition and their concern for them. Perceived uncertainty, loss of control, and feelings of dependency are common themes. Integrating patients' concerns into prescribing practice can enhance treatment. Combining and integrating psychotropic medication and psychosocial interventions are important aspects of oncological care.

6.1 Introduction

Medication has both pharmacological and symbolic effects, as the extensive literature on placebo response makes clear. Prescription is part of a therapeutic relationship in which meaning as well as medication is dispensed. Cancer patients are understandably sensitive to the implications of what their doctors say and do, looking for implications regarding their future and their doctors' concern for them. Anyone diagnosed with cancer is thrust into a whirlpool of experiences.

M. Kogon (✉)
Stanford Center for Integrative Medicine, Stanford University, Stanford, CA, USA
e-mail: mkogon@stanford.edu

D. Spiegel
Department of Psychiatry and Behavioral Sciences, Stanford University, Stanford, CA, USA
e-mail: dspiegel@stanford.edu

L. Grassi and M. Riba (eds.), *Psychopharmacology in Oncology and Palliative Care*,
DOI 10.1007/978-3-642-40134-3_6, © Springer-Verlag Berlin Heidelberg 2014

The shock of diagnosis plunges patients into existential fears at a time when levelheaded thinking is required to optimize treatment decisions. Patients' personal history, their belief system, and past exposure to traumatic events will also shape their approach to the illness and its treatment. The presence of valued family and social networks as well as the stage of life will influence their response to diagnosis and treatment. Any therapeutic avenue needs to address these problems in their individual and collective complexity.

To take symptoms seriously means to effectively manage them. But it also means to always view symptoms in the context of the person who experiences them and fashion the intervention accordingly. When blending psychopharmacological with psychosocial aid, the symbolic meaning of medication needs to be considered. Will the recommendation to take a medication for a particular symptom be experienced as dismissive, a turning away from real engagement? Or will a casual recommendation to seek counseling be viewed as not taking seriously the physical manifestation of a treatment side effects or a cancer-related symptom? While Chap. 4 provided a detailed overview over the psychosocial assessment in psychopharmaco-oncology, this chapter will focus on the integration of psychosocial treatments and medication. The question whether to use medication, psychosocial intervention, or both and how to organically integrate them will be a constant companion for the treating professional. We also need to stay open and flexible to changes and adjustments as the patients change and adjust during the illness.

The emotional experiences that come with cancer are a natural and expected aspect of having cancer. Usually, they are not an expression of psychopathology. It is thus important to differentiate symptoms in patients with preexisting mental health problems from symptoms that are part of the course of the experience with cancer. This differentiation will help lower the threshold toward getting patients the help they need. However, this requires the recognition of patients' symptoms as more than psychiatric: both the professional as well as the patient need to appreciate symptoms in the context of the patient's history, background, and belief system. Psychotropic medication should in general be symptom- and treatment-response focused. In general adjustment reactions to the understandable stresses associated with cancer can be handled with supportive psychotherapy. More severe symptoms of anxiety, depression, and other psychiatric problems that do not respond to psychotherapy may require medication even if they are new and clearly cancer related. Thus, the use of antidepressant and antianxiety medications implies an evaluation that symptoms are more serious and less amenable to psychotherapy alone. This message is often not lost on patients, who may appreciate or resist the addition of psychotropics to their usually large regimen of medications.

The careful integration of psychosocial and psychopharmacological treatment is fundamental for cancer patients. Depression and depressive symptoms have long been recognized in a considerable percentage of cancer patients (Derogatis et al. 1983; Chochinov 2001; Akechi et al. 2004). Treating depression is not just important to improve patients' well-being but because depression has been implicated in the progression of cancer (Lutgendorf and Sodd 2011; Giese-Davis et al. 2011). Diagnosing depression in cancer patients is a challenge in itself.

Sadness or distressed mood can be a normal reaction to illness circumstances. Also symptoms such as fatigue, anorexia, malaise, difficulty concentrating, and exhaustion, which are diagnostic for depression, are all symptoms associated with cancer and its treatment. As a result of these confounding factors, both under- and overdiagnosis of depressive symptoms and depression occur: reactive sadness that is a natural part of the experience of cancer might be misdiagnosed as depression, and conversely, depression might be misinterpreted as cancer blues (Evans et al. 2005). But even if there is agreement on a diagnosis, there are no clear guidelines about how to intervene. There is a considerable amount of data that indicates that psychosocial interventions improve depressive symptoms (Akechi et al. 2008) and that decreasing depressive symptoms might even prolong survival (Giese-Davis et al. 2011). Data on psychopharmacological interventions in cancer patients however are limited and conflicting. An initial meta-analysis indicated modest effectiveness of antidepressants among patients with medical illness, estimating the need to treat 4 patients to show significant improvement in one patient over placebo response (Gill and Hatcher 2000). Some earlier reviews on the use of antidepressants in cancer patients did not show effectiveness (Williams and Dale 2006). A more recent review suggested that these findings might be due to the heterogeneity of the data. Using more stringent inclusion criteria, Laoutidis and Mathiak (2013) suggested a helpful role for antidepressants among cancer patients.

Anxiety is also a common symptom in patients with cancer. It fluctuates during different phases of the illness, and it appears to be the more common problem in long-term cancer survivors than depression (Mitchell et al. 2013). Another area of interest is the assessment of distress and its impact on morbidity, suggesting using distress as a 6th vital sign. Cancer patients report distress at the time of diagnosis and distress, pain, and fatigue 1-year post-diagnosis (Carlson et al. 2013). Some reports indicate health-related distress, worry, or insomnia in up to 40 % of patients 8 years after successful treatment (Bill-Axelson et al. 2013). There is also a significant gap between patients' reports of significant distress and the percentage referred for services (Bultz personal communication). The National Comprehensive Cancer Network offers guidelines for palliative (Levy et al. 2012) and survivorship (Ligibel and Denlinger 2013) care, but there are currently no consistent guidelines about how to best integrate psychosocial and psychopharmacological treatment. An individualized approached is warranted. Treatment of symptoms is important regardless of their etiology. We will be more effective with a symptom-based approach if we also regard the patient as a whole, understanding patients' history, individuality, and idiosyncrasies in the context of their cancer experience.

The following recommendations are intended to help guide the integration of psychosocial and psychopharmacological treatment.

6.2 Major Considerations in Designing a Psychopharmacological Strategy

6.2.1 Preexisting Psychiatric Conditions, Mental Health, and Personal History

Assessing preexisting psychiatric conditions is crucial. Patients, family, friends, and professionals are often confused and stressed by the natural changes in the patients' emotions and tend to identify them as mental problems. Careful assessment will reduce the threshold to offering necessary help early and efficiently, also for patients without prior psychiatric conditions. It is, however, important to identify preexisting mental conditions. Cancer diagnosis and treatment itself often results in an activation of a stress response, possibly exacerbating earlier mental conditions requiring medication adjustment or even medication changes. Mental health conditions in cancer patients are associated with poorer outcomes (Fox et al. 2013; Giese-Davis et al. 2011). Cancer patients with a psychiatric disorder report less perceived social support than their nonpsychiatric peers, a perceived difference that disappears with psychopharmacological treatment (Costa-Requena et al. 2013). Effective treatment can prove clinically challenging during a time when most patients feel out of control and want stability. A necessary change or adjustment in medication may become the symbol for instability and may be adamantly rejected. If not addressed, such concerns carry the risk of jeopardizing the patient's health. In our clinical practice we were faced with a brain cancer patient who was adamant about not discontinuing the bupropion she had taken for depression for years. She preferred the increased risk of seizures to the trial of a different antidepressant medication. A gentleman with a longstanding history of bipolar disorder refused adjustments in his lithium dosage despite subtherapeutic levels to "not rock the boat." In a busy oncological setting, physicians are less likely to have the time and skill to detect the deeper meaning psychotropic medication can have for patients. The integration of psychotherapy and counseling into the process can facilitate the adjustment or change in medication by helping the patient discover the often unconscious root of their reluctance.

A traumatic past will also alter one's experience with cancer even if diagnostic criteria for PTSD are not met (Akechi et al. 2004). Psychological distress in cancer patients with a Holocaust experience is higher than in non-Holocaust counter parts (Peretz et al. 1994) and also affects how they cope with cancer (Baider et al. 1992). The treatment of cancer for a holocaust survivor can become the symbol of earlier abuse rather than the help it is intended to be. Anyone who has suffered through medical experimentation will be prone to misinterpret medical treatment and cannot freely trust its good intent. Psychosocial support will assist reframing one's experience probably more effectively than the suggestion to take a sedative during a required procedure or treatment. Patients with a history of sexual violence report more distress during a pelvic exam, experience fear and embarrassment, and have more maladaptive beliefs about the examination's necessity, safety, and utility. Not surprisingly the link is even stronger in women with concomitant

PTSD (Weitlauf et al. 2010). Since, therefore, a procedure with clear medical benefit may become a symbol of earlier violence, without correction of the distorted belief, the chances of avoidance coping increase, and with it the chances of poorer cancer surveillance and treatment.

Researchers have studied for decades what drives health and illness behavior (Cameron and Leventhal 2003). Data emerged that fear alone does not influence health behavior positively but needs to be paired with an action plan for people to act beneficially on their own behalf. The fear of breast cancer may not be sufficient to get a woman to have a screening of mammogram, but paired with a convenient appointment time and location it will be more likely obtained. We have learnt that somatic stimuli create fear states resulting in avoidance behavior unless they are paired with benign interpretations of the stimulus. People left to their own devices develop lay theories regarding health threats that are symptom based and often have little correspondence to medical science. Such convictions motivate avoidance behavior to reduce perceived danger rather than effectively searching for the cause of the symptom and a health promoting solution (Cameron and Leventhal 2003). Thus, linking fear to the potential for active coping and risk reduction can improve adherence to cancer screening and treatment, as well as psychotropic medication.

6.2.2   The Meaning of Cancer to Patients Influences Their View of Psychopharmacological Treatment

The same way medications have symbolic meaning, so has the use of the word "cancer." Despite great strides in cancer treatment and prolonged survival or even cure, many patients associate the word "cancer" with death and suffering, regardless of the actual prognosis. This historically rooted word association sets cancer apart from other chronic conditions that involve intermittent or gradual progression to possible death, such as multiple sclerosis or chronic heart failure. This experienced negativity will influence patients' perceptions during the course of their illness and thus alter how they view the use of psychotropic medication. Patients often view cancer as an enemy that they need to fight and conquer. The cancer becomes a personified entity separate from the patient, an experience that sets cancer apart from other illnesses. With chronic heart failure we treat a diseased organ and not the presumed enemy from within. Patients often feel ambivalent toward systemic chemotherapy because they want to only attack the cancer without collateral damage to themselves. When we prescribe psychotropics in that context whom are we treating: the patient or the cancer? Cancer covers a broad range of illnesses; as do the psychosocial issues associated with them. Some make psychopharmacological treatment more urgent or necessary, while others need to be approached with caution.

6.2.3   Disease Phase and Stage

Differentiate four phases: diagnosis, treatment and posttreatment/survivorship, and palliative care. The emotional experience in reaction to cancer differs during each stage, and thus the treatment will differ. At the time of diagnosis emotions of surprise, anger, and disappointment are more prominent than after treatment when fear and worry about the uncertainty of the future will be more prominent. During treatment physical challenges and treatment-related side effects tend to dominate the emotional reactions.

Phase of illness and the stage of the illness are factors in helping determine how to best integrate psychosocial treatments with medication. Since cancer covers a broad range of illnesses, someone with a curable form of breast cancer will respond differently emotionally than a patient with metastasized disease who is given 3 months to live. Treatment needs to be adjusted accordingly as can be illustrated with the common symptom of insomnia. Concerns about dependency should not be the primary reason to withhold benzodiazepines from patients in late stages of their illness. In patients with curable illness however stress reduction techniques for temporary insomnia at the time of diagnosis are effective tools when there is concern about dependency. Patients with metastatic disease face a different set of emotional and physical challenges than patients with curable illness. The fear of recurrence is usually replaced by the fear of progression. Patients need to adjust emotionally to living with their illness rather than worry about the illness returning. As metastatic patients become aware of the ineffectiveness of medical treatment their anxiety will increase. Metastatic patients often express a pronounced fear of suffering and dependency on others more so than death (Spiegel and Classen 2000). The role of psychotropics needs to be evaluated carefully. Many patients with advanced illness are on antidepressants, but data suggest limited efficacy (Lloyd-Williams et al. 2013), suggesting that combined psychotherapeutic support and medication may be more effective.

Considerations at the Time of Diagnosis

Sleep Disruption After the initial shock of diagnosis, patients will often look for optimal treatment and are faced with a variety of important choices for treatment as well as a suitable treating team. In this phase many patients are in cognitive overdrive, trying to optimize choices that they are usually not equipped to judge medically. This leads to thought intrusion and thought flooding and associated with it, insomnia. This is a phase when it is fundamental to facilitate sleep. Uninterrupted, restful sleep will result in better thinking and better decision-making ability. Exploring with patients the possibility that their intense thinking at night is an attempt at trying to find a solution to their malady and is not a sign of psychiatric illness can be just as useful as prescribing medication. Thinking takes the symbolic role of mastery and control; patients often do not recognize this purpose and may misinterpret it as random and intrusive. This is a time when professionals should not avoid targeted and time-limited integration of benzodiazepines into the treatment. The choice whether psychosocial support and the use of medication need to be combined or administered alone will reveal itself in collaborative explorations with the patient. For some patients it is important to take control over their treatment while others prefer to delegate it to their healthcare professionals. Limited treatment choices can result in distress and secondary insomnia because of patients' relative lack of choices and sense of helplessness. It is important to help patients understand the well-meant but maladaptive responses, particularly if the emotional and cognitive maladjustment influences treatment choices. To become aware that consulting with numerous doctors and searching the internet extensively is not intended primarily to gain knowledge about one's illness but rather to obtain a sense of control and mastery, the energy toward such pursuits can be used more effectively in other areas. Since motives to act are often hidden from awareness and compete with one another, patients' emotions and behavior can look erratic and might require intervention. If nonpharmacological psychosocial interventions or over the counter medications do not effectively treat insomnia, initial and temporary use of benzodiazepines or other hypnotics is indicated for brief periods of time. There are considerable individual differences with respect to onset and duration of action among patients as well as among different benzodiazepines. The choice of medication will depend on patients' individual response and their circumstances. Particular emphasis needs to be put on the meaning medication can have for patients in this phase. If patients feel that being medicated is the result of the treatment team not wanting to address the many questions and concerns the patients have, the relationship to the team and the well-being of the patient will suffer. By the same token, similar disappointment can be elicited by refusing to prescribe a sleeping pill when insomnia is a serious and worsening problem. A detailed interview will help unearth the patient's experience, interpretation, and expectations in this situation. Not feeling in control often creates a sense of dependency in which one feel less courageous about expressing specific needs as to not be experienced as demanding and critical. See Fig. 6.1.

Inappropriate Guilt Another symbolic source of anxiety and depression among recently diagnosed cancer patients is the common belief that some of the patients' behaviors might have caused cancer. Patients often do not have the ability to comprehend the complexity of cancer etiology and conclude cause and effect between a particular behavior and their cancer, even if the behavior itself is not clearly carcinogenic. In an attempt at comprehending, the incomprehensible patients create meaning that is not based in the reality of their illness. If stress is the presumed culprit of the cause of cancer, any stressfully experienced event will create additional distress and fear of being stressed. Thoughts about possible causality are often associated with feelings of guilt to the degree that some patients will regard their cancer as punishment. Many cancer patients would rather feel guilty than helpless, and there is ample support in the popular literature for the mistaken notion that cancer reflects some unconscious need for punishment (Siegel 1986) or a failure to properly image one's body fighting back (Simonton et al. 1978). If these often unconscious beliefs are not illuminated and discussed,

Fig. 6.1 Dynamics at the time of diagnosis

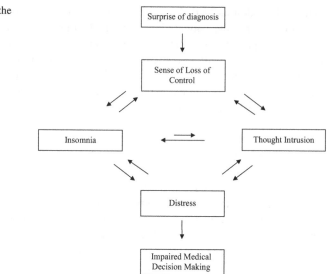

patients are at risk of making unsound choices with respect to treatment or may request psychotropics when they are not warranted. In this circumstance, clarification may supersede the need for prescription.

Considerations During Cancer Treatment

Treatment-related symptoms are often an important focus and might require some psychosocial or psychopharmacological intervention. Anxiety in women with breast cancer tends to be highest prior to the first chemotherapy infusion and higher among women who undergo mastectomy versus breast conserving therapy (Lim et al. 2011). Treating cancer therapy-related symptoms will often improve the patient's mood. Chemotherapy-related and anticipatory nausea are common in this phase. While hypnosis and acupuncture are effective (Richardson et al. 2007; Garcia et al. 2013), benzodiazepines are often necessary, not just to treat nausea but to alleviate stress, which often exacerbates nausea through adrenergic activation. The integration of psychotropic medication has a better chance of success when patients understand the impact distress has on their physical symptoms. They will experience a feeling of empowerment when stress reduction decreases physical symptoms, at times resulting in smaller dose of medication.

The same way prior trauma influences the patient's experience treatment itself can be traumatic even without prior trauma history (French-Rosas et al. 2011). Being strapped down as part of radiation treatment can be traumatic. Some patients interpret chemotherapy as poisonous rather than the help it is intended to be. If the experienced distress is not addressed to help understand its causes, patients who were fully functional before might doubt their coping competence or even their sanity. Deciphering the trigger for the distress will help alleviating it.

An exploration of the encountered or anticipatory distress will often bring relief when it is understood as a loss of control or the inability to take action while lying still. Benzodiazepines clearly have a role in alleviating disabling anxiety. Balancing preventive and therapeutic interventions such as self-hypnosis and guided imagery with medication is important, both to enhance the patient's sense of control and competence and to limit dependency on medication.

It is important to again obtain and act on a history of past trauma, as cancer treatment may reactivate trauma-related memories (Baider et al. 1992; Peretz et al. 1994). Combining the use of psychotropics and psychosocial interventions is important, but sometimes psychosocial intervention alone can also help decrease the need for medication including psychotropics during treatment: Women undergoing excisional biopsy or lumpectomy for breast cancer use less sedatives during surgery after receiving a 15-min presurgery hypnosis session (Montgomery et al. 2007). The implications are substantial, since that same study documented decreased—per patient—cost, mostly due to reduced surgical time. The same study demonstrated prevention of symptoms with the brief hypnosis intervention prior to breast cancer surgery, a decrease in the use of intraoperative analgesics and sedatives, and reduced postsurgical pain, nausea, and fatigue. Similarly, training in self-hypnosis can substantially reduce pain and anxiety during needle biopsy for breast cancer (Lang et al. 2006). Similar approaches involving the teaching of self-hypnosis produce comparable effects, including reduced procedure time and fewer complications, among patients undergoing invasive radiological procedures (Lang et al. 2000). These examples illustrate how organically blending the use of medication with use of other interventions can reduce medication use while improving medical outcome. Patients' expectancy and distress are contributing factors to the effectiveness of the intervention (Montgomery et al. 2010). As we explore further the psychology of patients' choices and the factors that facilitate learning symptom control techniques, such studies provide valuable opportunities for the development of future interventions.

Considerations for the Posttreatment/Survivorship Phase

The posttreatment/survivorship phase comes with its own set of challenges. Emotional responses need to be differentiated from emotional adjustment to treatment-related physical changes. Patients often have the expectation that a defined endpoint of treatment is the immediate beginning of feeling well. While patients often experience relief at the end of treatment, many patients underestimate the length of time required for recovery. Patients feel fatigue, a symptom that may last for months or even years after radio- and chemotherapy (Bower 2008). There are often other physical sequelae of treatment, some of which might be irreversible. Having to live with the uncertainty of cancer recurrence is hard enough, but the expectation and hope that dry mouth, dysphagia, pain, numbness, and tingling—to name only a few of the common symptoms—after treatment will resolve, add an emotional challenge, and may undermine patients' faith in the physicians. See Fig. 6.2.

Patients often have an altered sense of body image and self. When the hope of resuming normalcy posttreatment is reduced, patients often struggle to adjust.

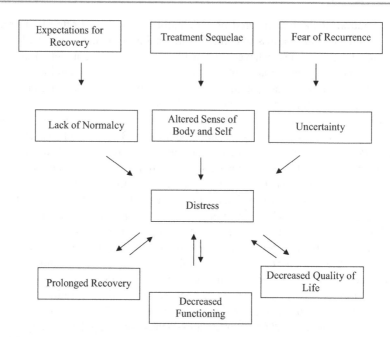

Fig. 6.2 Dynamics in the posttreatment/survivorship phase

The changed self becomes a source of disappointment and feelings of loss. Not being able to act as the old self feels like a personal failure. Patients often do not associate their symptoms with treatment but a lack of will power. It is important to help patients to understand and modulate their natural reaction to physical and life limitations related to cancer and its treatment.

The use of psychotropics in this phase will not just depend on the symptoms that need treatment but also on the side effect profile of the medication. Symptoms posttreatment are numerous. We want to minimize the chance of adding fatigue with a sedating medication if posttreatment fatigue is the major complaint. Individualization is key since issues involved include self-judgment and perceived judgment by the treating professional. Patients might misinterpret the suggestion to use medication to alleviate symptoms as lack of interest in their plight. On the other hand leaving the office without a prescription might be experienced as the same lack of interest by a different patient.

Emotions often fluctuate in the posttreatment/survivorship phase. Patients may feel stable or even happy as long as there are no reminders of their illness. However, as soon as scheduled surveillance scans or doctor visits loom, anxiety may trigger stressful thoughts and insomnia. Thought intrusions can reach taxing levels. Self-hypnosis or a short course of a benzodiazepine around stressful triggers often are effective if patients recognize the regularity and predictability of their reaction and understand that anxiety is the body's response to a perceived threat (Montgomery et al. 2013). Helping patients understand that the intermittent use of medication is temporary and that it is not a reflection of emotional weakness posttreatment can facilitate and even expedite recovery. As patients move further away from active treatment, their emotions will stabilize and using medication will naturally and gradually cease.

A careful history can reveal implications of treatments and their side effects that may impair adherence or response. To encourage breathing exercises in a patient with radiated sinuses or throat can backfire because of the dryness of their mucosa. Providing sedatives might be equally undesirable if a patient wants to wake up every two hours to minimize his mucosal membranes from drying out during the night. Whatever intervention is decided upon will have a higher chance at succeeding and being utilized by the patient if he or she feels understood. In other situations simple action is asked for: using a medication to treat neuropathy such as duloxetine, amytriptyline, or neurontin can improve emotional well-being just by treating the neuropathy. Problem solving can at times be as therapeutic as complex psychological analysis if it leads to improved well-being.

Changes in appearance and functioning that affect sexuality are a common occurrence in cancer. It is important to recognize this as part of treatment sequelae. Keeping these problems in mind may reduce reliance upon psychotropics that may worsen decreased libido, vaginal dryness, or erectile dysfunction. Many women with breast cancer present for treatment of symptoms that are believed to be tamoxifen or aromatase inhibitor related. Altered mood such as irritability is often cited as a reason for psychopharmacological or psychosocial intervention. Hot flashes triggering insomnia in already sleep-disturbed patients occur commonly. A medication such as venlafaxine is often helpful in this context, and evidence also exists for the effectiveness of gabapentin, citalopram, and clonidine (L'Esperance et al. 2013). Many patients experience relief when preventing a vicious cycle of irritability, hot flashes, and insomnia feeding on one another and potentially leading to depression. Recognizing that emotional symptoms might only be a reaction to physical symptoms facilitates treatment. Patients are unsettled by the emotional changes after treatment. To help patients recognize the source comes as such relief that the conversation that led to the insight might suffice as intervention. One caveat is patients' fixation on their physical symptoms. Finding solutions to resolving symptoms becomes a one-dimensional goal, at times at the expense of essential emotional adjustment to altered life circumstances. Living with symptoms may become an intolerable symbol for cancer's ongoing threat and the lack of normalcy. The at times unsuccessful pursuit of solutions for posttreatment symptoms can become a source of distress in itself. Supportive psychotherapy examining the patient's understandable frustration with the illness can be helpful. To explore both aspects—emotional adjustment to different circumstances and the desire to reduce symptoms to improve well-being needs to be balanced.

Another issue in the posttreatment/survivorship phase is control. Treatment can be traumatic (French-Rosas et al. 2011) and can alter health coping (Weitlauf et al. 2010). Avoiding a surveillance MRI or CT in an attempt to protect from the symptoms experienced during radiation treatment is protective emotionally but not desirable medically. The use of short-acting benzodiazepines is often indicated for controlled exposure during the surveillance scan. Also, giving patients some control over the timing or scheduling of their surveillance scans is often therapeutic for them. A patient from our practice with esophageal cancer had decided to forgo her surveillance scan arguing that she still felt traumatized from radiation. A combination of guided imagery and 2 mg of lorazepam however got her through the procedure smoothly. She felt empowered when she realized how radiation treatment and her fear of the surveillance scan were linked. She experienced no difficulty with later scans. In general facilitating a process that allows a patient to have more of a sense of control over the conduct of surveillance and treatment and deepen patients' understanding about themselves and their circumstances will help. In this regard, training in self-hypnosis for use during procedures can also be quite helpful (Spiegel 2013).

Fear of recurrence is a frequently reported problem among cancer survivors. A recent review reported 39 % to 97 % of cancer survivors having some degree of fear of recurrence. Fear of recurrence ranges from a normal reaction to clinically significant, and 20 % to 79 % of patients identify fear of recurrence as an unmet treatment need (Simard et al. 2013). Many long-term survivors experience fear of recurrence years after the end of treatment (Koch et al. 2013). Fear often leads to behavior that is not in the best interest of the patient. It can lead to avoidance coping, or, conversely, to overzealous quests for examinations and evaluations. Fear of recurrence can also lead to misinterpretations of everyday physical symptoms, patients believing that physical symptoms constitute recurrence. Such patients may lose their everyday health competence (Horlick-Jones 2011). Fear of recurrence leads to reassurance seeking behavior, such as increased visits to the ER (Lebel et al. 2013), reported higher frequency of unscheduled visits to the primary care physician, higher frequency of breast self-examination, and other forms of self-examination for cancer. On the other hand, fear of recurrence in breast cancer patients has also been shown to be associated with avoidance coping, for example, not seeking mammograms or ultrasounds (Thewes et al. 2012). Generally, non-pharmacological interventions are effective and desirable to facilitate the return to some sense of normalcy, but if behavior changes jeopardize health, pharmacological intervention can become necessary. It is important to investigate the deeper purpose of the behavior to tailor an effective intervention. The knowledge that health coping can cover opposing ends of the spectrum can support patients in the assessment if their own behavior is situationally appropriate. This knowledge is also helpful to illuminate patients' motive to request or reject psychotropic medication. Fear of recurrence is often not just about the fear of cancer coming back, but becomes a stand-in for difficulty with uncertainty, unpredictability, or even fears of death. Psychotherapy creates understanding that can improve health behavior.

Considerations for Palliative Care

Palliative care until recently has been associated with the idea of end-of-life care. The notion was that there is a trade-off between quality of life and quantity of life. Care traditionally was provided late in the course of illness to alleviate patients' at times uncontrolled symptoms and to improve quality of life. End-of-life care is addressed specifically in part III of this book. However, more recently the notion of palliative care as end-of-life care has shifted after a study demonstrated a survival advantage when palliation was delivered early to patients with metastatic non-small-cell lung cancer in addition to standard oncological care (Temel et al. 2010). Despite these data, a shift in perception about what constitutes palliative care has been slow in coming. The presentation of palliative care to patients still needs to be delivered gently since many patients are not familiar with the concept or have a negative association with the word palliation. Patients often feel as if their health professionals have given up on them if palliation is mentioned. Introducing an analgesic medication may imply to a cancer patient the end of treatment of curative intent and a withdrawal of medical "interest." To offer an antidepressant or anxiolytic when patients are faced with the somber decision, whether or not to pursue aggressive medical interventions that aim to prolong their life can easily be misinterpreted as substitution for "active" care. As patients feel abandoned by their doctors, stress-related emotions are a natural response. Patients themselves might feel that they are abandoning their loved ones if they do not continue aggressive treatment. Thoughts of death and dying coalesce with the desire to live moments to the fullest, creating an unfamiliar blend of perplexing emotions. Temel's study (Temel et al. 2010) is a clear illustration that palliative care to improve quality of life in cancer patients does more than merely coexist with treatments that aim to increase quantity of life. Palliative care might in fact help extend survival. Not surprisingly the percentage of patients with depressive symptoms was significantly lower in the palliation group. Interestingly, the percentage of patients receiving new prescriptions for antidepressants was similar in both groups. Thus, the effectiveness of the intervention was most likely not the result of medication but the intervention itself. It targeted physical and psychosocial symptoms, discussed goals of care, and assisted with decision-making regarding treatment and might also have helped optimize the delivery of anticancer therapy. While it makes sense that treatment emphasizes adequate symptom control, it is important to learn the meaning the use of psychotropic medications has for the individual patient and adjust prescribing accordingly. Patients often express concern that effective symptom management comes at the price of sedation, symbolizing the loss of control. Since many psychotropic medications are in fact sedating, a careful exploration of the patients' wishes and concerns is warranted. Feeling in control of the medication dosage helps patients balance symptom relief and side effects. This will help to address the concern about sedation at a time when patients have to relinquish control in other areas.

6.2.4 General Rules of Choice of Medication

Part II of this book contains recommendations for specific medications for various conditions. We want to discuss the concept of the meaning that taking medications can have and how to optimize the use of psychotropics in the light of symptom control and meaning. In general be guided by primary symptom, for example, insomnia. In such a case sedating antidepressants such as trazodone, doxepin, or quetiapine might be desired. Nausea is a common symptom in cancer patients; both treatment-related nausea as well as anticipatory nausea when thinking about treatment. Starting a course of hypnosis or acupuncture before chemotherapy will not just give patients a desired sense of control but also will reduce the need for antiemetic medication during treatment. However, always remember the meaning medication can have to patients. Ironically, patients at times do not want to take psychotropics during chemotherapy to "not to further poison" their body. Illuminating how the patients' belief system can result in detrimental choices will be helpful in making more informed choices. Informing patients about the medications and their mechanism of action is important. Many patients consult the Internet or other resources. There is danger of losing a patient's trust and adherence when the names of medications evoke fear about psychiatric illness because they were prescribed as a presumed "antipsychotic" or "antidepressant." The action the medication has is more relevant than the class it belongs to or the public image it has. Also try to minimize number of medications. If a patient suffers from hot flashes that result in insomnia and trigger secondary changes in mood, this patient will not need three different medications, but a choice of venlafaxine, gabapentin, or citalopram can address all three. Similarly to insomnia neuropathy will also affect sleep and mood. Using gabapentin or duloxetine to treat neuropathy will also have a good chance at improving concomitant insomnia and depression. When physicians pay attention to such details, patients feel protected and looked after. Patients often feel lost in the complexity of their situation. Simplifications of procedures, schedules, medications regimens, and improvement of coordination of care provide an anchor of safety during a time of uncertainty and unpredictability.

Polypharmacology is a potential problem with cancer patients, who often have multiple and intractable symptoms. Commonly experienced long-term symptoms after cancer treatment are insomnia, depression, pain, fatigue, and cognitive dysfunction. Patients understandably are frustrated when functionality does not reach the precancer baseline. It is tempting to treat insomnia at night with zolpidem and daytime fatigue with modafinil. But we need to consider interactions between many medications as well as counterbalancing effects medications often have. We recommend taking a thorough history of medication use before prescribing additional ones. Polypharmacology is not just the result of the physician's desire to eliminate symptoms but also related to patients' expectations. Patients' frustration and disappointment with symptoms after treatment can also lead to a simplistic and mechanistic approach to treatment. The disappointment that the end of treatment does not always mean the end of symptoms feeds an unrealistic expectation with respect to effectiveness of medication. There is the hope that medications will fix all symptoms since the realization of having to adjust to limitations post-cancer is yet unbearable. The medication becomes a symbol that patients might pursue exclusively to avoid the adjustment process to a life post-cancer. Taking medication becomes an attempt at recreating the pre-cancer reality. Frustration in treating anxiety or depression may come to symbolize patient reactions to the limitations of cancer treatment itself. When this happens it is not just the combination and integrations of medication and psychosocial intervention that matters but the gentle balancing to meet the patient's existential experience and concerns. In the same way patients search for the cause of their cancer at the time of diagnosis they will worry about causes that could possibly promote recurrence or progression. Much guilt centers on being stressed about being stressed. Bringing to light the fears will set a better stage for deciding on whether to use medication or psychotherapy or both to help decrease stress.

6.2.5 Medication Interactions

Many patients will have difficulty sleeping at the time of diagnosis. If the medication of choice for nausea at your Cancer Center is lorazepam, you can utilize its sedating effects for insomnia at the time of diagnosis and prescribe and declare its function it also has as a sleeping pill. Patients will be grateful for simplification of their medication regimen. Once patients start chemotherapy their insomnia is effectively treated and there is no need to add a medication for the treatment of nausea. It is not wise to force patients from one benzodiazepine to another if not necessary. If someone responds well to alprazolam for insomnia or anxiety at the time of diagnosis, the patient does not need to change to lorazepam as an adjunctive antiemetic because it is the hospital's default choice. It is important to consider and understand the patient's belief system during times of emotional fragility. Stress alters thinking negatively. Staying on the same medication even if the choice does not follow hospital protocol, but has the same efficacy will make patients feel supported and give them a sense of control. A patient in emotional alignment with the treating team will more likely follow the medical recommendations that medically matter.

Some SSRIs such as fluoxetine or paroxetine are strong CYP2D6 inhibitors affecting the efficacy of tamoxifen. While the drug-induced CYP2D6 inhibition by some SSRIs resulting in considerably reduced endoxifen formation affecting the efficacy of tamoxifen treatment have been long known there is still frequent use reported (Binkhorst et al. 2013). Starting women with breast cancer on paroxetine for insomnia or emotionality at the beginning of cancer treatment will require a change in medication if they are scheduled to start tamoxifen at a later point. While to the physician a medication change during the course of the illness might seem simple, it can be another unsettling experience for the patient during a time of perceived instability. Helping the patient to feel understood and supported can add a sense of stability and increase adherence to treatment. QT interval prolongation is another phenomenon requiring attention, as some chemotherapy is cardiotoxic. NSAIDs are frequently prescribed for pain in cancer patients but so are steroids and SSRIs, increasing the risk of gastrointestinal ulcers. Considering the possible medication interactions early on will instill trust and promote an effective working relationship between patient and healthcare professional. Prescribers also need to

remember cancer biology. A patient with a neuroendocrine tumor secreting serotonin cannot be casually prescribed an SSRI.

6.2.6 Individual Differences

It is important to acknowledge the wide range of individual responses patients can
experience in reaction to a cancer diagnosis and treatment. Patients who used to be
social and outgoing might now be more reflective and yearn for solitude. This
change in behavior is not necessarily an expression of depression but can indicate a
changed sense of self with setting different priorities. A prescription for an antidepressant in response to the patient expressing understandably sad mental content
regarding existential concerns may be experienced as dismissive. This will particularly be the case if the patient expressed not wanting to take medication. A patient
not feeling heard or not feeling taken seriously will be less likely to follow his or her
doctor's recommendation. Thoughts of death can be natural and do not necessarily
require an emergency psychiatric consultation. Patients differ in their ability to
express themselves. Physicians need to adjust their communication accordingly.
Another important different coping style that can help guide treatment choices is
expression versus suppression of emotion. Patients also have very different needs
with respect to their desire for pharmacological versus non-pharmacological treatment. Other relevant aspects of individuality are racial and ethnic differences
(Burroughs et al. 2002). Differences are relevant physically, regarding how patients
metabolize medication based on genetic differences. Race, culture, and ethnicity
will also influence how patients view medication. While some cultures have high
expectation for medication to be curative and thus often have a higher tolerance for
medication side effects, other cultures focus on medication profile safety. There are
also variations with respect to perception of healthcare professionals. In some
cultures a collaborative relationship is emphasized while others might be accus-
tomed to a more formal and directive relationship. Illness itself can be perceived as
personal and private, not wanting to share details. This need for privacy can result in
the patient not revealing information pivotal to treatment. Family involvement
varies widely among cultures. All these factors have to be gently explored when
searching for the best integration of medication with psychosocial intervention.

6.2.7 Symbolic Meaning of Medication

Physicians are trained about medication in concrete physiological ways and often
forget the symbolic meaning of their prescriptions. Prescribing psychotropics in
particular convey messages that are rooted in cultural and social context (Metzl and
Riba 2003). They also represent aspects of the physician–patient relationship.
Medications carry undeclared and implicit messages that are not always easy to
understand, and it takes trust and time to unearth them. Both patient and doctor
bring expectations into the relationship that will affect the perception of

medication. Medication can become a representation of autonomy or dependency. In the context of cancer this effect will be magnified, as living with cancer comes with perceived loss of autonomy and increased fear of dependency. While taking medication is perceived as welcome assistance in some cases, it becomes a sign of weakness in others. At times negative and positive meaning can coexist when a patient interprets the well-meant prescription as the doctor's need for control rather than the aid it is meant to be. Prescription of medication can on the one hand provide evidence to a cancer patient that the doctor is taking his or her symptoms seriously and is trying to help them. However, medication can also be experienced as an attempt to control distress without dealing with the underlying reasons for it. Using psychotropic medications can thus be seen as an attempt to suppress rather than understand emotion. Coupling medication prescription and management with supportive psychotherapy is a way of dealing with such concerns and getting beyond them. Also, some cancer patients feel overmedicated or receive medications that come with serious and uncomfortable side effects, making the idea of more medications less appealing. The meaning of medication is also a manifestation of culture and changes over time. Increased direct-to-consumer advertising has changed patients' expectations and requests to their physicians. While there is an increase in available information, which makes for more informed consumers, it also results in distortion of information for commercial purposes. An active patient participant in medication choice can both be a blessing as well as a burden, as consumers' lay opinions can lead to a misinterpretation of medical facts. The scientific community might be putting the controversy whether antidepressants are carcinogenic to rest (Frick and Rapanelli 2013) but enough conflicting data exist to confuse patients. Without the professional qualifications to interpret medical information, patients need to be able to rely on their doctors to help make medication choices. A high quality working relationship between the treating team and the patient is needed to integrate medication and other treatments optimally. Demands for medication and interventions cannot be based on erroneous beliefs and unrealistic expectations. Clarifying communication by asking the patient what they heard and understand is often helpful.

Conclusion/Summary

The effective use of psychotropic medications in oncological care involves attention to both pharmacology and symbolic communication. Numerous factors influence the meaning of medication, including preexisting psychiatric condition, disease phase, disease stage, individual and cultural differences, side effect profile, medication interactions, and cancer-specific symptoms. Exploration of the symbolic meaning of medications to the patient can usefully guide choices. Common themes include perceived uncertainty, loss of control, and feelings of dependency. Combining understanding of psychopharmacology with the importance of psychosocial support can potentiate treatment effects. Expectation enhances efficacy. Knowledgeably combining an understanding of the patient's concerns with the effects of medication can optimize psychopharmacological integration into oncological care.

References

Akechi T, Okuyama T, Sugawara Y, Nakano T, Shima Y, Uchitomi Y. Major depression, adjustment disorders, and post-traumatic stress disorder in terminally ill cancer patients: associated and predictive factors. J Clin Oncol. 2004;22(10):1957–65.

Akechi T, Okuyama T, Onishi J, Morita T, Furukawa TA. Psychotherapy for depression among incurable cancer patients. Cochrane Database Syst Rev. 2008; (2): CD005537.

Bill-Axelson A, Garmo H, Holmberg L, Johansson JE, Adami HO, Steineck G, Johansson E, Rider JR. Long-term distress after radical prostatectomy versus watchful waiting in prostate cancer: a longitudinal study from the Scandinavian prostate cancer group-4 randomized clinical trial. Eur Urol. 2013;64(6):920–8.

Baider L, Peretz T, Kaplan De-Nour A. Effect of the Holocaust on coping with cancer. Soc Sci Med. 1992;34(1):11–5.

Binkhorst L, Mathijssen RH, van Herk-Sukel MP, Bannink M, Jager A, Wiemer EA, van Gelder T. Unjustified prescribing of CYP2D6 inhibiting SSRIs in women treated with tamoxifen. Breast Cancer Res Treat. 2013;139(3):923–9.

Bower JE. Behavioral symptoms in patients with breast cancer and survivors. J Clin Oncol. 2008; 26(5):768–77.

Burroughs VJ, Maxey RW, Levy RA. Racial and ethnic differences in response to medicines: towards individualized pharmaceutical treatment. J Natl Med Assoc. 2002;94(10 Suppl):1–26.

Cameron L, Leventhal H. The self-regulation of health and illness behavior. London: Routledge; 2003.

Carlson LE, Waller A, Groff SL, Giese-Davis J, Bultz BD. What goes up does not always come down: patterns of distress, physical and psychosocial morbidity in people with cancer over a one year period. Psychooncology. 2013;22(1):168–76.

Chochinov HM. Depression in cancer patients. Lancet Oncol. 2001;2(8):499–505.

Costa-Requena G, Ballester Arnal R, Gil F. Perceived social support in Spanish cancer outpatients with psychiatric disorder. Stress Health. 2013;29(5):421–6.

Derogatis LR, Morrow GR, Fetting J, Penman D, Piasetsky S, Schmale AM, Henrichs M, Carnicke Jr CL. The prevalence of psychiatric disorders among cancer patients. JAMA. 1983;249(6):751–7.

Evans DL, Charney DS, Lewis L, Golden RN, Gorman JM, Krishnan KR, Nemeroff CB, Bremner JD, Carney RM, Coyne JC, Delong MR, Frasure-Smith N, Glassman AH, Gold PW, Grant I, Gwyther L, Ironson G, Johnson RL, Kanner AM, Katon WJ, Kaufmann PG, Keefe FJ, Ketter T, Laughren TP, Leserman J, Lyketsos CG, McDonald WM, McEwen BS, Miller AH, Musselman D, O'Connor C, Petitto JM, Pollock BG, Robinson RG, Roose SP, Rowland J, Sheline Y, Sheps DS, Simon G, Spiegel D, Stunkard A, Sunderland T, Tibbits Jr P, Valvo WJ. Mood disorders in the medically ill: scientific review and recommendations. Biol Psychiatry. 2005;58(3):175–89.

Fox JP, Philip EJ, Gross CP, Desai RA, Killelea B, Desai MM. Associations between mental health and surgical outcomes among women undergoing mastectomy for cancer. Breast J. 2013;19(3):276–84.

French-Rosas LN, Moye J, Naik AD. Improving the recognition and treatment of cancer-related posttraumatic stress disorder. J Psychiatr Pract. 2011;17(4):270–6.

Frick LR, Rapanelli M. Antidepressants: influence on cancer and immunity? Life Sci. 2013; 92(10):525–32.

Garcia MK, McQuade J, Haddad R, Patel S, Lee R, Yang P, Palmer JL, Cohen L. Systematic review of acupuncture in cancer care: a synthesis of the evidence. J Clin Oncol. 2013;31(7):952–60.

Giese-Davis J, Collie K, Rancourt KM, Neri E, Kraemer HC, Spiegel D. Decrease in depression symptoms is associated with longer survival in patients with metastatic breast cancer: a secondary analysis. J Clin Oncol. 2011;29(4):413–20.

Gill D, Hatcher S. Antidepressants for depression in people with physical illness. Cochrane Database Syst Rev. 2000; (2): CD001312.

Horlick-Jones T. Understanding fear of cancer recurrence in terms of damage to 'everyday health competence'. Sociol Health Illn. 2011;33(6):884–98.

Koch L, Jansen H, Brenner H, Arndt V. Fear of recurrence and disease progression in long-term (>/= 5 years) cancer survivors–a systematic review of quantitative studies. Psychooncology. 2013;22(1):1–11.

Lang EV, Benotsch EG, Fick LJ, Lutgendorf S, Berbaum ML, Berbaum KS, Logan H, Spiegel D. Adjunctive non-pharmacological analgesia for invasive medical procedures: a randomised trial. Lancet. 2000;355(9214):1486–90.

Lang EV, Berbaum KS, Faintuch S, Hatsiopoulou O, Halsey N, Li X, Berbaum ML, Laser E, Baum J. Adjunctive self-hypnotic relaxation for outpatient medical procedures: a prospective randomized trial with women undergoing large core breast biopsy. Pain. 2006;126(1–3): 155–64.

Laoutidis ZG, Mathiak K. Antidepressants in the treatment of depression/depressive symptoms in cancer patients: a systematic review and meta-analysis. BMC Psychiatry. 2013;13:140.

Lebel S, Tomei S, Feldstain A, Beattle S, McCallum M. Does fear of cancer recurrence predict cancer survivors' health care use? Support Care Cancer. 2013;21(3):901–6.

L'Esperance S, Frenette S, Dionne A, Dionne JY, Comite de l'evolution des pratiques en, oncologie. Pharmacological and non-hormonal treatment of hot flashes in breast cancer survivors: CEPO review and recommendations. Support Care Cancer. 2013;21(5):1461–74.

Levy MH, Adolph MD, Back A, Block S, Codada SN, Dalal S, Deshields TL, Dexter E, Dy SM, Knight SJ, Misra S, Ritchie CS, Sauer TM, Smith T, Spiegel D, Sutton L, Taylor RM, Temel J, Thomas J, Tickoo R, Urba SG, Von Roenn JH, Weems JL, Weinstein SM, Freedman-Cass DA, Bergman MA. Palliative care. J Natl Compr Canc Netw. 2012;10(10):1284–309.

Ligibel JA, Denlinger CS. New NCCN guidelines for survivorship care. J Natl Compr Canc Netw. 2013;11(5 Suppl):640–4.

Lim CC, Devi MK, Ang E. Anxiety in women with breast cancer undergoing treatment: a systematic review. Int J Evid Based Healthc. 2011;9(3):215–35.

Lloyd-Williams M, Payne S, Reeve J, Kolamunnage DR. Antidepressant medication in patients with advanced cancer–an observational study. QJM. 2013;106(11):995–1001.

Lutgendorf SK, Sodd AK. Biobehavioral factors and cancer progression: physiological pathways and mechanisms. Psychosom Med. 2011;73(9):724–30.

Metzl J, Riba M. Understanding the symbolic value of medications: A brief review. Primary Psychiatry. 2003;10(7):45–8.

Mitchell AJ, Ferguson DW, Gill J, Paul J, Symonds P. Depression and anxiety in long-term cancer survivors compared with spouses and healthy controls: a systematic review and meta-analysis. Lancet Oncol. 2013;14(8):721–32.

Montgomery GH, Bovbjerg DH, Schnur JB, David D, Goldfarb A, Weltz CR, Schechter C, Graff-Zivin J, Tatrow K, Price DD, Silverstein JH. A randomized clinical trial of a brief hypnosis intervention to control side effects in breast surgery patients. J Natl Cancer Inst. 2007;99(17): 1304–12.

Montgomery GH, Hallquist MN, Schnur JB, David D, Silverstein JH, Bovbjerg DH. Mediators of a brief hypnosis intervention to control side effects in breast surgery patients: response expectancies and emotional distress. J Consult Clin Psychol. 2010;78(1):80–8.

Montgomery GH, Schnur JB, Kravits K. Hypnosis for cancer care: over 200 years young. CA Cancer J Clin. 2013;63(1):31–44.

Peretz T, Baider L, Ever-Hardani P, De-Nour AK. Psychological distress in female cancer patients with Holocaust experience. Gen Hosp Psychiatry. 1994;16(6):413–8.

Richardson J, Smith JE, McCall G, Richardson A, Pilkington K, Kirsch I. Hypnosis for nausea and vomiting in cancer chemotherapy: a systematic review of the research evidence. Eur J Cancer Care (Engl). 2007;16(5):402–12.

Siegel B. Love, Medicine and Miracles. New York: Harper & Row; 1986.

Simard S, Thewes B, Humphris G, Dixon M, Hayden C, Mireskandari S, Ozakinci G. Fear of cancer recurrence in adult cancer survivors: a systematic review of quantitative studies. J Cancer Surviv. 2013;7(3):300–22.

Simonton OC, Mathews-Simonton S, Creighton J. Getting well again, Los Angeles, J.P. Inc: Tracher; 1978.

Spiegel D, Classen C. Group Therapy for Cancer Patients: A Research Based Handbook of Psychosocial Care. New York: Basic/Perseus Books; 2000.

Spiegel D. Tranceformations: hypnosis in brain and body. Depress Anxiety. 2013;30(4):342–52.

Temel JS, Greer JA, Muzikansky A, Gallagher ER, Admane S, Jackson VA, Dahlin CM, Blinderman CD, Jacobsen J, Pirl WF, Billings JA, Lynch TJ. Early palliative care for patients with metastatic non-small-cell lung cancer. N Engl J Med. 2010;363(8):733–42.

Thewes B, Butow P, Bell ML, Beith J, Stuart-Harris R, Grossi M, Capp A, Dalley D. Fear of cancer recurrence in young women with a history of early-stage breast cancer: a cross-sectional study of prevalence and association with health behaviours. Support Care Cancer. 2012;20(11): 2651–9.

Weitlauf JC, Frayne SM, Finney JW, Moos RH, Jones S, Hu K, Spiegel D. Sexual violence, posttraumatic stress disorder, and the pelvic examination: how do beliefs about the safety, necessity, and utility of the examination influence patient experiences? J Womens Health (Larchmt). 2010;19(7):1271–80.

Williams S, Dale J. The effectiveness of treatment for depression/depressive symptoms in adults with cancer: a systematic review. Br J Cancer. 2006;94(3):372–90.

Psychopharmacology and Complementary and Nonconventional Treatments in Oncology

7

Lili Tang and Richard Fielding

若人欲了知 三世一切佛 應觀法界性 一切唯心造

(華嚴經夜摩天宮品)

("If someone is to understand clearly and fully the temperament of Buddha of the past, present and future, or their individual ways to achieve betterment; He must ponder and reflect that the characteristic of everything, no matter good or evil, congenial or bitter, is all construed in his heart.")

A poem from Avatamsaka (Garland) Sutra.
"There is neither good nor bad, except thinking makes it so."
Epictetus.

Abstract

Cancer is a life-threatening disease, and cancer treatments are traumatic, mutilative, functionally impairing, and disruptive to family, work, and personal life, whereas patients often hope for resumption of as near normal a life as possible. Cancer survival outcomes are improving year after year, but treatments often fail to achieve the substantive cures that patients seek, or they may do so, but at significant cost to the patient's and their family's overall health and well-being.

Psychological therapies are intended to help patients deal with the emotional impacts, but may be seen as a symptomatic treatment, and where psycho-therapies are culturally established, many patients prefer alternatives, rejecting the implications that they are psychologically "disturbed". Even when psycho-therapeutic services are available patients often adopt complementary/

L. Tang (✉)
Department of Psycho-Oncology, Peking University Cancer Hospital, Beijing 100142, China
e-mail: tanglili2005@hotmail.com

R. Fielding
Centre for Psycho-Oncology Research and Training, School of Public Health, The University of Hong Kong, Hong Kong, China
e-mail: fielding@hku.hk

L. Grassi and M. Riba (eds.), *Psychopharmacology in Oncology and Palliative Care*,
DOI 10.1007/978-3-642-40134-3_7, © Springer-Verlag Berlin Heidelberg 2014

alternative (CAM) therapeutic methods, such as Traditional Chinese Medicine (TCM), Qi Gong, Yoga, Ayurveda, meditation, and a variety of others, warranting consideration of their potential psychological contributions in cancer.

In this chapter we first consider the evidence underpinning cancer-related distress and common symptoms. The complexity and comorbidity of many symptom clusters make symptom control difficult even when the cause is well understood. CAM can offer novel approaches to help manage some of these conditions. The remainder of the chapter continues this evidence-based approach by evaluating the evidence for two main Asian complementary approaches: TCM and Yoga to enhance the management of psychosocial distress, suffering, and other psychosocial demands associated with aspects of cancers and their treatments.

7.1   Introduction

Cancer survival outcomes are improving year after year, but treatments often fail to achieve the substantive cures that patients seek, or they may do so, but at significant cost to the patient's and their family's overall health and well-being. Cancer treatments are traumatic, mutilative, functionally impairing, and disruptive to family, work, and personal life, whereas patients often hope for resumption of as near normal a life as possible. Commonly, intrusive residual symptoms remain after disease and/or treatments are ended. Some may arise from treatments that must be followed for up to 5 years after primary therapy ceases. Persistence of these symptoms is a major source of ongoing emotional and psychological distress in a majority of cancer patients. Patients presenting with late-stage, disseminated, aggressive, or resistant disease also face the implications of advanced illness and dying. Psychological therapies intended to help patients deal with the emotional impacts and psychotropic medication can be beneficial, but may be seen as a symptomatic treatment, and where psychotherapies are culturally established, many patients prefer alternatives, rejecting the implications that they are psychologically "disturbed". Finally traditional networks are also influential with families often deciding on the patient's care, rather than the patient alone.

Despite notable advances, Western Medicine (WM) has yet to develop excellence in holistic cancer care, so robust, evidence-based equivalents in the Western medical tradition are limited to psychotherapeutic, cognitive-behavioral, and biofeedback/relaxation approaches. Even when such services are available patients often adopt complementary/alternative (CAM) therapeutic methods, such as Traditional Chinese Medicine (TCM), Qi Gong, Yoga, Ayurveda, meditation, and a variety of others. Often they do not tell their clinicians of this, with between half to two-thirds not reporting (Ndao et al. 2013; Singendonk et al. 2013). These play an important role for managing cancer-related issues and many users find them very helpful. Stress management approaches are among the most popular, with mindbody therapies dominating, with almost 60 % of youth/young adults reporting use in parts of the USA (Ndao et al. 2013), and among adults, most (44–61 %) reported spiritual practices including prayer, but only 1.2 % reported using acupuncture 12–24 months after treatment ended (Gansler et al. 2008); 42 % of Dutch pediatric patients reported using CAM, mostly homeopathy and diet supplements (Singendonk et al. 2013). In Canadian pediatric cancer patients, less than 30 % reported some CAM use (Tomlinson et al. 2011). One in two Singaporean adult cancer patients reported CAM use and told their doctors (51 %), but most oncologists were unaware of concurrent CAM use during chemotherapy in (Chow et al. 2010); almost one in two Turkish cancer patients reported some CAM use, mostly (95 %) herbal agents (Tas et al. 2005). CAM seems to be most popular among female compared to male cancer patients (Paltiel et al. 2001). Many CAM approaches are receiving active attention from researchers. We have chosen here to evaluate the evidence for two main Asian complementary approaches: TCM and Yoga to enhance the management of psychosocial distress, suffering, and other psychosocial demands associated with aspects of cancers and their treatments.

7.2 Cancer-Related Distress

Distress in cancer arises from multiple sources but can be broadly classified as follows: avoidance anxiety/fear about undesired outcomes; attachment loss linked to goal or other desired outcomes, applied to self or concern for others, especially vulnerable surviving family members; existential, spiritual, meaning-related issues; and critical decisions, such as deciding treatments. Many of these issues develop from and interact to enhance the disruptiveness of physical symptoms, mostly fatigue, pain, insomnia, and functional impairments, which restrict working capacity, stamina, and in some cases mobility in earlier disease, and in more advanced disease dyspnea, dysphagia, anorexia, constipation, anemia, neurological and metabolic symptoms, and pain. If these symptoms are well managed and relieved as much as possible, the patient's quality of life will be much improved. As a result, psychological distress should decline.

A crucial component to effective cancer care is, then, superlative symptom management. All too often symptoms persist, either because treatment is ineffective, or suitable services are unavailable, are inaccessible, or lack comprehensive symptom assessment. For example, fatigue is notoriously difficult to ameliorate using pharmacological approaches. Its generalized nature is poorly understood and includes anemia, anorexia, mood disorders, and physical deconditioning, among others. Evidence now exists that insomnia which itself may have complex causes, including poorly controlled pain, anxiety, or depressed mood, and external factors, such as noisy or bright nocturnal environments, precedes fatigue, which in turn precedes depression (Jim et al. 2013). Psychopharmacology approaches to such problems alone are in general less effective than when combined with practical therapies, such as problem-oriented approaches like cognitive therapy (Blackburn et al. 1981; Van Balkom et al. 1997).

While distress tends to decline over time, this trajectory is by no means uniform or universal. Probably far fewer patients than previously thought have high levels of persistent distress, and a majority of patients are quite resilient when facing cancer (Helgeson et al. 2004; Deshields et al. 2006; Henselmans et al. 2010; Lam et al. 2010, 2011, 2012a, b; Bonanno et al. 2011). Most resilient patients are able to cope with periodic spikes of distress, but many of these might benefit substantially from non-medication interventions that build self-efficacy and help to deal with demands and perhaps manage the low-level anxiety common in cancer (Mitchell et al. 2013). A subset of patients, around 10–20 %, seem to have more sustained coping difficulties and these patients would seem most likely to benefit the most from more intensive interventions.

The complexity and comorbidity of many of these symptom complexes make symptom control difficult even when the cause is well understood. CAM can offer novel approaches to help manage some of these conditions and do so more effectively than standardized psychopharmacological approaches alone may always do. However, many patients would appreciate guidance from clinicians on which to use, and many CAMs have little, if any, evidence for efficacy, and some are harmful.

7.3   Traditional Chinese Medicine

7.3.1   Symptom Management

TCM activities potentially beneficial in cancer include herbal formulations, acupuncture, and activity-based interventions—Qigong and Tai Chi Chuan. The evidence base for most herbal interventions used in TCM remains to be fully established (Zhang et al. 2011).

Pain and fatigue are intrusive and distress-inducing symptoms. In a systematic review of 52 studies pain prevalence was 33 % (95 % Confidence interval 21–46 %) after curative treatment; 59 % (44–73 %) during anticancer treatment, and 64 % (58–69 %) in advanced/metastatic and terminal disease. The overall prevalence of patients at all disease stages who reported pain was 53 % (43–63 %) (Van den Beuken-van Everdingen et al. 2007). Among 5,084 participants in 11 European countries and Israel 56 % suffered moderate-to-severe pain at least monthly (Breivik et al. 2009). In China, among 1,555 cancer patients 61 % reported pain, mostly associated with advanced disease (Liu et al. 2001). Similarly, the U.S. National Comprehensive Cancer Network (NCCN) has reported that 70–100 % of patients with cancer experienced fatigue. When fatigue and pain are moderate to severe, they become disabling and are the main obstacles to effective rehabilitation. In TCM, pain and fatigue are symptomatic of Qi and Xu stagnation and blockages or disordered flow of Qi in the $Jing$-Luo system (Qi meridians). Reviewing 115 articles, including 41 Randomized Clinical Trials (RCTs), Xu et al. (2007) suggested that TCM may be effective for cancer pain, generating effects similar to those of Western analgesics. The review concluded TCM has many potentially useful methods, including external application, oral administration, intravenous infusion, inhalation, and enema for symptomatic treatment of pain. These methods might be particularly useful if patients refuse opiates for fear of dependency, a common problem in Asian countries, for example (Liu et al. 2001), or to supplement opioid analgesics in intractable pain (Zhang et al. 2006).

Acupuncture for Symptom Control Acupuncture research faces methodological difficulties and disagreements principally over the nature of appropriate study controls and methodological heterogeneity. A recent Cochrane review (Madsen et al. 2009) examined 13 acupuncture trials on 3,025 patients with a variety of pain symptoms. In eight of those trials treatment allocation was adequately concealed, enabling control of placebo effect, but none of the clinicians administering the treatments were blinded. When pooled, results indicated there was a small, probably clinically insignificant, difference of 4 mm (2–6 mm) on a 100 mm scale in favor of the acupuncture group compared to sham acupuncture controls. Larger differences in pain ratings are observed in trials comparing acupuncture and no-treatment controls. At this time there is insufficient evidence of a clear, clinically significant analgesic effect beyond that attributable to known nonspecific effects.

Reviewing 11 pooled studies using data on postoperative nausea and vomiting Ezzo et al. (2011) concluded there was evidence of a biologic effect from acupuncture-point stimulation. A single-blind RCT compared effects of once-weekly traditional acupuncture, pericardium (P6) acupuncture, sham acupuncture, and no-treatment control for four weeks on nausea and vomiting in 593 pregnant women (Smith et al. 2002). Women receiving traditional acupuncture, P6 acupuncture, and sham acupuncture reported significantly less nausea and dry retching than women in the no acupuncture group, but there were no differences in actual vomiting. Real acupuncture was associated with earlier reduction in nausea and retching than in the sham group. Another study found Deqi acupuncture no more effective than sham acupuncture in preventing radiotherapy-associated nausea, though both interventions were associated with reduced nausea over time (Enblom et al. 2012).

Similar claims for acupuncture benefit in cancer-related fatigue and quality of life have been made (e.g., Molassiotis et al. 2007, 2012). However, again these studies failed to eliminate potential for bias from attributing improved outcomes to knowledge of having had acupuncture in the absence of a suitable sham control group (Azad and John 2013). A recent systematic review of acupuncture for cancer-related fatigue concluded that four of seven RCTs showed effectiveness of acupuncture over sham acupuncture and usual care, but it has not been proved clearly that the observed outcomes were due to specific effects of acupuncture or nonspecific effects of care due to methodological flaws in the studies (Posadzki et al. 2013).

7.3.2 The Psychological in TCM

The holistic nature of TCM does not clearly distinguish between physical and psychological aspects of experience, unlike Western Cartesian systems. So while TCM approaches to psychology can also be dated thousands of years ago, they are not easily separated from physical health issues. Early medicine texts describe the etiology, mechanisms, and treatments for psychosomatic diseases. TCM recognizes seven emotions: joy, anger, sorrow, sadness, fear, surprise, and thought. Excesses of these emotions are believed to damage specific *Zang-Fu* organs (heart, lung, kidney, spleen, liver—these are functional rather than anatomic "organs"). The correspondence between these emotions and *Zang-Fu* organs is seen in *Jutong* theory of Suwen (Fig. 7.1). This described how emotions could disrupt the *Qi* (life energy) balance: rage leading to *Qi* ascending; excessive joy leading to *Qi* loss; excessive sorrow leading to *Qi* consumption; fear leading to *Qi* sinking; and fright leading to *Qi* turbulence. This emotional theory is considered not only an important explanation for psychosomatic diseases in TCM, but also the core content in traditional Chinese health care and health maintenance through moderation in emotions. Leung (1998) reviews these and other Chinese concepts of emotion in more detail.

Acupuncture for Anxiety Auricular acupuncture for anxiety (AAA) has been studied in noncancer conditions. Pre-surgical anxiety in 91 elective surgery patients was compared with auricular acupuncture for relaxation (AAR) and acupuncture in non-active auricular points (ANA). Groups were comparable on baseline trait anxiety (State-Trait Anxiety Inventory). After, the AAR relaxation group reported significantly lower STAI scores than ANA controls, but the AAA anxiety acupuncture group had scores comparable to the ANA control group (Wang et al. 2001). Similarly, a head-to-head comparison of auricular acupuncture with intranasal midazolam and sham acupuncture against a no acupuncture control for dental extraction anxiety reported greater reductions in anxiety scores in both the auricular acupuncture and midazolam groups relative to control (Karst et al. 2007). A systematic review of 10 RCTs and two other trials of acupuncture in anxiety disorders and perioperative anxiety concluded insufficient methodological detail was provided to confidently conclude acupuncture was effective in anxiety (Pilkington et al. 2007).

Insomnia, Anxiety, Depression Insomnia, anxiety, and depression are the three most prevalent psychological problems in cancer patients. These significantly interact with physical symptoms and lower the patients' quality of life. These are often comorbid with fatigue and pain (Wong and Fielding 2012), and, in American cancer populations, are associated with poorer outcomes (Brintzenhofe-Szoc et al. 2009). In a consecutive sample of 8,265 outpatients 12 % had mixed anxiety/depression, 18 % depressive symptoms, and 24 % anxiety symptoms (Brintzenhofe-Szoc et al. 2009). Among 10,000 Canadian cancer outpatients screen-detected anxiety was 19 % for clinical symptoms and 23 % for subclinical

Fig. 7.1 Jutong theory of
Suwen Model of Emotions
in TCM

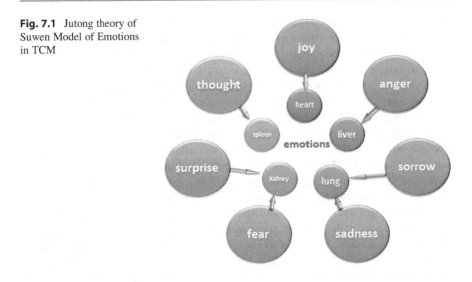

symptoms while clinical depression symptoms were present in 13 % and subclinical symptoms in 16 % (Linden et al. 2012). In over 1,000 Australian patients assessed at 6 and 12 months following diagnosis, anxiety prevalence was 22 % and 21 %, respectively, while depression prevalence was 13 % at both time points (Boyes et al. 2013). A meta-analysis of 43 studies indicated that anxiety prevalence in cancer patients and their spouses respectively at 18 % (95%CI 17.8–23.6 %) vs. 14 % (9.8–18.5 %) was slightly more prevalent than depression at 12 % (7.7–16.2 %) vs. 10 % (8–10.6 %) (Mitchell et al. 2013). These recent reviews are consistent with reports showing that a majority of cancer patients are mostly resilient to cancer-related distress (Lam et al. 2010, 2011, 2012a, 2013). A well-designed RCT over 6 weeks in which acupuncture plus paroxetine was compared to paroxetine alone found improved response in the combined group in moderately depressed patients (Qu et al. 2013). However, the paroxetine-only group was not given sham acupuncture and so placebo effects cannot be excluded (Van Haselen and Jütte 2013). Particularly in non-Euro-American cultural groups a common barrier for cancer patients with depression and anxiety is worry about facing the dual stigma of being labeled a cancer patient and "crazy" or mentally ill. Both cancer and mental illness are often strongly stigmatized conditions which make patients extremely reluctant to accept mainstream psychiatric interventions, such as medication and psychotherapy. However, much anxiety experienced about cancer following treatment cessation has to do with the meaning of symptoms and uncertainty regarding future outcomes (Lam and Fielding 2003; Lam et al. 2012b). Insomnia is a more prevalent problem for cancer patients and often occurs comorbid with depression and anxiety. Again, laying awake at night and wondering what the future holds for yourself and family or difficulty sleeping because of pain or other symptoms (Desai et al. 2013) can become a chronic problem. Among 991 Canadian cancer patients, perioperatively 28 % met diagnostic criteria for insomnia syndrome, and 34 % had insomnia symptoms, decreasing to 26 % and 22 % respectively 2 months after surgery (Savard et al. 2009). Feng et al. (2011) reported greater improvements in sleep quality and lower depression scores in a group of cancer patients receiving acupuncture versus a group receiving fluoxetine. However, the study was not blinded to treatment. An RCT comparison of 71 cases on insomnia randomized to head acupuncture for insomnia or standard acupuncture produced significantly better sleep quality after 30 days in the head insomnia group (Dong et al. 2008). A recent systematic review (Yeung et al. 2012) suggested that Chinese herbs could be effective for insomnia after totally 227 studies, 17,916 subjects, and 87 TCM patterns were collected and analyzed. The meta-analysis suggested that Chaihu-Shugan-San (柴胡疏肝散), a traditional Chinese medicine formula, was effective and safe in treating depressed patients (Wang et al. 2012). However the quality of studies included in the review and meta-analysis were, again, considered inadequate. So, more well-designed RCTs are needed to examine whether mainstream TCM interventions including acupuncture and herbal preparations can offer any benefit in depressed patients and others with anxiety and insomnia. However, in Taiwan, during 2002, 29,800 prescriptions for herbs to treat insomnia were issued through the Taiwan National Health Insurance system (Chen et al. 2011). There appears to be a significant market for these interventions in Asia.

7.3.3 Activity-Based TCM Interventions: Qigong and Tai Chi

Qigong and *Tai Chi Chuan* (TCC) are the two most widely practiced physical activity-based interventions of TCM.

Qigong Medical *Qigong* for health and healing consists primarily of meditative, slow, repetitive physical movements coordinated with breathing exercises (Sancier 1996). It is considered in TCM to be an energy-healing intervention used to prevent and cure ailments and to improve health through regular practice. *Qigong* comes in two main forms: external *Qigong* and internal *Qigong*. External *Qigong* (External *Qi* Therapy (EQT)) refers to *Qigong* practitioners who have mastered the technique, directing or emitting *Qi* energy to help patients clear *Qi* blockages, move bad *Qi* out of the body, and balance the *Qi* flow in order to relieve pain or other illnesses. Internal *Qigong* refers to a self-practice of *Qigong* to achieve optimal health for mind and body (Lee and Jang 2005). Although neither *Qi* therapy itself nor the mechanism of its effects is understandable or explicable within any paradigm of modern science, its effects on the human body are claimed to be beneficial in many clinical and psychological illnesses (Lee et al. 2003). In 1998 two types of *Qigong* were recommended by the Chinese government for therapeutic benefit in treating cancer: Guo-Lin new *Qigong* and Chinese Taiji Five-Element *Qigong* (Chen and Yeung 2002). Guo-Lin New *Qigong* is characterized by a slow walking exercise accompanied by arm movements coordinated with slight twisting movements of the waist (Jones 2001). It was reported that some cases achieved complete remission from cancer after practicing Guo-Lin New *Qigong* (Chen and Yeung 2002). However, most practitioners used *Qigong* as a supplementary therapy to conventional treatments or other therapy (Huang 1996). Taiji Five-Element *Qigong* was developed by He Binhui. The main focus of Taiji Five-Element *Qigong* is to activate the patients' deteriorated immune system, suppressed self-recovery power, and concealed self-regeneration capabilities (He and Chen 2002). A randomized controlled trial showed that the External *Qi* of Taiji Five-Element *Qigong* could inhibit the liver cancer cell growth in mice (Chen et al. 1997). Most research studies of Qigong therapy for cancer patients have examined internal Qigong, whereas most research on Qigong therapy for cancer in animals or culture cells has involved EQT (external Qigong) (Chen and Yeung 2002). The molecular and cellular mechanisms underlying claimed antitumor effect of EQT was also explored in some studies; for example, External Qi of Yan Xin Qigong has been reported to differentially regulate apoptosis and survival pathways in cancer versus normal cells and exert cytotoxic effects preferentially on cancer cells (Yan et al. 2006). However, as with TCM studies generally, most Qigong research lacks the use of randomized controlled design, faces difficulties in blinding participants and investigators, and lacks large sample sizes, which pose difficulties when it comes to excluding alternative explanations for observed effects. Study findings also require replication.

Tai Chi Chuan (TCC) TCC involves sets of physical activities derived from the Chinese martial arts tradition, comprising linked, choreographed slow movements coordinated with deep and regular breath. TCC has been practiced for centuries by Chinese people of all age groups to maintain health and wellness. Some studies have indicated that TCC may have therapeutic effects and that it might benefit cancer patients (Mansky et al. 2006). TCC is considered a "moving meditation" because it is said to endow its practitioners with great calm and mental tranquility (Taylor-Piliae et al. 2006; Wang et al. 2009). A recent literature review concluded that TCC brings psychological benefits with regard to the quality of life of the participants. In particular improved emotional well-being (general mood, stress, anxiety, depression, and anger-tension), self-perception (self-efficacy and fear of failure), and bodily well-being (reduced sleep disorders) are reported (Jimenez et al. 2012).

Some studies have suggested that TCC might help improve both psychological and physical outcomes in cancer patients and survivors. Following TCC improvements have been reported for cancer patients' self-esteem (Mustian et al. 2004) and self-efficacy (Seoung 2008) and favorable effects on mood and psychological adaption (Eom 2007). Outcomes in TCC were similar to those seen for aerobic activity, which has been recommended for relieving common somatic symptoms of cancer, including vomiting, nausea, and fatigue (Lee et al. 2007). An RCT suggested significant improvements in hand grip strength and flexibility in extension and horizontal abduction, but not in a 6-min walking distance, or in range of flexion abduction, and horizontal adduction in breast cancer patients (Mustian et al. 2004). However, a recent systematic review indicated that all existing RCTs were of poor quality because they had a high risk of bias. Collectively, the existing trial evidence does not show convincingly that TCC is uniquely effective for supportive care in breast and other forms of cancer over and above other activity-based interventions. Future studies should use RCTs designs and be of high methodological quality, with a particular emphasis on including an adequate control intervention (Lee et al. 2010).

7.3.4   Summary of TCM Interventions

TCM applications in clinical oncology potentially offer many contributions: some TCM herbs have direct anticancer effects; herbs or manipulations may help relieve both common physical or mental symptoms and adverse reactions induced by conventional anticancer therapies; others may indirectly increase the sensitivity of the body to chemotherapy drugs or radiotherapy. However, with most of these possibilities robust clinical trial standard evidence of effectiveness remains rare. The quality of existing evidence is poor and so caution is warranted. While TCM may appear to contribute to overall improvements of the quality of life in cancer patients the mechanisms by which this is achieved remain obscure. TCM is widely integrated with WM in most Chinese hospitals, and many small and uncontrolled studies indicate possible benefit. Although increasingly popular with clinical staff, patients, and families, comprehensive application of TCM in conventional anti-cancer treatments both in and outside China needs more standardized procedures. For herbal preparations, good agricultural, manufacturing quality control, laboratory standards, and clinical practice are necessary to guarantee standardized conditions for quality control in the use of TCM herbs (Konkimalla and Efferth 2008). Many clinical trials of different TCM elements can be found in medical databases. However, almost all systematic reviews and meta-analyses of this literature conclude that most of these clinical trials have serious methodological defects (sample limitations; lack of multicenter involvement and lack of or inadequate control conditions and allocation concealment). Moreover, because most TCM prescriptions involve combinations of treatments, and herbal preparations are often several different components, and their use changes as *Zhang* (TCM diagnostic syndrome) changes over the course of the disease, so quantifying the active component(s) becomes a massively complex task. Conversely, isolating a single active ingredient removes much of the "contextual" basis behind TCM, so that it effectively ceases to be TCM and becomes pharmacology or physiology. Nevertheless, TCM has begun to show its unique characteristics and considerable potential to contribute in cancer care. Further, more methodologically rigorous research and integrative approaches combining WM and TCM together offer great promise to create more treatment options for cancer patients and their families.

7.4 Yoga

Yoga refers to a wide set of practices derived from Indian philosophical roots. Patanjali (Yoga Sutras) specified eight limbs (*Ashtangas*) of yoga: Yamas (morality), Niyamas (personal obligations), Asanas (body postures), Pranayama (breathing practices), Pratyahara (sense control), Dharana (concentration and inner awareness), Dhyana (meditation), and Samahdi (union with the divine). Of these, meditation, asana, and pranayama have received the most therapeutic interest.

7.4.1 The Psychological in Indian Philosophy

Indian philosophy's insight to psychological processes is wonderfully rich. Both the Buddhist and the yogic tradition from which it derives conceive very similar processes. In Advaita Vedanta, the subjective mind is classically considered to emerge from three components—*Manas*, *Chitta*, and *Buddhi*. *Manas*, the perceiving-judgmental-acting (thinking and willing) components of lower mind supervises the senses and organs of action (body and speech) and thus universalizes experience; *Chitta* assimilates impressions and is the cumulative faculty of mind; *Buddhi* approximates to intelligent self-awareness. The cumulative impressions in *Chitta* give rise to *Ahamkara* (ego) which drives the activity of *Manas*. A key function of *Buddhi* is *viveka*, or clarity of discrimination between the functions of mind and of consciousness to achieve what both yoga and Buddhism call *vidya*, or true sight. *Vidya* reveals the superficiality of everyday subjective "reality." All activities of mind functions are called *Vrittis*.

Chitta's tendency is to acquire mental "stuff" from which emerges individual identity, whereas the spiritual objective is to learn that individual identity is both a major contributor to suffering and cloak to truer insight or discrimination. Hence a clouded *Buddhi* thinks of the mind and all it perceived and generates, including the ego as real, whereas *viveka* reveals it to be like the reflection in a mirror. In contrast to Western spiritual traditions centering on Judeo-Christian beliefs, in both Buddhism and yoga suffering occurs when the belief in the separate *Chitta*-derived ego-self drives attachment to specific outcomes, which may or may not eventuate, rather than being equally accepting of all outcomes. This valuably informs both therapeutic practices for adaptation to cancer through the practice of acceptance, and in terminal illness can be helpful in building identification with more than just the body and ego. Hence, how we think about things determines the quality of the experience; lacking *viveka* we see ourselves as separate (*Avidya*), and hence suffer attachments and losses; with *viveka*, we achieve *vidya* and see separation as illusionary, and hence nothing can be gained or lost, and therein suffering ceases.

Diet and activity alter physical health and mental state. For example, certain foods, alcohol, for example, will dull *Buddhi* and create a lethargic mind, whereas strongly seasoned foods are believed to stimulate *Manas* and *Buddhi*, obscuring *viveka*, as waves on a lake obscure the view of the bottom. Diets that are calming facilitate *viveka*. In yoga the mind is likened to a drunken monkey, or a curious rat, always poking its nose into holes to see what lies there. All yoga practices are, therefore, ultimately directed towards the restraint of this drunken monkey mind. Hence Patanjali's aphorism *Yoga Chitta vritti nirodha* defines Yoga as the stilling of the disturbances of the mind. When this happens then the seer rests in his true self.

7.4.2 Yoga Practices for Improving Psychological Well-being in Cancer

Psychotherapeutic yoga practices that offer potential benefit during cancer are *Seva*, or selfless service—serving others with no expectation of return; *Asana*, or physical postures that strengthen and maintain the body; *Pranayama* breathing exercises to improve *prana* (life energy) control, thereby improving energy levels; and *Dhyana*, meditation, to quieten the mind, create a peaceful inner state, and improve *viveka*.

Most published studies have examined yoga as combinations of *asana*, *pranayama*, and *meditation*, and not the separate components (Levine and Balk 2012). Moreover, different streams of yoga (*Hatha, Raja, Bhakti*, for example) exist having different emphases (asana vs. meditation, vs. seva, for example). While the spirit of *yoga* is integrated practice, this complicates the identification of specific effects, for example, separating the known physiological effects of any form of exercise/physical activity from specific asana (or, for example, *Tai Chi chuan* and *Qigong*) practice and adjusting the known effects of physical relaxation from meditation. Finally, quantifying the relative contributions of these components to observed effects can help to tailor interventions based on yoga principles.

Seva Seva is a spiritual practice whereby the aspirant undertakes tasks without expectation of return. This requires putting aside the ego and personal desires and focuses on the action for its own sake rather than its consequences. Volunteering is a similar, pro-social behavior that increases social contact and provides distraction and the opportunities for social comparisons that can help recalibrate relative evaluations of advantage and disadvantage. Evidence is building for the benefits of volunteering. Volunteering apparently offers more psychological benefits in terms of life satisfaction to older adults rather than younger, but this might reflect differences in the nature of the voluntary activities undertaken (Van Willigen 2000). Volunteers tend to report lower rates of depression (Musick and Wilson 2003), while a prospective study found volunteers reported greater life satisfaction and control over life and physical health three years later compared to a matched group of non-volunteer controls (Thoits and Hewitt 2001). Finally, several prospective longitudinal studies suggest that after adjustment for age, gender, socioeconomic status, and prior health, volunteers are more likely to be alive at follow-up than non-volunteers (Musick et al. 1999). It has been claimed that providing social support is more beneficial than receiving it (Brown et al. 2003), despite the substantial work on the protective roles of social support in cancer. However, volunteering studies most exclude explanations due to healthy worker effects

(Shah 2009). If confirmed, volunteering may offer a potentially significant supplement to cancer patients with psychological difficulties over and above mainstream WM approaches.

Asana (Hatha Yoga) Hatha yoga comprises static (Asana) and dynamic exercises aimed at improving health by building bodily strength, flexibility, and stamina, enabling prolonged meditation that facilitates spiritual development. Hatha yoga has become extraordinarily popular in Western cultures over the past 30 years practiced by millions worldwide as a form of exercise and recreation or for stress reduction and spiritual practice.

Evaluating the benefits of *asana* practice requires separating specific effects of *asana* from those of general physical activity, which has substantial positive psychological benefits in its own right (Szabo 2003; Johnson and Kreuger 2007). A recent systematic review of yoga asana for cancer-related fatigue identified 10 RCTs involving 583 mostly breast cancer patients who met selection criteria. In four of these studies a positive effect claiming fatigue reduction was reported, and three studies reported a dose–response effect linked to the number of yoga classes attended (Sadja and Mills 2013). A study of 82 medical students used as their own controls and taught asana practice reported significant improvement on their General Health Questionnaire scores over one month of community practice (Bansal et al. 2013). Bankar et al. (2013) in a non-blinded trial of 65 older healthy community-dwelling adults in India found the practice of several asanas on a daily basis was associated with improved sleep quality scores on the Pittsburg Sleep Quality Index and better quality of life scores. Asana practice has been associated with increases in brain GABA levels by 27 % compared to a passive reading control and hence may offer benefit as an intervention for GABA-deficit disorders, such as anxiety and depression (Streeter et al. 2007). A small feasibility study of combining asana and pranayama in Dutch informal caregivers found increases in physical strength, aerobic endurance, and flexibility along with enhanced coping after 8 weeks, though dropout was high (Van Puymbroeck et al. 2007). A systematic review of RCT yoga intervention that included an asana component compared against no exercise or waitlist controls identified 16 studies from 13 RCTs; all but one (on lymphoma) involved breast cancer patients. Studies were evaluated as being of medium-to-good quality on average (67 %, range 22–89 %). The review concluded there was evidence supporting large reductions in anxiety, depression, and distress; moderate reductions in fatigue; and moderate increases in QoL and emotional and social functioning, but only small increases in functional well-being (Buffart et al. 2012). Another systematic review looking at clinical significance of patient reported outcomes for yoga interventions on QoL, psychological state, or symptoms reached similar conclusions for potential effectiveness (Culos-Reed et al. 2012).

Studies of specific styles of hatha yoga practice are reported. Iyengar yoga is a graded series of exercises utilizing props such as blocks (Iyengar 1979). A basic Iyengar program was reported to result in reduced symptoms of fatigue, depression, and perceived stress in women reporting persistent fatigue after breast cancer treatment, but the small sample size and no-treatment control group detract from the findings (Bower et al. 2012). A small systematic review reported similar effects of hatha yoga on fatigue, but cautioned against the small number of robust studies available (Cramer et al. 2012). Another small study of Iyengar yoga reported reduced 5 am salivary cortisol secretion and improved emotional well-being in nine women following 90-min, twice-weekly yoga for 8 weeks compared to waitlist controls (Banasik et al. 2011). However, none of these studies used an activity-based control intervention.

Pranayama Few studies have examined the effects of pranayama independent of other yoga components in cancer patients. Dhruva et al. (2012) randomized 16 patients receiving chemotherapy to pranayama or usual care. Pranayama dose (intervention attendance plus home practice) was associated with improved symptom and QoL scores. However, the small size of this pilot study limits its relevance. A small study of changes in stress-signaling gene expression reported upregulation 16-fold in 69 genes, and twofold in 4,428 genes, and increased expression of antiapoptotic agents and COX2 gene expression in lymphocytes, plus hormones associated with prolonged WBC survival in pranayama practitioners. Pranayama may offer particular benefit to patients with dyspnea or other breathing difficulties, by helping to improve subjective functional performance and exercise tolerance (Doneskey-Cuenco et al. 2009) particularly in older institutionalized and frail elderly patients (Cebrià et al. 2014). This latter point is of particular importance as a significant fraction of older cancer patients and those in late stages of their illness may be unable to perform other exercises. So pranayama exercises may have very specific benefits as an aid to dyspnea in late-stage cancer.

Meditation Meditation as a mind-body practice has become increasingly popular in Western culture. Mind-body interventions are considered among the most preferred and helpful complementary choices for cancer patients. Meditative techniques are not limited to Eastern religious or spiritual traditions, but are core practices of yoga and Buddhism. With an estimated 10 million practitioners in the USA and hundreds of millions worldwide, meditation is now one of the world's most widely practiced, enduring, and researched psychological disciplines (Walsh and Shapiro 2006).

There is no consensus definition of meditation. Cardoso et al. emphasized that, in order to be characterized as meditation, the procedure should encompass the following requirements: (1) the use of a specific technique (clearly defined); (2) muscle relaxation at some point; (3) "logic relaxation"; (4) it must necessarily be a self-induced state; and (5) use "self-focus" skill, or "anchoring" (Cardoso et al. 2004). From a cognitive and psychological perspective, meditation also has been defined as a family of self-regulation practices that aim to bring mental processes under voluntary control through focusing attention and awareness (Walsh and Shapiro 2006). More generally meditation can be considered as a discrete and well-defined experience of a state of "thoughtless awareness" or mental silence, in which the activity of the mind is minimized without reducing the level of alertness (Manocha 2000). This comes close to Patanjali's definition of stilling the disturbances of the mind. Meditation has been described as the attainment of a restful yet fully alert physical and mental state practiced by many as a self-regulatory approach to emotion management (Takahashi et al. 2005). Used in this way, meditation can be described to patients as a psychological tool. This may make it acceptable to patients who might feel it threatens their religious values to adopt practices associated with other religions. Meditative practices are found throughout cultures and achieved in a variety of ways.

Meditation forms include mantra meditation (comprising Transcendental Meditation, Relaxation Response, and Clinically Standardized Meditation), mindfulness meditation, and "active" meditation involving sustained movements often repetitive, such as Yoga, Tai Chi, Qi Gong (Ospina et al. 2007), and Sema in Sufism. The practice of meditation is divided into four components: form, object, attitude, and behavior of the mind (Dunn et al. 1999). Tacón (2003) suggested meditation practiced has two basic forms: exclusive/restrictive/concentration meditation or inclusive/mindfulness meditation. Concentration meditation emphasizes active focus on an internal or external object, such as the breath or a mantra, while restricting or minimizing distractions from other stimuli. If distracted, a practitioner of concentration meditation redirects attention to the mediation object. A widely practiced form of this meditation is transcendental meditation(TM) developed by Maharishi Mahesh Yogi in 1958 (Hussain and Bhushan 2010).

Mindfulness meditation involves including rather than excluding stimuli from the field of consciousness. Unlike concentration meditation, awareness is not focused on any single object. An operational working definition of mindfulness is the awareness that emerges through paying attention on purpose, in the present moment, and nonjudgmentally to the unfolding of experience moment by moment (Kabat-Zinn 2003). Vipassana, Zen meditation, Mindfulness-based Stress Reduction (MBSR), and Mindfulness-based Cognitive Therapy (MBCT) belong to this category. The most widely used mindfulness program today is the MBSR program developed by Kabat-Zinn and colleagues (Kabat-Zinn 1982, 2003). This program involves a structured, group-formatted, 8–10 week course comprising three mindfulness meditation practices that include the body scan, which involves "sweeping" through the body mentally from feet to head; mindfulness of breath and other perceptions; and Hatha yoga postures, designed to develop mindfulness during movement (Kabat-Zinn 1982). Meditation, in general, and MBSR, in particular, have been proposed to be potentially beneficial throughout the cancer experience (Carlson 2010). Most published studies of MBSR were conducted with breast and prostate cancer patients.

Studies examining the effects of mindfulness-based stress reduction approaches in cancer patients compared the MBSR intervention against an usual care group and mostly reported superior benefits or improvements in the MBSR groups. For example, Lengacher et al. (2012) found reductions in symptom intensity, particularly fatigue and sleep problems, in breast cancer patients over the 6-week study period. However, there were only modest advantages in the BCSR group relative to the controls. Carlson et al. (2013) compared 18-hour mindfulness meditation and "mild yoga" against 18 hour expressive group therapy and a 1-day stress management control condition in an RCT of 271 distressed women with breast cancer. The authors concluded the mindfulness group produced superior psychological outcomes but that both intervention groups had comparable normative cortisol profiles relative to controls; however, differences in the duration of control training raise concerns about possible exposure bias. Monti et al (2013) examined 191 women with breast cancer stratified by age and stress level and randomized to MBST or education intervention of equal duration (8-weeks). Both groups improved equally over the intervention period, but those women with higher stress levels improved significantly only in the mindfulness group, immediately and 6 months after completing the intervention. However, an RCT of 64 women with chronic fatigue after breast cancer chemotherapy underwent a mindfulness-style program with added physical activity (Spahn et al. 2013). While both groups reported reduced fatigue and better QoL, the mindfulness group did not show any additional improvement over the control activity (walking) group.

A randomized controlled trial, which evaluated the impact of the Transcendental Meditation program plus standard care as compared with standard care alone with experimental ($n = 64$) or control ($n = 66$) groups, reported that following a TM program resulted in improved evaluations on quality of life (QOL) and affect in older women ($\geq$55 years) with stages II to IV breast cancer (Nidich et al. 2009). Another study of the effects of Zen meditation practice on tumor progression claimed that the growth of prostate cancer cells could be reduced through the application of Zen meditation alone without any drug treatment (Yu et al. 2003).

A meta-analysis of ten studies, only four of which were RCTs, suggested that MBSR may be helpful for the mental health of cancer patients (Ledesma and Kumano 2008). Specifically, MBSR aids patients in relieving anxiety, stress, fatigue, and general mood and sleep disturbance and helps in improving the psychological aspects of their quality of life. Recruited patients were predominantly women with early-stage breast cancer (either in active treatment or in remission), having a high level of education, which suggests the kinds of cancer patients most willing to try MBSR therapy. Another review concluded that the effects of mindfulness-based therapy (MBT), including MBCT and MBSR on depression and anxiety in cancer, might be smaller because patients may experience physical symptoms listed on depression or anxiety scales as a result of their physical condition or as potential side effects of medical treatments; effect sizes for depression and anxiety symptoms in populations with cancer may be smaller than effect sizes in populations with anxiety or mood disorders due to a floor effect (Hofmann et al. 2010). This latter review points to the importance of careful design and measurement in studies of complementary approaches in cancer care.

Neuroimaging studies using functional MRI with techniques such as EEG to assess meditative state have begun to explore the neural mechanisms underlying mindfulness meditation practice. Experienced meditators demonstrate increased alpha and theta EEG power during meditation and reduced or enhanced autonomic response to external stimuli (Travis 2001; Takahashi et al. 2005). A controlled longitudinal study suggests that MBSR is associated with changes in gray matter concentration in brain regions involved in learning and memory processes, emotion regulation, self-referential processing, and perspective taking (Hölzel et al. 2011).

Combined Yoga Practice Most studies of yoga have utilized meditation in different proportions in combination with asanas and/or pranayama. Harder et al. (2012) reviewed 18 RCTs of yoga interventions and concluded there was moderate-to-good evidence of benefit for treatment-related side effects in breast cancer. Similarly, Boehm et al. (2012) in a systematic review of 19 clinical studies concluded that there was a mild effect of yoga on fatigue across a spectrum of chronically ill patient and healthy groups. Another systematic review following Cochrane guidelines found a small beneficial effect on QoL but not on specific symptoms in non-treatment controlled RCTs of women with breast cancer (Zhang et al. 2012). Again, quality of most studies was poor. A systematic review of RCTs with outcomes measuring depression concluded that yoga interventions and combined interventions for depression in cancer patients were associated with improvement in depressive symptoms and reduced depression scores (D'Silva et al. 2012). In 28 Japanese cancer patients undergoing antineoplastic chemotherapy who undertook MBSR, yoga and breathing exercises scores on the Hospital Anxiety and Depression Scale (HADS) declined significantly while the Spirituality scale of the FACIT QoL measure increased (Ando et al. 2009). Though they have not been evaluated for effectiveness in cancer care, specific yogic practices of bodily cleansing may also have benefit for specific symptoms.

Summary Meditation-based interventions are receiving more attention as complementary choices for cancer patients. A growing body of literature suggests that meditation may offer an effective supplement in reducing symptoms of a number of particularly stress-related disorders and for improving QOL. Study quality is improving, but outstanding questions remain as to the unique contributions of meditation compared with, for example, whole body relaxation.

▶ **Key Points**

- Application of CAM in clinical oncology has potentially broad prospects: (1) direct anticancer effects; (2) indirectly increase the sensitivity of chemotherapy drugs or radiotherapy; (3) improve both common physical or mental symptoms and adverse reactions induced by conventional anticancer therapies; (4) psychosocial considerations in TCM could enrich humanistic care in oncology.
- However, most CAM interventions have weak or mixed evidence of effectiveness and further high-quality research is needed to rule out methodological and generalized nonspecific effects such as placebo, and healthy worker effects as explanations for study findings.
- The research evidence supporting use and benefits of qigong and TCC in cancer patients remains weak. Both qigong and TCC remain to be proven to have

therapeutic value as complementary therapies for cancer patients over and above other exercise activities.

- Yoga-based therapies show promise for interventions. In particular specific symptoms may be helped using these, for example, pranayama in dyspnea. As with TCM activity-based therapies, asana needs to be clearly shown to have effects over and above those known to be associated with exercise and increased activity, distraction, and relaxation.
- Meditation is basically the self-regulation of attention and awareness.
- Meditation, in general, or MBSR, in particular, has potential to be beneficial throughout a cancer experience.
- Spiritual care and intervention should be available to cancer patients. These may offer valuable complementary benefits for cancer patients.

7.5 Concluding Comments

7.5.1 Methodological Issues

There has been an explosion in studies on a range of complementary therapeutic approaches for use in cancer. For example, PubMed searches of cancer and mindfulness generated 180 papers, the majority of which were published since 2010. These have mostly focused on mindfulness-based and mixed yoga interventions. Many are pilot or feasibility studies, reviews of earlier trials, plus a smaller number of larger-scale RCTs. A number of methodological issues need addressing. Earlier studies are of lower quality, using smaller samples and lacking suitable control conditions. The vast majority of available studies have compared an active intervention with an usual treatment or wait-list control. These control groups allow for assessment of change due to passage of time, but they fail to match for the exposure and attention that intervention group participants receive, or, for example, in activity-based interventions, nonspecific exercise effects. When they have been used comparable active control groups often also show improvements of similar magnitude to the intervention conditions. This raises the strong suspicion that there is a lot of nonspecific activity which can generate improvements in outcomes but which is not necessarily tied to any one, or type of intervention. These methodological issues urgently need resolving. Future studies should compare active interventions with an equally active, control condition matched for duration of exposure. Allocation concealment and intention-to-treat analyses are also required.

Regarding the greater focus on yoga and mindfulness, this may be as much a reflection of fashion and popularity, as of effectiveness. There are many more teachers of yoga and mindfulness than of *Qi gong* in Western countries, where most of the psycho-oncology interventional research is carried out, and so this emphasis in the literature most probably simply reflects this practical fact. Chinese and Indian literatures are replete with small studies of yoga and Qigong effectiveness, but these tend to be small, poorly controlled, and hence open to risk of significant bias.

One great value of complementary interventions seems to lie in their integrated and gentle nature, and it is this that appeals to many patients. Moreover, the main practices reviewed above tend to be nontoxic and easily performed without specialist equipment. Nonetheless, there is a case for examining and identifying therapeutic components so that they can be combined in the most efficacious manner to optimize benefit.

7.5.2 Which Interventions?

With the foregoing methodological note in mind, the decision is about which, if any, of the complementary treatments reviewed to recommend clinically as a supplement or adjunct for the management of psychologically relevant symptoms. Most currently lack a robust evidence base. However, some studies have compared the relative evidence for different physical interventions (*Qigong*, *Taiji*, *asana*, meditation). One review of studies of these different interventions for the most intensively studied group, breast cancer patients, concluded that there was reasonably robust evidence of psychological benefit from yoga, particularly mindfulness-type interventions, but insufficient research to conclude if *Qigong*, *Taiji*, or Pilates are beneficial (Stan et al. 2012). However, a substantial systematic review by the Cochrane collaboration of a broad range of exercise-based interventions in cancer patients on active treatment ranging from walking through to *Qigong* and yoga concluded that benefits were seen with almost all activity-based interventions (Mishra et al. 2012a), and this suggests that at least some of the observed effects in non-controlled or no-treatment control studies can be attributed to exercise effects. One interesting finding from this study of 56 trials on 4,826 participants is that most psychological benefits (QoL, mood, fatigue, sleep, emotional well-being, social function) were greater for cancer survivors other than those with breast cancer, except regarding anxiety, where breast cancer patients benefitted more. More vigorous interventions were associated with greater benefits, suggesting a dose–response effect. However, the authors caution against the high risk of performance, selection, and attrition biases, in the reviewed studies. A comparable review by the same authors on studies of the impacts on HRQoL of activity-based interventions in cancer survivors (Mishra et al. 2012b) concluded that lower levels of depression, body image disturbance, and cancer-related concerns, sleep, pain, anxiety, and social functioning were present in interventions groups doing activity-based interventions. However, authors caution against heterogeneity of interventions and outcome measures and the smaller number of studies examining some outcomes.

Thus it would seem that there is good evidence that exercise activity-based interventions are associated with generalized improvements in both symptom profiles and psychosocial well-being. So the first line of action for the clinician seeking to facilitate the management of psychological and symptom distress may be to help a patient select a course of physical activity that best suits them: that may be gardening, for others brisk walking, whereas others may favor a yoga-style exercise program, or other combined Body-mind-spirit interventions. Graded activity of increasing intensity, particularly those that engage the attention, seems to be most effective and has both physical conditioning and psychological benefits improving fatigue, sleep quality, pain reporting, anorexia, stamina, as well as mood, anxiety, generalized emotional well-being, social functioning, and QoL. Many such interventions also provide a distraction from thoughts and worries about cancer.

Meditative interventions are probably beneficial, are harmless, and may help to build greater self-efficacy and acceptance, and this can improve well-being in cancer patients at all stages of the illness trajectory. There is a type of activity or meditation for almost everyone. Meditation may have unique benefits in terms of spiritual and existential well-being.

For patients unable to do physical activities, then meditative interventions such as mindfulness-based approaches seem to be most likely to offer benefit. Some may benefit specific symptom difficulties. There is some evidence that pranayama techniques can improve respiratory function for those unable to perform normal activity-based interventions and with breathing difficulties (Cebrià et al. 2014), and nausea may be helped by acupuncture, though the evidence base remains weak (Ezzo et al. 2011). Again, however, it might be most effective to encourage or collaborate with the patient to identify an approach that suits their values and expectations. Many of the published studies of interventions have used either self-selected patients or have high dropout rates, and this suggests that matching the patients to the right intervention is critical to their adherence, consistent with evidence from treatment decision-making (TDM) studies where patients report greatest satisfaction when their actual level of TDM involvement matches that of their preferred involvement (Lam and Fielding 2003). Finally, consider recommending supplementing activity-based interventions with pro-social activities aimed at assisting or benefitting others (voluntary work), which has increasingly good evidence for comprehensive benefit to psychological and physical well-being and can be added to recommendations to assist patients who do not have jobs, households, or dependent family to fill their time.

References

Ando M, Morita T, Akechi T, et al. The efficacy of mindfulness-based meditation therapy on anxiety, depression, and spirituality in Japanese patients with cancer. J Palliat Med. 2009; 12(12):1091–4. doi:10.1089/jpm.2009.0143.

Azad A, John T. Do randomized acupuncture studies in patients with cancer need a sham acupuncture control arm? J Clin Oncol. 2013;31(16):2057–8.

Banasik J, Williams H, Haberman M, et al. Effect of Iyengar yoga practice on fatigue and diurnal salivary cortisol concentration in breast cancer survivors. J Am Acad Nurse Pract. 2011;23(3): 135–42. doi:10.1111/j.1745-7599.2010.00573.x.

Bankar MA, Chaudhari SK, Chaudhari KD. Impact of long term Yoga practice on sleep quality and quality of life in the elderly. J Ayurveda Integr Med. 2013;4(1):28–32. doi:10.4103/0975-9476.109548.

Bansal R, Gupta M, Agarwal B, et al. Impact of short term yoga intervention on mental well being of medical students posted in community medicine: a pilot study. Indian J Community Med. 2013;38(2):105–8. doi:10.4103/0970-0218.112445.

Blackburn IM, Bishop S, Glen AIM, Whalley MJ, Christie JA. The efficacy of cognitive therapy in depression: a treatment trial using cognitive therapy and pharmacotherapy, each alone and in combination. Br J Psychiatry. 1981;139:181–9.

Boehm K, Ostermann T, Milazzo S, et al. Effects of yoga interventions on fatigue: a meta-analysis. Evid Based Complement Alternat Med. 2012;2012:124703.

Bonanno G, Westphal M, Mancini AD. Resilience to loss and potential trauma. Annu Rev Clin Psychol. 2011;7:511–35.

Bower JE, Garet D, Sternlieb B, et al. Yoga for persistent fatigue in breast cancer survivors: a randomized controlled trial. Cancer. 2012;118(15):3766–75. doi:10.1002/cncr.26702.

Boyes AW, Girgis A, D'Este CA, et al. Prevalence and predictors of the short-term trajectory of anxiety and depression in the first year after a cancer diagnosis: a population-based longitudinal study. J Clin Oncol. 2013;31(21):2724–9. doi:10.1200/JCO.2012.44.7540.

Breivik H, Cherny N, Collett B, et al. Cancer-related pain: a pan-European survey of prevalence, treatment, and patient attitudes. Ann Oncol. 2009;20(8):1420–33.

Brintzenhofe-Szoc KM, Levin TT, Li Y, et al. Mixed anxiety/depression symptoms in a large cancer cohort: prevalence by cancer type. Psychosomatics. 2009;50(4):383–91. doi:10.1176/appi.psy.50.4.383.

Brown SL, Nesse RM, Vinokur AD, et al. Providing social support may be more beneficial than receiving it results from a prospective study of mortality. Psychol Sci. 2003;14(4):320–7.

Buffart LM, van Uffelen JG, Riphagen II, et al. Physical and psychosocial benefits of yoga in cancer patients and survivors, a systematic review and meta-analysis of randomized controlled trials. BMC Cancer. 2012;27(12):559. doi:10.1186/1471-2407-12-559.

Carlson LE. Meditation and yoga. In: Holland JC, Breitbart WS, Jacobson PB, et al., editors. Psycho-Oncology. 2nd ed. New York, NY: Oxford University Press; 2010. p. 429–39.

Carlson LE, Doll R, Stephen J, et al. Randomized controlled trial of mindfulness-based cancer recovery versus supportive expressive group therapy for distressed survivors of breast cancer (MINDSET). J Clin Oncol. 2013;31(25):3119–26.

Cardoso R, De Souza E, Camano L, et al. Meditation in health: an operational definition. Brain Res Brain Res Protoc. 2004;14(1):58–60.

Cebrià I, Iranzo MD, Arnall DA, Igual Camacho C, et al. Effects of inspiratory muscle training and yoga breathing exercises on respiratory muscle function in institutionalized frail older adults: a randomized controlled trial. J Geriatr Phys Ther. 2014;37(2):65–75.

Chen FP, Jong MS, Chen YC, et al. Prescriptions of Chinese herbal medicines for insomnia in Taiwan during 2002. Evid Based Complement Alternat Med. 2011;2011:236341. doi:10.1093/ecam/nep018.

Chen K, Yeung R. Exploratory Studies of Qigong Therapy for Cancer in China. Integr Cancer Ther. 2002;1(4):345–70.

Chen XJ, Liu GQ, He BH. The study on the inhibition effect of Taiji five-element Qigong on liver cancer cells growth in mice [in Chinese]. Chin Qigong Sci. 1997;6:8–9.

Chow WH, Chang P, Lee SC, et al. Complementary and alternative medicine among Singapore cancer patients. Ann Acad Med Singapore. 2010;39(2):129–35.

Culos-Reed SN, Mackenzie MJ, Sohl SJ, et al. Yoga & cancer interventions: a review of the clinical significance of patient reported outcomes for cancer survivors. Evid Based Complement Alternat Med. 2012;2012:642576. doi:10.1155/2012/642576. Epub 2012 Oct 17.

Cramer H, Lange S, Klose P, et al. Can yoga improve fatigue in breast cancer patients? A systematic review. Acta Oncol. 2012;51(5):559–60.

Deshields T, Tibbs T, Fan M, et al. Differences in patterns of depression after treatment for breast cancer. Psycho-Oncology. 2006;15:398–406.

Desai K, Mao JJ, Su I, et al. Prevalence and risk factors for insomnia among breast cancer patients on aromatase inhibitors. Support Care Cancer. 2013;21(1):43–51. doi:10.1007/s00520-012-1490-z.

Dhruva A, Miaskowski C, Abrams D, et al. Yoga breathing for cancer chemotherapy-associated symptoms and quality of life: results of a pilot randomized controlled trial. J Altern Complement Med. 2012;18(5):473–9. doi:10.1089/acm.2011.0555.

Doneskey-Cuenco D, Nguyen HQ, Paul S, et al. Yoga therapy decreases dyspnea-related distress and improves functional performance in people with chronic obstructive pulmonary disease: a pilot study. J Altern Complement Med. 2009;15(3):225–34. doi:10.1089/acm.2008.0389.

Dong JP, Wang S, Sun WY, et al. Randomized controlled observation on head point-through-point therapy for treatment of insomnia. Zhongguo Zhen Jiu. 2008;28(3):159–62 [in Chinese].

D'Silva S, Poscablo C, Habousha R, et al. Mind-body medicine therapies for a range of depression severity: a systematic review. Psychosomatics. 2012;53(5):407–23. doi:10.1016/j.psym.2012.04.006.

Dunn BR, Hartigan JA, Mikulas WL. Concentration and mindfulness meditations: unique forms of consciousness? Appl Psychophysiol Biofeedback. 1999;24(3):147–65.

Enblom A, Johnsson A, Hammar M, et al. Acupuncture compared with placebo acupuncture in radiotherapy-induced nausea–a randomized controlled study. Ann Oncol. 2012;23(5):1353–61. doi:10.1093/annonc/mdr402.

Eom A. Effects of a tai chi program for early mastectomy patients. Korean J Women Health Nurs. 2007;13:43–50.

Ezzo J, Richardson MA, Vickers A et al. Acupuncture-point stimulation for chemotherapy-induced nausea or vomiting. Cochrane Collab. 2011; (3): 1–29

Feng Y, Wang XY, Li SD, et al. Clinical research of acupuncture on malignant tumor patients for improving depression and sleep quality. J Tradit Chin Med. 2011;31(3):199–202.

Gansler T, Kaw C, Crammer C, et al. A population-based study of prevalence of complementary methods use by cancer survivors: a report from the American Cancer Society's studies of cancer survivors. Cancer. 2008;113(5):1048–57. doi:10.1002/cncr.23659.

Harder H, Parlour L, Jenkins V. Randomised controlled trials of yoga interventions for women with breast cancer: a systematic literature review. Support Care Cancer. 2012;20(12):3055–64. doi:10.1007/s00520-012-1611-8.

He B, Chen K. Qigong analysis. Integr Can Care. 2002;1(2):200–2.

Helgeson VS, Snyder P, Seltman H. Psychological and physical adjustment to breast cancer over 4 years: identifying distinct trajectories of change. Health Psychol. 2004;23:3–15.

Henselmans I, Helgeson VS, Seltman H, et al. Identification and prediction of distress trajectories in the first year after a breast cancer diagnosis. Health Psychol. 2010;29:160–8.

Hofmann SG, Sawyer AT, Witt AA, et al. The effect of mindfulness-based therapy on anxiety and depression: A meta-analytic review. J Consult Clin Psychol. 2010;78(2):169–83.

Hölzel BK, Carmody J, Vangel M, et al. Mindfulness practice leads to increases in regional brain gray matter density. Psychiat Res: Neuroimaging. 2011;191(1):36–43.

Huang NQ. Influnce of Guo-Lin Qigong on the lung function microcirculation in cancer. Chin J Som Sci. 1996;6(2):51–4 [In Chinese].

Hussain D, Bhushan B. Psychology of meditation and health: present status and future directions. Int J Psychol Psychol Ther. 2010;10(3):439–51.

Iyengar BKS. Light on yoga: The bible of modern yoga – its philosophy and practice. New York: Schocken Books, Inc.; 1979.

Jim HSL, Jacobson PB, Phillips KM, et al. Lagged relationships among sleep disturbance, fatigue and depressed mood during chemotherapy. Health Psychol. 2013;32:768–74.

Jimenez PJ, Melendez A, Albers U. Psychological effects of Tai Chi Chuan. Arch Gerontol Geriatr. 2012;55:460–7.

Johnson W, Kreuger RF. The psychological benefits of vigorous exercise: a study of discordant MZ twin pairs. Twin Res Hum Genet. 2007;2:275–83.

Jones BM. Changes in cytokine production in healthy subjects practicing Guolin Qigong: a pilot study. BMC Complement Altern Med. 2001;1:8.

Kabat-Zinn J. An outpatient program in behavioral medicine for chronic pain patients based on the practice of mindfulness meditation: theoretical considerations and preliminary results. Gen Hosp Psychiatr. 1982;4:33–47.

Kabat-Zinn J. Mindfulness-based interventions in context: past, present, and future. Clin Psychol: Sci Pract. 2003;10(2):144–56.

Karst M, Winterhalter M, Munte S, et al. Auricular acupuncture for dental anxiety: a randomized controlled trial. Anaesth Analg. 2007;104:295–300.

Konkimalla VB, Efferth T. Evidence-based Chinese medicine for cancer therapy. J Ethnopharmacol. 2008;116(2):207–10.

Lam WWT, Fielding R. The evolving experience of illness for Chinese women with breast cancer: A qualitative study. Psycho-Oncology. 2003;12:127–40.

Lam WWT, Chan M, Hung WK, et al. Resilience to distress among Chinese women diagnosed with breast cancer. Psycho-Oncology. 2010;19:1044–51.

Lam WWT, Yee TS, Bonanno GA, et al. Distress trajectories during the first year following diagnosis of breast cancer in relation to 6-years survivorship. Psycho-Oncology. 2011;21:90–9.

Lam WWT, Li WWY, Bonanno GA, et al. Trajectories of body image and sexuality during the first year following diagnosis of breast cancer and their relationship to 6 years psychosocial outcomes. Breast Cancer Res Treat. 2012a;131:957–67.

Lam WWT, Ye M, Fielding R. Trajectories of quality of life among Chinese patients diagnosed with nasopharyngeal cancer. PLoS One. 2012b;7(9):e44022.

Lam WWT, Soong I, Yau TK, et al. The evolution of psychological distress trajectories in women diagnosed with advanced breast cancer: a longitudinal study. Psychooncology. 2013;22(12): 2831–9.

Ledesma D, Kumano H. Mindfulness-based stress reduction and cancer: A meta-analysis. Psychooncology. 2008;18:571–9.

Lee MS, Lee MS, Kim HJ, et al. Qigong reduced blood pressure and catecholamine levels of patients with essential hypertension. Int J Neurosci. 2003;113:1691–701.

Lee MS, Jang HS. Two case reports of the acute effects of Qi therapy (external Qigong) on symptoms of cancer: short report. Complement Ther Clin Pract. 2005;11:211–3.

Lee MS, Pittler MH, Ernst E. Is Tai chi an effective adjunct in cancer care? A systematic review of controlled clinical trials. Support Care Cancer. 2007;15:597–601.

Lee MS, Choi TY, Ernst E. Tai chi for breast cancer patients: a systematic review. Breast Cancer Res Treat. 2010;120:309–16.

Lengacher CA, Reich RR, Post-White J, et al. Mindfulness based stress reduction in post-treatment breast cancer patients: an examination of symptoms and symptom clusters. J Behav Med. 2012;35(1):86–94. doi:10.1007/s10865-011-9346-4.

Leung JP. Emotions and mental health in Chinese people. J Ch Fam Stud. 1998;7(2):115–28.

Levine AS, Balk JL. Yoga and quality-of-life improvement in patients with breast cancer: a literature review. International journal of yoga therapy. 2012;22(1):95–100.

Linden W, Vodermaier A, Mackenzie R, et al. Anxiety and depression after cancer diagnosis: prevalence rates by cancer type, gender, and age. J Affect Disord. 2012;141(2–3):343–51. doi:10.1016/j.jad.2012.03.025.

Liu Z, Lian Z, Zhou W, et al. National survey on prevalence of cancer pain. Chin Med Sci J. 2001;16(3):175–8.

Madsen MV, Gøtzsche PC, Hróbjartsson A. Acupuncture treatment for pain: systematic review of randomised clinical trials with acupuncture, placebo acupuncture, and no acupuncture groups. BMJ. 2009;338:a3115. doi:10.1136/bmj.a3115.

Manocha R. Why meditation? Aust Fam Physician. 2000;29(12):1135–8.

Mansky P, Sanners T, Wallerstedt D, et al. Tai Chi Chuan: mind-body practice or exercise intervention? Studying the benefit for cancer survivors. Integr Cancer Ther. 2006;5:192–201.

Mishra SI, Scherer RW, Snyder C, et al. Exercise interventions on health-related quality of life for people with cancer during active treatment. Cochrane Database Syst Rev. 2012a;8, CD008465. doi:10.1002/14651858.CD008465.pub2.

Mishra SI, Scherer RW, Geigle PM, et al. Exercise interventions on health-related quality of life for cancer survivors. Cochrane Database Syst Rev. 2012b;8, CD007566. doi:10.1002/14651858.CD007566.pub2.

Mitchell AJ, Ferguson DW, Gill J, et al. Depression and anxiety in long-term cancer survivors compared with spouses and healthy controls: a systematic review and meta-analysis. Lancet Oncol. 2013;14(8):721–32. Published online June 5, http://dx.doi.org/10.1016/S1470-2045(13)70244-4.

Molassiotis A, Bardy J, Finnegan-John J, et al. Acupuncture for cancer related fatigue in patients with breast cancer: A pragmatic randomized controlled trial. J Clin Oncol. 2012;30:4470–6.

Molassiotis A, Sylt P, Diggins H. The management of cancer-related fatigue after chemotherapy with acupuncture and acupressure: A randomized controlled trial. Complement Ther Med. 2007;15:228–37.

Monti DA, Kash KM, Kunkel EJ, et al. Psychosocial benefits of a novel mindfulness intervention versus standard support in distressed women with breast cancer. Psychooncology. 2013;22(11):2565–75. doi:10.1002/pon.3320.

Musick M, Herzog AR, House JS. Volunteering and mortality among older adults: findings from a national sample. J Gerontol Ser B: Psychol Sci Soc Sci. 1999;54(3):S173–80.

Musick M, Wilson J. Volunteering and depression: The role of psychological and social resources in different age groups. Soc Sci Med. 2003;56(2):259–69.

Mustian KM, Roscoe JA, Katula JA, et al. Tai Chi Chuan, health-related quality of life and self-esteem: a randomized trial with breast cancer survivors. Support Care Cancer. 2004;12:871–6.

Ndao DH, Ladas EJ, Bao Y, et al. Use of complementary and alternative medicine among children, adolescent, and young adult cancer survivors: a survey study. J Pediatr Hematol Oncol. 2013;35(4):281–8. doi:10.1097/MPH.0b013e318290c5d6.

Nidich SI, Fields JZ, Rainforth MV, et al. A randomized controlled trial of the effects of transcendental meditation on quality of life in older breast cancer patients. Integr Cancer Ther. 2009;8(3):228–34.

Ospina MB, Bond TK, Karkhaneh M et al. Meditation practices for health: state of the research. Rockville, MD: Agency for Healthcare Research and Quality; Evidence Report/Technology Assessment No. 155; 2007

Paltiel O, Avitzour M, Peretz T, et al. Determinants of the use of complementary therapies by patients with cancer. J Clin Oncol. 2001;19(9):2439–48.

Pilkington K, Kirkwood G, Rampes H, et al. Acupuncture for anxiety and anxiety disorders–a systematic literature review. Acupunct Med. 2007;25(1–2):1–10.

Posadzki P, Moon TW, Choi TY, et al. Acupuncture for cancer-related fatigue: a systematic review of randomized clinical trials. Support Care Cancer. 2013;21(7):2067–73.

Qu SS, Huang Y, Zhang ZJ, et al. A 6-week randomized controlled trial with 4-week follow-up of acupuncture combined with paroxetine in patients with major depressive disorder. J Psychiatr Res. 2013;47(6):726–32.

Sadja J, Mills PJ. Effects of yoga interventions on fatigue in cancer patients and survivors: a systematic review of randomized controlled trials. Explore (NY). 2013;9(4):232–43.

Sancier KM. Medical applications of qigong. Altern Ther Health Med. 1996;2:40–6.

Savard J, Villa J, Ivers H, et al. Prevalence, natural course, and risk factors of insomnia comorbid with cancer over a 2-month period. J Clin Oncol. 2009;27(31):5233–9. doi:10.1200/JCO.2008.21.6333.

Seoung MY. Effect of tai chi exercise program on physical functioning and psychological problems of breast cancer patients after surgery. MS thesis, Department of Nursing, Chungnam National University, Daejeon; 2008

Shah D. Healthy worker effect phenomenon. Indian J Occup Environ Med. 2009;13(2):77–9. doi:10.4103/0019-5278.55123.

Singendonk M, Kaspers GJ, Naafs-Wilstra M, et al. High prevalence of complementary and alternative medicine use in the Dutch pediatric oncology population: a multicenter survey. Eur J Pediatr. 2013;172(1):31–7. doi:10.1007/s00431-012-1821-6.

Smith C, Crowther C, Beilby J. Acupuncture to treat nausea and vomiting in early pregnancy: a randomized controlled trial. Birth. 2002;29(1):1–9.

Spahn G, Choi KE, Kennemann C, et al. Can a multimodal mind-body program enhance the treatment effects of physical activity in breast cancer survivors with chronic tumor-associated fatigue? A randomized controlled trial. Integr Cancer Ther. 2013;12(4):291–300. doi:10.1177/1534735413492727.

Stan DL, Collins NM, Olsen MM, et al. The evolution of mindfulness-based physical interventions in breast cancer survivors. Evid Based Complement Alternat Med. 2012;2012:758641.

Streeter CC, Jensen JE, Perlmutter RM, et al. Yoga Asana sessions increase brain GABA levels: a pilot study. J Altern Complement Med. 2007;13(4):419–26.

Szabo A. Acute psychological benefits of exercise performed at self-selected workloads: Implications for theory and practice. J Sports Sci Med. 2003;2:77–87.

Tacón AM. Meditation as a complementary therapy in cancer. Fam Community Health. 2003; 26(1):64–73.

Takahashi T, Murata T, Hamada T, et al. Changes in EEG and autonomic nervous activity during meditation and their association with personality traits. Int J Psychophysiol. 2005;55(2): 199–207.

Tas F, Ustuner Z, Can G, et al. The prevalence and determinants of the use of complementary and alternative medicine in adult Turkish cancer patients. Acta Oncol. 2005;44(2):161–7.

Taylor-Piliae RE, Haskell WL, Waters CM, et al. Change in perceived psychosocial status following a 12-week Tai Chi exercise programme. J Adv Nurs. 2006;54:313–29.

Thoits PA, Hewitt LN. Volunteer work and well-being. J Health Soc Behav. 2001;42(2):115–31.

Tomlinson D, Hesser T, Ethier MC, et al. Complementary and alternative medicine use in pediatric cancer reported during palliative phase of disease. Support Care Cancer. 2011;19(11):1857–63. doi:10.1007/s00520-010-1029-0.

Travis F. Autonomic and EEG patterns distinguish transcending from other experiences during transcendental meditation practice. Int J Psychophysiol. 2001;42(1):1–9.

Van Balkom AJLM, Bakker A, Spinhoeven P. A meta-analysis of the treatment of panic disorder with or without agoraphobia: a comparison of psychopharmacological, cognitive-behavioral, and combination treatments. J Nerv Mental Dis. 1997;185:510–6.

Van den Beuken-van Everdingen MHJ, De Rijke JM, Kessels AG, et al. Prevalence of pain in patients with cancer: a systematic review of the past 40 years. Ann Oncol. 2007;18(9): 1437–49.

Van Puymbroeck M, Payne LL, Hsieh PC. A phase I feasibility study of yoga on the physical health and coping of informal caregivers. Evid Based Complement Alternat Med. 2007;4(4): 519–29. doi:10.1093/ecam/nem075.

Van Haselen R, Jütte R. The placebo effect and its ramifications for clinical practice and research. Villa La Collina at Lake Como, Italy, 4–6 May 2012. Complement Ther Med. 2013;21(2): 85–93. doi:10.1016/j.ctim.2012.11.005.

Van Willigen M. Differential Benefits of Volunteering Across the Life Course. J Gerontol B Psychol Sci Soc Sci. 2000;55(5):S308–18. doi:10.1093/geronb/55.5.S308.

Walsh R, Shapiro SL. The meeting of meditative disciplines and Western psychology: a mutually enriching dialogue. Am Psychol. 2006;61(3):227–39.

Wang WC, Zhang AL, Rasmussen B, et al. The effect of Tai Chi on psychosocial well-being: a systematic review of randomized controlled trials. J Acupunct Meridian Stud. 2009;2:171–81.

Wang SM, Peloquin C, Kain ZN. The use of auricular acupuncture to reduce anxiety. Anaesth Analg. 2001;93:1178–80.

Wong WS, Fielding R. The co-morbidity of chronic pain, insomnia, and fatigue in the general adult population of Hong Kong: prevalence and associated factors. J Psychosomatic Res. 2012;73(1):28–34. doi:10.1016/j.jpsychores.2012.04.011.

Wang Y, Fan R, Huang X. Meta-analysis of the clinical effectiveness of traditional Chinese medicine formula Chaihu-Shugan-San in depression. J Ethnopharmacol. 2012;141(2):571–7.

Xu L, Lao LX, Ge A, et al. Chinese herbal medicine for cancer pain. Integr Cancer Ther. 2007; 6(3):208–34.

Yan X, Shen H, Jiang HJ, et al. External Qi of Yan Xin Qigong differentially regulates the Akt and extracellular signal-regulated kinase pathways and is cytotoxic to cancer cells but not to normal cells. Int J Biochem Cell Biol. 2006;38:2102–13.

Yeung WF, Chung KF, Man-Ki Poon N, et al. Chinese herbal medicine for insomnia: a systematic review of randomized controlled trials. Sleep Med Rev. 2012;16(6):497–507.

Yu T, Tsai HL, Hwang ML. Suppressing tumor progression of in vitro prostate cancer cells by emitted psychosomatic power through Zen meditation. Am J Chin Med. 2003;31(03):499–507.

Zhang T, Ma SL, Xie GR, et al. Clinical research on nourishing yin and unblocking meridians recipe combined with opioid analgesics in cancer pain management. Chin J Integr Med. 2006; 12(3):180–4.

Zhang AL, Changli Xue C, Fong HHS. Integration of herbal medicine into evidence-based clinical practice: current status and issues. In: Benzie IFF, Wachtel-Galor S, editors. Herbal medicine: biomolecular and clinical aspects. 2nd ed. Boca Raton (FL): CRC Press; 2011. Chapter 22.

Zhang J, Yang KH, Tian JH, et al. Effects of yoga on psychologic function and quality of life in women with breast cancer: a meta-analysis of randomized controlled trials. J Altern Complement Med. 2012;18(11):994–1002. doi:10.1089/acm.2011.0514.

Part II

Psychotropic Drug Use in Clinical Oncology and Palliative Care Settings

Treatment of Anxiety and Stress-Related Disorders

Ken Shimizu, Kazuhiro Yoshiuchi, and Hideki Onishi

Abstract

In the majority of patients, anxiety is an adaptive reaction, promoting appropriate attitudes toward treatment, but sometimes anxiety persists beyond a certain level, involving distress and negative influences. Among the diagnostic criterion, "Anxiety Disorders" and "Trauma- and Stressor-Related Disorders" of DSM-5, previous studies reported about 15 % of cancer patients were affected with Adjustment Disorder, and small percent of patients were with more severe and chronic psychopathology such as Panic Disorder, Posttraumatic Stress Disorder (PTSD), and so on. In pharmacotherapy for anxiety, antidepressants, benzodiazepine-, and non-benzodiazepine-class, antianxiety drugs are generally used. Adverse events and drug interactions can easily occur, and it is important to know the profile of each drug, which could reduce the possibility of adverse events and provide favorable effects on specific physical symptoms.

K. Shimizu (✉)
Psycho-oncology Division, National Cancer Center Hospital, 5-1-1 Tsukiji, Chuou-ku, Tokyo, Japan
e-mail: keshimiz@ncc.go.jp

K. Yoshiuchi
Department of Stress Sciences and Psychosomatic Medicine, Graduate School of Medicine, The University of Tokyo, 7-3-1 Hongo, Bunkyo-ku, Tokyo, Japan
e-mail: kyoshiuc-tky@umin.ac.jp

H. Onishi
Department of Psycho-Oncology, Saitama Medical University International Medical Center, 1397-1 Yamane, Hidaka City, Saitama 350-1298, Japan
e-mail: honishi@saitama-med.ac.jp

L. Grassi and M. Riba (eds.), *Psychopharmacology in Oncology and Palliative Care*,   129
DOI 10.1007/978-3-642-40134-3_8, © Springer-Verlag Berlin Heidelberg 2014

8.1   Introduction

Anxiety is a general term for uncomfortable emotional phenomena due to being threatened by future uncertainties, categorized into two aspects: psychological and physical. While psychological anxiety refers to unpleasant emotions which are frequently expressed as "worried," "scared," "need help," and "want to escape," it should be noted that the feelings and manifestations of psychological anxiety vary among individuals. On the other hand, physical anxiety refers to autonomic symptoms, involving diverse physical conditions, including: palpitation; a feeling of breathing difficulty; chest tightness; perspiration; dry mouth; tremors in extremities; diarrhea; frequent urination; and pupillary dilatation. Although fear is considered a similar psychiatric symptom, it has traditionally been differentiated from anxiety in respect of known and clearly limited causes of the threat. However, in current psychiatric settings, the terms "anxiety," "fear," "worry," and "concern" are regarded as almost compatible with each other; for example, in the nosological classification phobias are usually included in the category of anxiety disorder despite the presence of clear causes (House and Stark 2002).

The presence of cancer is a life-threatening condition, and anxiety is very common among cancer patients. It is observed throughout the course of the disease, from diagnosis and treatment to recurrence and withdrawal from active treatment. In addition to threat of death, patients have various concerns such as physical discomforts, bodily dysfunction, alteration in appearance, changes in social role, and so on. During the initial cancer notification, patients receive diverse information, including: the stage of cancer; possibility of complete healing; treatment goals; treatment options, such as chemotherapy, surgical procedures, and radiotherapy, and their side effects; and the necessity of hospitalization, in addition to the development of cancer. Anxiety is triggered by such overwhelming information (Stark and House 2000).

In the majority of patients, anxiety is an adaptive reaction, promoting appropriate attitudes toward treatment. In some cases, however, anxiety persists beyond a certain level, involving distress and negative influences. In previous studies, excessive anxiety was reported to interfere with normal functions, lead to inappropriate treatment options (Latini et al. 2007), involve severe, subjective physical symptoms (Andrykowski 1990), and be associated with a decrease in the general QOL on some occasions (Brown et al. 2010).

8.2   Pathophysiology of Anxiety

While the neurophysiological mechanism of anxiety has not yet been fully clarified, it has been suggested that noradrenergic and serotonergic nerve activity in the brain may be excessive in patients with anxiety, as shown in Fig. 8.1. Noradrenergic nerve cell bodies are mainly located in the locus coeruleus above the pons, and the majority of those activated by serotonin are observed in the raphe nucleus. It has been reported that anxiety as a type of emotion occurs in a network created through

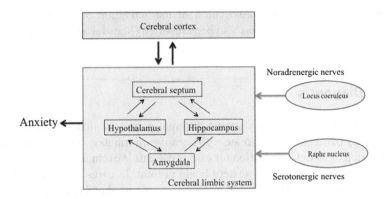

Fig. 8.1 Mechanism of anxiety

neural connections between noradrenergic and serotonergic nerves and a region called the limbic system, consisting of the hypothalamus, amygdala, nucleus, and hippocampus. A number of reports have pointed out that the morphological characteristics of the hippocampus and amygdala are associated with anxiety disorder. In line with this, there may be noradrenergic and serotonergic nervous input in this network, or the network itself may be created by these monoamine nerves (Tanaka et al. 2000).

In patients with anxiety disorder, the association of norepinephrine has been suggested in relation to unstable noradrenaline regulation and the frequent occurrence of severe panic attacks in those with panic disorder after the administration of β-adrenergic antagonists, such as isoproterenol (Pohl et al. 1988), and α2-adrenergic antagonists, such as yohimbine (Vasa et al. 2009). Clonidine as an α2-adrenergic drug is known to reduce anxiety symptoms (Hood et al. 2011). Furthermore, decreased norepinephrine metabolites in the cerebrospinal fluid and urine have been reported in patients with anxiety disorder (Geracioti et al. 2008).

The hypothesis that serotonergic nerves are associated with the occurrence of anxiety is based on the results of studies in the field of basic medicine, suggesting that the activation of serotonergic nerves with stress as stimulation induces anxiety (Blazevic et al. 2012), while the suppression of serotonergic nervous activity by stimulating serotonergic proprioceptors (5-HT1A receptors) creates antianxiety effects (Yamaguchi et al. 2012). These results also suggested an association with subtypes of serotonin receptors in human genes (Munafo et al. 2005), in addition to the therapeutic effects of clomipramine as a serotonergic antidepressant in some types of anxiety disorder, such as obsessive–compulsive and panic disorders (Bakker et al. 1999). The association between serotonin and anxiety has also been suggested in other previous studies, reporting the effectiveness of 5-HT1A receptor agonists, such as buspirone and tandospirone, to treat anxiety disorder (Jacobson et al. 1985).

Furthermore, it is widely known that γ-aminobutyric acid (GABA) is associated with anxiety disorder, based on the therapeutic effects of benzodiazepines

(Stephens et al. 1987). The association of the activation of the hypothalamic-pituitary-adrenal (HPA) axis has also been reported (Matsuoka et al. 2003; Nakano et al. 2002).

8.3   Diagnosis

The symptoms of anxiety vary among different periods of time even in the same patient; they particularly deteriorate with negative information. The important point and first step of anxiety evaluation for cancer patients is excluding the possibility of organic or substance-induced anxiety being present. In cases involving cognitive dysfunction, patients' unbelievable remarks, or patients showing different psychological reactions from those previously presented, the presence of organic or substance-induced anxiety should be actively suspected. Once the possibility of organic or substance-induced anxiety is ruled out, it is possible to diagnose patients showing severe anxiety with one of the several categories in which anxiety can be present and that, in oncology and palliative care settings, involve, according to the DSM5, anxiety disorder or trauma and stressor-related disorders.

8.4   Prevalence of Anxiety and Related Factors

In previous studies, the prevalence of anxiety symptoms widely varied: 6–49 % (Kissane et al. 2004; Stark et al. 2002; Salvo et al. 2012). It depends on whether the adopted evaluation method is self-administered, such as the Hospital Anxiety and Depression Scale (HADS), or structured interview-based. For example, one study examining anxiety symptoms using the HADS anxiety with a cutoff of more than seven reported that anxiety was present in 49 % of the patients with lung cancer (Stark et al. 2002). On the other hand, those evaluating anxiety in patients with advanced cancer in different stages using the Edmonton Symptom Assessment System (ESAS) reported that anxiety was observed in 37 % (Salvo et al. 2012). Another study reported the trajectory of anxiety and point prevalence assessed by HADS was 22 % at 6 months and 21 % at 1 year, after diagnosis (Boyes et al. 2013). Considering that a tendency to overdiagnose common anxiety has been pointed out, the results of questionnaire surveys should be carefully discussed (Hall et al. 1999).

The prevalence of anxiety has also been examined by performing meta-analysis, based on the DSM or International Classification of Disease (ICD), in the following two settings: (1) palliative care and (2) oncological and hematological. In such studies, the prevalence of adjustment disorder was 15.4 % in palliative care and 19.4 % in oncological and hematological settings. Similarly, those of anxiety disorder were 9.8 and 10.3 %, respectively, suggesting that the prevalence of these disorders may not markedly vary between palliative care and oncological and hematological settings (Mitchell et al. 2011).

In a hypothesis, factors associated with the occurrence of anxiety are classified as follows: predisposing: such as anxiety disorder, personality traits, and social isolation; cancer-related: such as the severity of pathological conditions and physical activity levels; treatment-related: such as side effects, the invasion of the central nervous system, and circulatory and respiratory disturbance; and symptom burdens: such as malaise and a feeling of breathing difficulty (Traeger et al. 2012). On the other hand, in the case of anxiety, while it has been suggested that patients' recognition of its presence before coping with it may be associated with its persistence—whether the disease persists, involving long-term distress, or it is just a short-term problem, and heals early, empirical studies to comprehensively confirm such an association have not yet been sufficiently conducted. Amongst previous studies, a survey of mixed cancer patients examined the importance of sex, cancer site, and social support and showed that a female sex and low social support were associated with significant anxiety (Stark et al. 2002). Another study also examined the contribution of age, sex, cancer site, and physical symptoms, and a younger age, a female gender, nausea, drowsiness, dyspnea, and overall well-being remained as factors that were significantly associated with anxiety (Salvo et al. 2012). These exploratory studies analyzed the factors that were associated with anxiety, but a conceptual model explaining anxiety in cancer patients has not been fully established. Furthermore, in a study using a large database of lung cancer patients, developed by the authors of this chapter, the association between pathological anxiety exceeding the cutoff for the HADS-anxiety subscale and predisposing, cancer-, and treatment-related factors, as well as symptom burdens, was comprehensively examined (Nakaya et al. 2006). The results showed that personality traits, such as neurotic tendencies, and coping styles were closely associated, while cancer- and treatment-related factors and symptom burdens were less closely associated.

When analyzing the single data regarding anxiety in cancer settings, it is necessary however to distinguish the syndromes subsumed under the category of anxiety disorders with respect to those subsumed under the category of trauma- and stressor-related disorders.

8.5 Anxiety Disorders in Cancer Settings

Case

Mr. A was a 44-year-old man who was hospitalized to undergo chemotherapy for advanced lung cancer. He strongly worried about the progression of the disease and always has a feeling of breathing difficulty after being pointed out of the pleural effusion. Three days after his admission, he suddenly began screaming, "I am being strangled!! I am dying!!" He had concomitant symptoms of palpitation, sweating, sensations of shortness of breath, feeling of choking, and simultaneous fear of losing control, and his episodes met the criteria for panic attack.

8.5.1 Generalized Anxiety Disorder

In patients with generalized anxiety disorder, excessive and anticipatory anxiety about multiple events and activities persists for 6 months or more. In such cases, anxiety is difficult to control and involves symptoms such as uneasiness, frequent fatigue, difficulty concentrating, irritation, muscle tension, and sleep disorder. Patients who continually complain of concerns over cancer may be classified into this category; it is difficult for them to concentrate on relevant activities (APA 2000). In clinical environments, some patients temporarily present with generalized anxiety disorder, without meeting the criterion that the symptoms should persist for 6 months or more.

8.5.2 Panic Disorder

When panic attacks, involving a rapid pulse, *trepidatio cordis*, perspiration, tremors, and feelings of suffocation, suddenly and repeatedly occur over 1 month or more, leading to excessive anxiety about their relapse or behavioral changes, panic disorder is diagnosed. In some patients with panic disorder, avoidance of activities possibly causing an elevated heart rate or breathing difficulty is occasionally observed. The prevalence of panic disorder was reported as 3.0 % in advanced cancer patients (Spencer et al. 2010), and psychiatric physicians must often treat patients who have experienced clinically significant panic attacks in clinical oncology settings; such patients must receive immediate treatment, as marked fear could lead to a discontinuation of cancer treatment (Slaughter et al. 2000). Panic attacks can occur in the context of several medical conditions (e.g., cardiac, respiratory, vestibular, or gastrointestinal disorders), and certain types of cancer patients may be at risk for panic attacks. Panic attacks also occur in cancer patients, triggered by a feeling of breathing difficulty due to pleural effusion in those with lung cancer and zonesthesia in the cervical region in those with head and neck cancer (Shimizu et al. 2007).

8.5.3 Agoraphobia and Specific Phobias

This category refers to phobias of specific objects or situations or severe and persistent anticipatory fears. Anxiety is triggered as severe reactions, such as panic attacks, to such situations. Claustrophobia prevents some cancer patients from undergoing MRI examination.

8.5.4 Social Anxiety Disorder

Social anxiety disorder is caused by marked and persistent fears of social environments possibly leading to exposure to unknown people or situations forcing a person to act in front of others. Being exposed to such situations, anxiety as severe reactions, such as panic attacks, occurs. Prevalence of Social anxiety disorder in cancer patients was reported from 3 to 4.8 % (Kadan-Lottick et al. 2005; Spencer et al. 2010). Patients with social anxiety disorder may show severe anxiety when communicating with medical professionals.

8.6   Trauma- and Stressor-Related Disorders

Case
Ms. A was a 34-year-old woman with early stage breast cancer. She has a little bit nervous temperament by nature and was dumbstruck when she was informed having cancer. She had successfully underwent surgery, but she looked restless and uncomfortable as the discharge date nears. She strongly worried about recurrence of the disease, although the physician explained that very low rate of recurrence was estimated. She tended to interpret everyday bodily symptoms as indicative of recurrence, asked physician or nurses about the symptoms, and sought reassurances from them. She was referred to a psychiatrist and diagnosed as adjustment disorder.

8.6.1   Acute Stress Disorder

Acute stress disorder is diagnosed when symptoms, such as emotional paralysis, loss of reality, depersonalization, and dissociative amnesia, are observed for 2 days or more after exposure to traumatic events. In cancer patients, dissociative amnesia and emotional paralysis are occasionally observed immediately after cancer notification. Full-blown acute stress disorder may affect from 2.5 % to 25 % of cancer patients, with negative consequences in terms of elevated dissociative responses, trait anxiety, preoccupation with one's diagnosis, and a decline in cognitive functioning (Kangas et al. 2007; Mehnert and Koch 2007). Recent data in oncohematology indicate that about 15 % of patients with leukemia suffer from acute stress disorders and another 15 % from subsyndromal acute stress disorders (Rodin et al. 2013).

8.6.2   Posttraumatic Stress Disorder

According to the DSM5, Posttraumatic Stress Disorder (PTSD) is diagnosed when symptoms are observed for 1 month or more in the following four domains after exposure to traumatic events: intrusion and reexperiencing the event; persistent avoidance of related stimuli; negative thoughts and mood or feelings (e.g., detachment from other; exaggerated expectation about oneself); heightened arousal (e.g., persistent hyper vigilance). A bulk of data are available regarding the prevalence of

PTSD in cancer settings (Rustad et al. 2012). A recent large prospective study indicates a high prevalence of PTSD among breast cancer patients (23 % at the first interview, 12 % at 6-month follow-up) (Vin-Raviv et al. 2013). Subsyndromal PTSD is also highly prevalent among cancer patients (Gold et al. 2012), and acute stress disorder is a risk factor for later development of PTSD (Kangas et al. 2005). It is well known that these symptoms are observed for a long term in pediatric cancer survivors and their families (Landolt et al. 2012). Difficulty in revisiting the hospital where cancer was diagnosed or talking about cancer-related events with others is also observed on some occasions. Persistent hypervigilance occurring after traumatic events may involve mental uneasiness and persistent sleeplessness.

8.6.3 Adjustment Disorder Involving Anxiety

Adjustment disorder is a diagnosis that bridges normality and pathology and has an indefinite symptomatology and an essential place in psychiatric taxonomy. It enables clinicians to differentiate adjustment disorder from normal (non-pathological) distress or from more severe and chronic psychopathology such as PTSD.

Adjustment disorders are extremely common in oncology (Mitchell et al. 2011). Previous study indicates a high prevalence of adjustment disorder among recurrent breast cancer patients (35 %) (Okamura et al. 2000), hematologic cancer patients receiving stem cell transplantation (22.7 %) (Prieto et al. 2002), terminally ill cancer patients (19 %) (Akechi et al. 2004).

Normal adjustment to cancer can be defined as an ongoing process of trying to gain mastery or control over cancer-related events. (Schuyler 2004). On the other hand, in adjustment disorder, anxiety is a response to a stressor (i.e., cancer) occurred within 3 months; its severity is markedly higher than the stress level; it severely interferes with daily activities; and it involves severe distress. Such anxiety generally disappears within 6 months after the removal of stress factors; therefore, if anxiety symptoms persist for more than 6 months, the diagnosis should be changed to one of the anxiety spectrum disorders. On the other hand, if stressors are recurrent or continuous, as frequently it occurs in cancer, adjustment disorders can be persistent. It has been reported that the prognosis of adjustment disorder in cancer patients improves relatively early (Shimizu et al. 2011), but there are forms that, if not properly treated, can become chronic and change in more severe psychiatric disorders (Grassi et al. 2007).

8.7   Treatment

8.7.1 Non-pharmacotherapy

As shown in Table 8.1, the effect varied in previous studies, depending on the type and period of intervention (Traeger et al. 2012).

Table 8.1 Evidence-based recommendations by cancer treatment status for use of psychosocial interventions to prevent or reduce anxiety

Disease or treatment status	RCT evidence	Psychiatric study entry criteria	Evidence level[a]
Cognitive and cognitive behavioral interventions			
Newly diagnosed	Trask et al. (2003)	Psychological distress	II
Undergoing radiotherapy	Evans and Connis (1995)	–	II
Completion of treatment	Savard et al. (2005)	Insomnia	I
	Espie et al. (2008)	Insomnia	
	Dolbeault et al. (2009)	–	
Terminal phase of illness	Moorey et al. (2009)	Anxiety or depression	II
Mixed status	Telch and Telch (1986)	Psychosocial distress	I
	Greer et al. (1992)	–	
	Strong et al. (2008)	Depression	
Relaxation training			
Newly diagnosed	Bindemann et al. (1991)	–	II
Postsurgery	Petersen and Quinlivan (2002)	–	I
	Cheung et al. (2003)	–	
Prebrachytherapy	Leon-Pizarro et al. (2007)	–	II
Undergoing chemotherapy	Burish and Lyles (1981)	–	I
	Burish et al. (1987)	–	
	Arakawa (1997)	–	
	Jacobsen et al. (2002)	–	
Undergoing radiotherapy	Decker et al. (1992)	–	II
Completion of treatment	Elsesser et al. (1994)	–	II
	Hidderley and Holt (2004)	–	
Supportive counseling			
Newly diagnosed	White et al. (2012)	–	II
Undergoing radiotherapy	Evans and Connis (1995)	–	II
Metastatic disease	Spiegel et al. (1981)	–	II
Education			
Newly diagnosed	McQuellon et al. (1998)	–	I
	Thomas et al. (2000)	–	
	Katz et al. (2004)	–	

(continued)

Table 8.1 (continued)

Disease or treatment status	RCT evidence	Psychiatric study entry criteria	Evidence level[a]
Presurgery	Ali and Khalil (1989)	–	II
Undergoing chemotherapy	**Jacobs et al.** (1983)	–	**II**

Adapted from Traeger et al. (2012)
RCT randomized controlled trial
RCTs demonstrating significant anxiety reduction in the intervention group relative to control group
[a]Evidence level: I, multiple RCTs with adequate sample sizes; II, at least one RCT with adequate sample size

8.7.2   Pharmacotherapy (Table 8.2)

In pharmacotherapy for anxiety, antidepressants, benzodiazepine-, and non-benzo-diazepine-class antianxiety drugs are generally used. In cancer treatment, benzo-diazepines are frequently used to treat anxiety, such as panic attacks, nausea, and sleeplessness. However, it should be noted that benzodiazepine-class antianxiety drugs may cause malaise and decreased concentration or negatively affect alcohol abuse. In the elderly, it may also lead to paradoxical reactions. As anxiety is time-dependent and intermittent in general, the dose of benzodiazepines, administered to obtain early effects, should be carefully reduced (Traeger et al. 2012).

To treat anxiety for a long period of time, drugs with a different action are frequently more appropriate. In the treatment of PTSD, panic, generalized anxiety, and social anxiety disorders in the general population, selective serotonin (SSRIs) and serotonin-norepinephrine reuptake inhibitors (SNRIs) are considered as first-line drugs.

In oncology settings, adverse events and drug interactions can easily occur. Therefore, it is important to know the profile of each drug, which could reduce the possibility of adverse events and provide favorable effects on specific physical symptoms (see "Antidepressants"). For example, as SSRIs, such as fluoxetine, fluvoxamine, and paroxetine, may decrease the blood concentration of tamoxifen, other drugs, including sertraline, citalopram, escitalopram, and venlafaxine, should be considered. It has recently been pointed out that, when using citalopram in combination with drugs metabolized by CYP2CIP, such as omeprazole, a prolonged QT interval and arrhythmia may occur. In addition, considering their anticholinergic effects, tricyclic antidepressants (TCAs) should be carefully used in patients with constipation and disturbance of consciousness. The elderly have been reported to be generally vulnerable to the anticholinergic effect of TCAs and nausea due to SSRIs.

Among other drugs showing an antidepressant action, mirtazapine is also used to treat anxiety, particularly in patients with sleeplessness and appetite loss, in con-sideration of its sedative and weight-gaining actions. Otherwise, olanzapine and quetiapine (particularly in patients at a risk of delirium) as atypical antipsychotics and gabapentin, as an anticonvulsant, are also frequently used; however, the effects of antipsychotics and anticonvulsants to treat anxiety in cancer patients have not yet been systematically confirmed.

Table 8.2 Anxiety Outcomes of Pharmacologic Interventions in Adults With Cancer. Adapted from Traeger et al. (2012)

Medications	References	Psychiatric study entry criteria	Positive	Negative	Evidence level[a]
			Trials		
Anxiolytics					
Alprazolam	Holland et al. (1991)	Anxiety or depression	X		II
	Wald et al. (1993)	Anxiety		X	
Lorazepam	Clerico et al. (1993)	–	X		I
	Gonzalez Baron et al. (1991)	–	X		
Antidepressants					
Fluoxetine	Holland et al. (1998)	Depression	X		II
	Razavi et al. (1996)	Depression		X	
Paroxetine	Musselman et al. (2001)		X		II
	Musselman et al. (2006)	Depression		X	
Sertraline	Stockler et al. (2007)	Symptoms of anxiety, subthreshold depression, fatigue, or low energy		X	II
Desipramine	Holland et al. (1998)	Depression	X		II
	Musselman et al. (2006)	Depression		X	
Imipramine	Cankurtaran et al. (2008)	Anxiety or depression		X	III
Mirtazapine	Cankurtaran et al. (2008)	Anxiety or depression	X		III

RCT randomized controlled trial

[a]Evidence level: I, multiple RCTs with adequate sample sizes (preferably placebo controlled); II, at least one RCT with adequate sample size (preferably placebo controlled); III, nonrandomized controlled prospective studies, case series, or high-quality retrospective studies

Conclusion

In some cancer patients, anxiety persists beyond a certain level, involving distress and negative influences. Adjustment Disorder is the most prevalent diagnosis, and some patients were with more severe and chronic psychopathology such as Panic Disorder, PTSD, and so on. Although pharmacotherapy for anxiety is effective for cancer patients, adverse events and drug interactions can easily occur, and it is important to know the profile of each drug.

References

Akechi T, Okuyama T, Sugawara Y, Nakano T, Shima Y, Uchitomi Y. Major depression, adjustment disorders, and post-traumatic stress disorder in terminally ill cancer patients: associated and predictive factors. J Clin Oncol. 2004;22:1957–65.

Ali NS, Khalil HZ. Effect of psychoeducational intervention on anxiety among Egyptian bladder cancer patients. Cancer Nurs. 1989;12(4):236–42.

Andrykowski MA. The role of anxiety in the development of anticipatory nausea in cancer chemotherapy: a review and synthesis. Psychosom Med. 1990;52(4):458–75.

APA. Diagnostic and statistical manual of mental disorders. 4th ed. text revision. Washington, DC: American Psychiatric Press; 2000

Arakawa S. Relaxation to reduce nausea, vomiting, and anxiety induced by chemotherapy in Japanese patients. Cancer Nurs. 1997;20(5):342–9.

Bakker A, van Dyck R, Spinhoven P, van Balkom AJ. Paroxetine, clomipramine, and cognitive therapy in the treatment of panic disorder. J Clin Psychiatry. 1999;60(12):831–8.

Bindemann S, Soukop M, Kaye SB. Randomised controlled study of relaxation training. Eur J Cancer. 1991;27(2):170–4.

Blazevic S, Colic L, Culig L, Hranilovic D. Anxiety-like behavior and cognitive flexibility in adult rats perinatally exposed to increased serotonin concentrations. Behav Brain Res. 2012;230(1): 175–81.

Boyes AW, Girgis A, D'Este CA, Zucca AC, Lecathelinais C, Carey ML. Prevalence and predictors of the short-term trajectory of anxiety and depression in the first year after a cancer diagnosis: a population-based longitudinal study. J Clin Oncol. 2013;31:2724–9.

Brown LF, Kroenke K, Theobald DE, Wu J, Tu W. The association of depression and anxiety with health-related quality of life in cancer patients with depression and/or pain. Psychooncology. 2010;19(7):734–41.

Burish TG, Lyles JN. Effectiveness of relaxation training in reducing adverse reactions to cancer chemotherapy. J Behav Med. 1981;4(1):65–78.

Burish TG, Carey MP, Krozely MG, Greco FA. Conditioned side effects induced by cancer chemotherapy: prevention through behavioral treatment. J Consult Clin Psychol. 1987;55(1): 42–8.

Cankurtaran ES, Ozalp E, Soygur H, Akbiyik DI, Turhan L, Alkis N. Mirtazapine improves sleep and lowers anxiety and depression in cancer patients: superiority over imipramine. Support Care Cancer. 2008;16(11):1291–8.

Cheung YL, Molassiotis A, Chang AM. The effect of progressive muscle relaxation training on anxiety and quality of life after stoma surgery in colorectal cancer patients. Psychooncology. 2003;12(3):254–66.

Clerico M, Bertetto O, Morandini MP, Cardinali C, Giaccone G. Antiemetic activity of oral lorazepam in addition to methylprednisolone and metoclopramide in the prophylactic treatment of vomiting induced by cisplatin. A double-blind, placebo-controlled study with cross-over design. Tumori. 1993;79(2):119–22.

Decker TW, Cline-Elsen J, Gallagher M. Relaxation therapy as an adjunct in radiation oncology. J Clin Psychol. 1992;48(3):388–93.

Dolbeault S, Cayrou S, Bredart A, Viala AL, Desclaux B, Saltel P, Gauvain-Piquard A, Hardy P, Dickes P. The effectiveness of a psycho-educational group after early-stage breast cancer treatment: results of a randomized French study. Psychooncology. 2009;18(6):647–56.

Elsesser K, van Berkel M, Sartory G, Biermann-Göcke W, Öhl S. The effects of anxiety management training on psychological variables and immune parameters in cancer patients: a pilot study. Behav Cogn Psychother. 1994;22(1):13–23.

Espie CA, Fleming L, Cassidy J, Samuel L, Taylor LM, White CA, Douglas NJ, Engleman HM, Kelly HL, Paul J. Randomized controlled clinical effectiveness trial of cognitive behavior therapy compared with treatment as usual for persistent insomnia in patients with cancer. J Clin Oncol. 2008;26(28):4651–8.

Evans RL, Connis RT. Comparison of brief group therapies for depressed cancer patients receiving radiation treatment. Public Health Rep. 1995;110(3):306–11.

Grassi L, Mangelli L, Fava GA, Grandi S, Ottolini F, Porcelli P, Rafanelli C, Rigatelli M, Sonino N. Psychosomatic characterization of adjustment disorders in the medical setting: some suggestions for DSM-V. J Affect Disord. 2007;101:251–4.

Geracioti Jr TD, Baker DG, Kasckow JW, Strawn JR, Jeffrey Mulchahey J, Dashevsky BA, Horn PS, Ekhator NN. Effects of trauma-related audiovisual stimulation on cerebrospinal fluid norepinephrine and corticotropin-releasing hormone concentrations in post-traumatic stress disorder. Psychoneuroendocrinology. 2008;33(4):416–24.

Gold JI, Douglas MK, Thomas ML, Elliott JE, Rao SM, Miaskowski C. The relationship between posttraumatic stress disorder, mood states, functional status, and quality of life in oncology outpatients. J Pain Symptom Manage. 2012;44:520–31.

Gonzalez Baron M, Chacon JI, Garcia Giron C, Ordonez Gallego A, Garcia de Paredes ML, Feliu J, Zamora P, Herranz C, Garrido P, Artal A. Antiemetic regimens in outpatients receiving cisplatin and non-cisplatin chemotherapy. A randomized trial comparing high-dose metoclopramide plus methylprednisolone with and without lorazepam. Acta Oncol. 1991;30(5):623–7.

Greer S, Moorey S, Baruch JD, Watson M, Robertson BM, Mason A, Rowden L, Law MG, Bliss JM. Adjuvant psychological therapy for patients with cancer: a prospective randomised trial. BMJ. 1992;304(6828):675–80.

Hall A, A'Hern R, Fallowfield L. Are we using appropriate self-report questionnaires for detecting anxiety and depression in women with early breast cancer? Eur J Cancer. 1999;35(1):79–85.

Hidderley M, Holt M. A pilot randomized trial assessing the effects of autogenic training in early stage cancer patients in relation to psychological status and immune system responses. Eur J Oncol Nurs. 2004;8(1):61–5.

Holland JC, Morrow GR, Schmale A, Derogatis L, Stefanek M, Berenson S, Carpenter PJ, Breitbart W, Feldstein M. A randomized clinical trial of alprazolam versus progressive muscle relaxation in cancer patients with anxiety and depressive symptoms. J Clin Oncol. 1991;9(6):1004–11.

Holland JC, Romano SJ, Heiligenstein JH, Tepner RG, Wilson MG. A controlled trial of fluoxetine and desipramine in depressed women with advanced cancer. Psychooncology. 1998;7(4):291–300.

Hood SD, Melichar JK, Taylor LG, Kalk N, Edwards TR, Hince DA, Lenox-Smith A, Lingford-Hughes AR, Nutt DJ. Noradrenergic function in generalized anxiety disorder: impact of treatment with venlafaxine on the physiological and psychological responses to clonidine challenge. J Psychopharmacol. 2011;25(1):78–86.

House A, Stark D. Anxiety in medical patients. BMJ. 2002;325(7357):207–9.

Jacobs C, Ross RD, Walker IM, Stockdale FE. Behavior of cancer patients: a randomized study of the effects of education and peer support groups. Am J Clin Oncol. 1983;6(3):347–53.

Jacobsen PB, Meade CD, Stein KD, Chirikos TN, Small BJ, Ruckdeschel JC. Efficacy and costs of two forms of stress management training for cancer patients undergoing chemotherapy. J Clin Oncol. 2002;20(12):2851–62.

Jacobson AF, Dominguez RA, Goldstein BJ, Steinbook RM. Comparison of buspirone and diazepam in generalized anxiety disorder. Pharmacotherapy. 1985;5(5):290–6.

Kadan-Lottick NS, Vanderwerker LC, Block SD, Zhang B, Prigerson HG. Psychiatric disorders and mental health service use in patients with advanced cancer: a report from the coping with cancer study. Cancer. 2005;104:2872–81.

Kangas M, Henry JL, Bryant RA. Predictors of posttraumatic stress disorder following cancer. Health Psychol. 2005;24(6):579–85.

Kangas M, Henry JL, Bryant RA. Correlates of acute stress disorder in cancer patients. J Trauma Stress. 2007;20:325–34.

Katz MR, Irish JC, Devins GM. Development and pilot testing of a psychoeducational intervention for oral cancer patients. Psychooncology. 2004;13(9):642–53.

Kissane DW, Grabsch B, Love A, Clarke DM, Bloch S, Smith GC. Psychiatric disorder in women with early stage and advanced breast cancer: a comparative analysis. Aust N Z J Psychiatry. 2004;38(5):320–6.

Landolt MA, Ystrom E, Sennhauser FH, Gnehm HE, Vollrath ME. The mutual prospective influence of child and parental post-traumatic stress symptoms in pediatric patients. J Child Psychol Psychiatry. 2012;53(7):767–74.

Latini DM, Hart SL, Knight SJ, Cowan JE, Ross PL, Duchane J, Carroll PR. The relationship between anxiety and time to treatment for patients with prostate cancer on surveillance. J Urol. 2007;178(3 Pt 1):826–31. discussion 831-822.

Leon-Pizarro C, Gich I, Barthe E, Rovirosa A, Farrus B, Casas F, Verger E, Biete A, Craven-Bartle J, Sierra J, Arcusa A. A randomized trial of the effect of training in relaxation and guided imagery techniques in improving psychological and quality-of-life indices for gynecologic and breast brachytherapy patients. Psychooncology. 2007;16(11):971–9.

Matsuoka Y, Yamawaki S, Inagaki M, Akechi T, Uchitomi Y. A volumetric study of amygdala in cancer survivors with intrusive recollections. Biol Psychiatry. 2003;54(7):736–43.

McQuellon RP, Wells M, Hoffman S, Craven B, Russell G, Cruz J, Hurt G, DeChatelet P, Andrykowski MA, Savage P. Reducing distress in cancer patients with an orientation program. Psychooncology. 1998;7(3):207–17.

Mehnert A, Koch U. Prevalence of acute and post-traumatic stress disorder and comorbid mental disorders in breast cancer patients during primary cancer care: a prospective study. Psychooncology. 2007;16(3):181–8.

Mitchell AJ, Chan M, Bhatti H, Halton M, Grassi L, Johansen C, Meader N. Prevalence of depression, anxiety, and adjustment disorder in oncological, haematological, and palliative-care settings: a meta-analysis of 94 interview-based studies. Lancet Oncol. 2011;12(2):160–74.

Moorey S, Cort E, Kapari M, Monroe B, Hansford P, Mannix K, Henderson M, Fisher L, Hotopf M. A cluster randomized controlled trial of cognitive behaviour therapy for common mental disorders in patients with advanced cancer. Psychol Med. 2009;39(5):713–23.

Munafo MR, Clark T, Flint J. Does measurement instrument moderate the association between the serotonin transporter gene and anxiety-related personality traits? A meta-analysis. Mol Psychiatry. 2005;10(4):415–9.

Musselman DL, Lawson DH, Gumnick JF, Manatunga AK, Penna S, Goodkin RS, Greiner K, Nemeroff CB, Miller AH. Paroxetine for the prevention of depression induced by high-dose interferon alfa. N Engl J Med. 2001;344(13):961–6.

Musselman DL, Somerset WI, Guo Y, Manatunga AK, Porter M, Penna S, Lewison B, Goodkin R, Lawson K, Lawson D, Evans DL, Nemeroff CB. A double-blind, multicenter, parallel-group study of paroxetine, desipramine, or placebo in breast cancer patients (stages I, II, III, and IV) with major depression. J Clin Psychiatry. 2006;67(2):288–96.

Nakano T, Wenner M, Inagaki M, Kugaya A, Akechi T, Matsuoka Y, Sugahara Y, Imoto S, Murakami K, Uchitomi Y. Relationship between distressing cancer-related recollections and hippocampal volume in cancer survivors. Am J Psychiatry. 2002;159(12):2087–93.

Nakaya N, Goto K, Saito-Nakaya K, Inagaki M, Otani T, Akechi T, Nagai K, Hojo F, Uchitomi Y, Tsugane S, Nishiwaki Y. The lung cancer database project at the National Cancer Center, Japan: study design, corresponding rate and profiles of cohort. Jpn J Clin Oncol. 2006;36(5):280–4.

Okamura H, Yamamoto N, Watanabe T, Katsumata N, Takashima S, Adachi I, Kugaya A, Akechi T, Uchitomi Y. Psychological distress following first recurrence of disease in patients with breast cancer: prevalence and risk factors. Breast Cancer Res Treat. 2000;61:131–7.

Petersen RW, Quinlivan JA. Preventing anxiety and depression in gynaecological cancer: a randomised controlled trial. BJOG. 2002;109(4):386–94.

Pohl R, Yeragani VK, Balon R, Rainey JM, Lycaki H, Ortiz A, Berchou R, Weinberg P. Isoproterenol-induced panic attacks. Biol Psychiatry. 1988;24(8):891–902.

Prieto JM, Blanch J, Atala J, Carreras E, Rovira M, Cirera E, Gastó C. Psychiatric morbidity and impact on hospital length of stay among hematologic cancer patients receiving stem-cell transplantation. J Clin Oncol. 2002;20:1907–17.

Razavi D, Allilaire JF, Smith M, Salimpour A, Verra M, Desclaux B, Saltel P, Piollet I, Gauvain-Piquard A, Trichard C, Cordier B, Fresco R, Guillibert E, Sechter D, Orth JP, Bouhassira M, Mesters P, Blin P. The effect of fluoxetine on anxiety and depression symptoms in cancer patients. Acta Psychiatr Scand. 1996;94(3):205–10.

Rodin G, Yuen D, Mischitelle A, Minden MD, Brandwein J, Schimmer A, Marmar C, Gagliese L, Lo C, Rydall A, Zimmermann C. Traumatic stress in acute leukemia. Psychooncology. 2013; 22:299–307.

Rustad JK, David D, Currier MB. Cancer and post-traumatic stress disorder: diagnosis, pathogenesis and treatment considerations. Palliat Support Care. 2012;10(3):213–23.

Salvo N, Zeng L, Zhang L, Leung M, Khan L, Presutti R, Nguyen J, Holden L, Culleton S, Chow E. Frequency of reporting and predictive factors for anxiety and depression in patients with advanced cancer. Clin Oncol. 2012;24(2):139–48.

Savard J, Simard S, Ivers H, Morin CM. Randomized study on the efficacy of cognitive-behavioral therapy for insomnia secondary to breast cancer, part I: Sleep and psychological effects. J Clin Oncol. 2005;23(25):6083–96.

Schuyler D. Cognitive therapy for adjustment disorder in cancer patients. Psychiatry (Edgmont). 2004;1:20–3.

Shimizu K, Kinoshita H, Akechi T, Uchitomi Y, Andoh M. First panic attack episodes in head and neck cancer patients who have undergone radical neck surgery. J Pain Symptom Manag. 2007; 34(6):575–8.

Shimizu K, Akizuki N, Nakaya N, Fujimori M, Fujisawa D, Ogawa A, Uchitomi Y. Treatment response to psychiatric intervention and predictors of response among cancer patients with adjustment disorders. J Pain Symptom Manag. 2011;41(4):684–91.

Slaughter JR, Jain A, Holmes S, Reid JC, Bobo W, Sherrod NB. Panic disorder in hospitalized cancer patients. Psychooncology. 2000;9:253–8.

Spencer R, Nilsson M, Wright A, Pirl W, Prigerson H. Anxiety disorders in advanced cancer patients: correlates and predictors of end-of-life outcomes. Cancer. 2010;116:1810–9.

Spiegel D, Bloom JR, Yalom I. Group support for patients with metastatic cancer. A randomized outcome study. Arch Gen Psychiatry. 1981;38(5):527–33.

Stark DP, House A. Anxiety in cancer patients. Br J Cancer. 2000;83(10):1261–7.

Stark D, Kiely M, Smith A, Velikova G, House A, Selby P. Anxiety disorders in cancer patients: their nature, associations, and relation to quality of life. J Clin Oncol Off J Am Soc Clin Oncol. 2002;20(14):3137–48.

Stephens DN, Schneider HH, Kehr W, Jensen LH, Petersen E, Honore T. Modulation of anxiety by beta-carbolines and other benzodiazepine receptor ligands: relationship of pharmacological to biochemical measures of efficacy. Brain Res Bull. 1987;19(3):309–18.

Stockler MR, O'Connell R, Nowak AK, Goldstein D, Turner J, Wilcken NR, Wyld D, Abdi EA, Glasgow A, Beale PJ, Jefford M, Dhillon H, Heritier S, Carter C, Hickie IB, Simes RJ. Effect of sertraline on symptoms and survival in patients with advanced cancer, but without major depression: a placebo-controlled double-blind randomised trial. Lancet Oncol. 2007;8(7): 603–12.

Strong V, Waters R, Hibberd C, Murray G, Wall L, Walker J, McHugh G, Walker A, Sharpe M. Management of depression for people with cancer (SMaRT oncology 1): a randomised trial. Lancet. 2008;372(9632):40–8.

Tanaka M, Yoshida M, Emoto H, Ishii H. Noradrenaline systems in the hypothalamus, amygdala and locus coeruleus are involved in the provocation of anxiety: basic studies. Eur J Pharmacol. 2000;405(1–3):397–406.

Telch CF, Telch MJ. Group coping skills instruction and supportive group therapy for cancer patients: a comparison of strategies. J Consult Clin Psychol. 1986;54(6):802–8.

Thomas R, Daly M, Perryman B, Stockton D. Forewarned is forearmed-benefits of preparatory information on video cassette for patients receiving chemotherapy or radiotherapy–a randomised controlled trial. Eur J Cancer. 2000;36(12):1536–43.

Traeger L, Greer JA, Fernandez-Robles C, Temel JS, Pirl WF. Evidence-based treatment of anxiety in patients with cancer. J Clin Oncol. 2012;30:1197–205.

Trask PC, Paterson AG, Griffith KA, Riba MB, Schwartz JL. Cognitive-behavioral intervention for distress in patients with melanoma: comparison with standard medical care and impact on quality of life. Cancer. 2003;98(4):854–64.

Vasa RA, Pine DS, Masten CL, Vythilingam M, Collin C, Charney DS, Neumeister A, Mogg K, Bradley BP, Bruck M, Monk CS. Effects of yohimbine and hydrocortisone on panic symptoms, autonomic responses, and attention to threat in healthy adults. Psychopharmacology. 2009; 204(3):445–55.

Vin-Raviv N, Hillyer GC, Hershman DL, Galea S, Leoce N, Bovbjerg DH, Kushi LH, Kroenke C, Lamerato L, Ambrosone CB, Valdimorsdottir H, Jandorf L, Mandelblatt JS, Tsai WY, Neugut AI. Racial disparities in posttraumatic stress after diagnosis of localized breast cancer: the BQUAL study. J Natl Cancer Inst. 2013;105:563–72.

Wald TG, Kathol RG, Noyes Jr R, Carroll BT, Clamon GH. Rapid relief of anxiety in cancer patients with both alprazolam and placebo. Psychosomatics. 1993;34(4):324–32.

White VM, Macvean ML, Grogan S, D'Este C, Akkerman D, Ieropoli S, Hill DJ, Sanson-Fisher R. Can a tailored telephone intervention delivered by volunteers reduce the supportive care needs, anxiety and depression of people with colorectal cancer? A randomised controlled trial. Psychooncology. 2012;21(10):1053–62.

Yamaguchi T, Tsujimatsu A, Kumamoto H, Izumi T, Ohmura Y, Yoshida T, Yoshioka M. Anxiolytic effects of yokukansan, a traditional Japanese medicine, via serotonin 5-HT1A receptors on anxiety-related behaviors in rats experienced aversive stress. J Ethnopharmacol. 2012;143(2):533–9.

Pharmacotherapy of Depression in Cancer Patients

9

Peter Fitzgerald, Madeline Li, Luigi Grassi, and Gary Rodin

Abstract

Pharmacotherapy is an important component of treatment for more severe and persistent depression in patients with cancer and advanced disease. The initiation of such treatment should follow a careful diagnostic assessment, and the choice of an antidepressant should be based upon the symptom profile of the patient, the antidepressant side-effect profile, and the least potential for interaction with chemotherapy and other medications. Although an antidepressant medication with a rapid onset of action is desirable in this population, psychostimulants and other such agents have not been shown to be effective. Psychotherapy should typically be provided in conjunction with pharmacotherapy and, in the case of minor depression, may be the sole therapeutic modality. This includes attentive psychoeducation on common concerns about antidepressants expressed by medical patients, in order to ensure safety and enhance compliance.

9.1   Introduction

Clinically significant depression in cancer patients is at least three times as common as in the general population. Major depression has been found to occur in approximately 16 % of patients with cancer, with minor depression and dysthymia

P. Fitzgerald (✉) • M. Li • G. Rodin
Department of Psychosocial Oncology & Palliative Care, Princess Margaret Cancer Centre, University Health Network, 610 University Avenue, Toronto, Ontario, M5G 2M9
e-mail: Peter.Fitzgerald@uhn.ca; Madeline.Li@uhn.ca; Gary.Rodin@uhn.ca

L. Grassi
Institute of Psychiatry, Department of Biomedical and Speciality Surgical Sciences, University of Ferrara, Ferrara, Italy
e-mail: luigi.grassi@unife.it

L. Grassi and M. Riba (eds.), *Psychopharmacology in Oncology and Palliative Care*,   145
DOI 10.1007/978-3-642-40134-3_9, © Springer-Verlag Berlin Heidelberg 2014

combined reported to be present in almost 22 % of patients (Mitchell et al. 2011). A majority of patients with subthreshold depression do not progress to major depression, although both major and minor depression are associated with significant impairment of well-being (Rowe and Rapaport 2006). Depression in cancer has been associated with poorer quality of life (Grassi et al. 1996), greater physical symptom burden (Fitzgerald et al. 2013), poorer treatment compliance (Colleoni et al. 2000), and an elevated rate of suicide and desire for hastened death (Chochinov et al. 1998; Rodin et al. 2007).

While the focus of this chapter is on the pharmacotherapy of depression, it is important that treatment in cancer patients address not only the target symptoms but also the disease-related and psychosocial factors that contribute to the emergence of depression in this context. Such treatment includes addressing pain and other distressing physical symptoms, the relationship with oncologists and other healthcare providers, the social support system, and the individual experience of illness (Li et al. 2012). Pharmacotherapy is most effective in those with more severe depression (Fournier et al. 2010), whereas psychotherapeutic approaches are of value in both milder and more severe cases (Driessen et al. 2010).

9.2 Screening and Diagnosis of Depression in Cancer

The first step in treating depression in cancer patients is the timely recognition and diagnosis of this disturbance. A common barrier to the diagnosis in oncology and other medical settings is the failure of healthcare providers to inquire about symptoms (Taylor et al. 2011a). Screening tools can improve the detection of depression in the clinic setting, although the evidence that this results in improved depression outcomes in cancer patients is still mixed (Mitchell 2013). Such improvement will, of course, depend upon the resources that are applied to the treatment of depression in individuals in whom it is identified.

Clinicians should routinely inquire about mood in clinical assessments, but depression rating scales may be used beforehand to identify those at highest risk (Mitchell et al. 2012). These include brief screening tools, such as those with one or two stem questions, which have good sensitivity. Longer depression rating scales with better construct validity, such as the Patient Health Questionnaire-9 (PHQ-9) (Thekkumpurath et al. 2011), Hospital Anxiety and Depression Scale (HADS) (Mitchell et al. 2010), or Beck Depression Inventory II (BDI-II) (Hopko et al. 2008) (see Table 9.1), may be used when this is feasible.

Positive screening results should be followed by a diagnostic clinical assessment. It is important in this assessment to consider the comorbid conditions and potential etiological factors contributing to the depressive symptoms. These include delirium, dementia, adverse drug effects (e.g. steroids, interferons), drug or alcohol withdrawal states, brain metastases with pseudobulbar affect, and Parkinsonism with masked facies. Other psychiatric disorders such as psychosis, and particularly anxiety disorders, can also present with depressive symptoms. Psychosis is marked by disorganised thinking and the presence of hallucinations and delusions. Restlessness and overwhelming anxiety are often the primary complaints in anxiety

Table 9.1 Validated depression screening scales in cancer

Measure	Sensitivity[a]	Specificity[a]
One stem		
"Are you depressed?"	68.3 %	88.1 %
Distress thermometer	80.2 %	75.6 %
Two stem		
"During the last month, have you been bothered by…	95.6 %	88.9 %
…feeling down, depressed, or hopeless?"		
…having little interest or pleasure in doing things?"		
Patient Health Questionnaire-9 (PHQ-9)		
• 9 items, concordant with diagnostic criteria	93 %	81 %
Hospital Anxiety and Depression Scale (HADS)		
• 14 items, excludes somatic symptoms	76.4 %	79.4 %
• HADS-Depression item subscale	66.6 %	80.9 %
Beck Depression Inventory II (BDI-II)		
• 21 items, preponderance of somatic symptoms	83.6 %	87.4 %

[a]Weighted results from pooled meta-analysis (Mitchell et al. 2012) except for PHQ-9 (Thekkumpurath et al. 2011)

disorders, in contrast to the flattened affect and dysphoria of depression. The diagnostic criteria for major depression (Table 9.2-I) should be used to inform and categorise the diagnosis of a depressive disorder. Pharmacotherapy should generally be reserved for patients who meet diagnostic criteria for a major depressive episode.

Distinguishing the somatic symptoms of depression from cancer-related symptoms can be challenging, since symptoms such as anorexia and fatigue may arise from the effects of cancer and its treatment and/or to comorbid depression. Clinicians must rely more heavily on the psychological symptoms of sadness, such as loss of interest, feelings of worthlessness, and the presence of suicidal ideation in order to diagnose depression. Although there is clinical subtlety in distinguishing realistic sadness in this context from clinical depression, persistent and pervasive sadness in association with symptoms such as hopelessness and excessive guilt is most likely to reflect the presence of a depressive disorder (Table 9.2-II).

9.3   Antidepressants: An Overview of Prescribing Practices

Several counselling steps should be taken prior to initiating antidepressant medication to a cancer patient. Potential side effects of the selected medication should be discussed, informing the patient that most side effects (especially the gastrointestinal (GI) disturbances, nausea, headache, and anxiety) are mild and transient and that if they do occur, tend to resolve within the first week or so of treatment. To manage expectations and to prevent premature discontinuation of the medication, it

Table 9.2 Diagnosis of major depression in cancer

I. DSM-5 diagnostic criteria for a major depressive episode (A and B criteria only)[a]

    A. At least five of the following symptoms, present during the same 2-week period, representing a change from previous functioning, each present nearly every day; at least one of the symptoms is either (1) or (2). Note: Do not include symptoms that are clearly attributable to another medical condition

      1. Depressed mood most of the day

      2. Markedly diminished interest or pleasure in almost all activities most of the day

      3. Significant weight loss or gain (change of >5 % in a month), or decrease or increase in appetite

      4. Insomnia or hypersomnia

      5. Psychomotor agitation or retardation

      6. Fatigue or loss of energy

      7. Feelings of worthlessness or excessive or inappropriate guilt

      8. Diminished ability to think or concentrate, or indecisiveness

      9. Recurrent thoughts of death (not just fear of dying), recurrent suicidal ideation, or a suicide attempt or plan

    B. Symptoms cause clinically significant distress or impairment in social, occupational, or other important areas of functioning

II. Psychological features of major depression vs. normative sadness[b]

Major depression	Normative sadness
• Feels isolated	• Maintains intimacy and connection
• Feeling of permanence	• Belief things will get better
• Excessive guilt and regret	• Can enjoy happy memories
• Self-critical ruminations/loathing	• Sense of self-worth
• Constant and pervasive	• Fluctuates with thoughts of cancer
• Sense of hopelessness	• Looks forward to the future
• Loss of interest in activities	• Retains capacity for pleasure
• Suicidal thoughts/behaviour	• Maintains will to live

[a]Condensed from the Diagnostic and Statistical Manual of Mental Disorders, 5th Edition (American Psychiatric Association (APA) 2013)
[b]Adapted from Rayner et al. (2011)

should be explained that side effects may occur before there is any therapeutic benefit.

Antidepressant medications usually start to take effect within 2–4 weeks of their initiation, though the full effect at a particular dosage may not be achieved for more than 4–6 weeks. Patients can be reassured that dependence or tolerance does not occur with these medications and that it is important to take them as prescribed, continuing even after remission of depressive symptoms. Patients should also be advised that all antidepressants have the potential to cause discontinuation symptoms, especially when discontinued abruptly and when they have been administered in higher doses (Blier and Tremblay 2006). Such symptoms include general malaise, dizziness, insomnia, headache, agitation, and in some, fleeting "shock like" sensations in the extremities. Though the discontinuation syndrome is transient and self-limiting, it can be distressing and, rarely, is prolonged. It typically lasts less than one week and is most likely to occur with antidepressants that have short half-lives (such as paroxetine or venlafaxine). To avoid this discontinuation

Table 9.3 Important factors to consider in choosing an antidepressant for a depressed cancer patient

- Past psychiatric history (e.g. assess for past positive treatment responses to an antidepressant)
- Concurrent medications (e.g. assess for potential drug–drug interactions)
- Somatic symptom profile (e.g. a sedating antidepressant may be preferable for those with prominent insomnia; cachectic patients may benefit from antidepressants that stimulate weight gain)
- Potential for dual benefit (e.g. duloxetine for neuropathic pain, venlafaxine for hot flashes)
- Type of cancer (e.g. avoid bupropion in those with central nervous system (CNS) cancers due to elevated seizure risk)
- Co-morbidities (e.g. avoid psychostimulants or tricyclic antidepressants (TCAs) in those with symptomatic cardiac disease)
- Cancer prognosis (e.g. in setting of terminal disease, the rapid onset of action of psychostimulants may be preferable)

syndrome, antidepressants should be gradually reduced, if possible, over the course of several weeks.

All antidepressants have been associated with an increased risk of suicidal thoughts and acts, particularly in adolescents and young adults (Stone et al. 2009; Schneeweiss et al. 2010). Although the absolute risk of suicidality risk in this context is very small and suicidality in general is greatly reduced by the use of antidepressants (Isacsson et al. 2010), it is now recommended that patients should be warned of this potential adverse effect prior to commencing treatment and be made aware of how to seek help if this occurs. Patients at higher risk of suicidality should be prescribed a limited quantity of antidepressant medications and monitored in follow-up more frequently.

There are other general considerations that are important to take into account when prescribing antidepressants. There should be screening for medical co-morbidities, such as hypothyroidism and vitamin B12 deficiency, which may be contributing to depression. It is advisable to start patients on a low dose, in order to assess for tolerability and the emergence of side effects, and subsequently, to titrate upwards, after one week, to a therapeutic dose. The choice of antidepressant requires a careful consideration of such factors (see Table 9.3) as the symptom profile of the patient, the type of cancer, concurrent medications, and co-morbidities (Okamura et al. 2008). Until the therapeutic effect of the antidepressant has become evident, it can be helpful to consider short-term use of benzodiazepines for anxiety/agitation or hypnotics for insomnia, if required.

A single episode of major depression that responds to antidepressant medication should be treated for at least 6–9 months after full remission, in the same dose as was used for acute treatment. This continuation of treatment after remission is necessary because termination of antidepressant therapy is associated with a return of depressive symptoms within 3–6 months (Anderson et al. 2008). Patients who have a history of recurrent depressive disorder should be advised to continue maintenance antidepressant treatment for at least 2 years, and in some cases, indefinite treatment is advisable (NICE Guidelines UK 2009; APA Guidelines 2010).

Case Example: Choosing an Antidepressant

Ms. A is a 45-year-old married female with locally advanced tonsillar cancer, who has recently commenced combined chemo-radiation treatment. She presented with elevated depression and anxiety scores on routine screening for psychological distress performed when she attended the oncology clinic. Ms. A then disclosed to her oncologist prominent feelings of sadness and marked fear about her future. In addition, she described distress about intrusive symptoms of nausea and pain, which were side effects of her radiation treatment, and she reported marked sleep disturbance.

The oncologist listened empathically, explained to Ms. A what he believed to be the sources of her symptoms and proposed a treatment plan. This included optimising her anti-nausea and analgesic regime and referring her to the psycho-oncology service for a more detailed assessment of mood and support needs. During that assessment, she disclosed a 4 week history of pervasive low mood, pessimism, and tearfulness, with reduced motivation and enjoyment levels. She also described impaired sleep, with predominant initial and middle insomnia, and a pattern of nocturnal rumination. Ms. A confided concerns related to loss of her occupational and social roles, due to illness and treatment effects, and she described difficulty tolerating the uncertainty about whether her disease would progress and be fatal. Her pain had improved since adjustment of her analgesic regime by her oncologist, though she was still experiencing some fluctuant nausea and prominent odynophagia, with difficulty swallowing. She was due to have a g-tube inserted shortly, to ensure adequate nutritional intake.

Ms. A was diagnosed by the psychiatrist as suffering from a major depressive episode with prominent anxiety. She agreed to commence antidepressant medication, in combination with ongoing psychotherapeutic support, to help her cope with the stresses of her illness. Mirtazapine was chosen as the antidepressant agent because it would not interact with the patient's chemotherapy or other medications and because of its sleep-promoting and anti-nauseant properties. Finally, the availability of this medication as an orodispersible formulation would allow consistent adherence, despite the patient's swallowing difficulties.

9.4 Potential Adverse Effects of Antidepressants

Antidepressant medications have potential serious adverse effects that are important to consider prior to treatment initiation and on an ongoing basis. There is evidence that they are associated with an increased incidence of osteoporosis and with bone fractures in the elderly (Coupland et al. 2011). Antidepressants also are associated with a slightly increased bleeding risk, particularly in the gastrointestinal tract (Looper 2007). Such bone-related and haematological effects arise through altered serotonergic activity within bone cells and platelets, respectively.

Hyponatraemia is another important potential adverse effect of antidepressant use, especially in serotonergic medications, although all classes of antidepressants have been implicated. Onset usually occurs within a few weeks of treatment initiation or dose adjustment and normalises once the causative agent has been withdrawn (Egger et al. 2006). All patients taking antidepressants should be monitored for potential signs of low sodium, such as dizziness, nausea, lethargy, confusion, cramps, and seizures. Risk factors include advanced age, female gender, low body weight, co-morbid medical conditions (including hypothyroidism, congestive cardiac disease, pneumonia, small cell lung cancer), and concomitant medications, including diuretics, NSAIDS, and chemotherapeutic agents. Routine monitoring of serum sodium is advisable, especially in cancer patients, who have additional risk factors for hyponatraemia. Educating patients about the signs and symptoms of hyponatraemia and the importance of seeking medical assessment if they develop is important.

Very rarely, antidepressants can cause serotonergic toxicity in the central nervous system, a complication referred to as serotonin syndrome (Boyer and Shannon 2005). The signs of this syndrome include acute autonomic instability (e.g. fluctuations in heart rate and blood pressure and also development of pyrexia), reduced cognitive acuity, tremor, and neuromuscular features, including clonus, myoclonus, and hyper-reflexia. In extreme cases convulsions, coma, and death can ensue. While serotonin syndrome predominantly arises when several serotonergic agents have been prescribed concurrently, it can occur idiosyncratically in response to a single serotonergic agent. Therefore, vigilance is important regarding its possible occurrence when any of its core signs or symptoms becomes apparent. Other serotonergic drugs that may increase the risk of serotonin toxicity include analgesics such as fentanyl and tramadol, the antibiotic linezolid, which has monoamine oxidase inhibition activity, and antiemetic medications such as metoclopramide and ondansetron. When suspected, it is important to discontinue all potential offending agents, monitor closely, and provide supportive care until symptoms resolve.

9.5 Efficacy of Antidepressants in Cancer Patients

Although a large body of research demonstrates the efficacy of antidepressant medications in the treatment of depressive disorders in a general population or psychiatric setting, there remains a dearth of randomised controlled trials specifically in people with cancer (Li et al. 2012). Those studies of pharmacologic treatment of depression in cancer that have been reported have provided mixed results, in part due to methodological limitations. These include small sample sizes, heterogeneity regarding the severity of depression, inclusion criteria, and demographic, disease-related, and treatment characteristics of the study samples (Massie 2004; Li et al. 2012). Three meta-analyses on the effectiveness of pharmacotherapy for depression in patients with general medical conditions have provided more robust positive findings (Taylor et al. 2011b; Rayner et al. 2011; Iovieno et al. 2011). All three studies found a significant advantage for antidepressant use in terms of depression remission and response compared with placebo.

The efficacy of antidepressants in the treatment of subthreshold or minor depression is still unclear with mixed findings in the literature. Rayner and colleagues (2011) demonstrated a greater effect size in the treatment of minor compared with major depression in their meta-analysis, and a more recent meta-analysis of depressed cancer patients found a significant and comparable positive effect of antidepressant treatment, irrespective of whether patients had clinical depression or subthreshold depressive symptoms (Laoutidis and Mathiak 2013). However, recent meta-analyses and systematic and narrative reviews of the evidence (Baumeister 2012; Hegerl et al. 2012; Barbui et al. 2011) suggest that antidepressant medications are not effective in the treatment of subthreshold and minor depression. Barbui et al. (2011) suggest that despite the extensive use of antidepressant medication for emotional complaints, antidepressants should not be used in the initial treatment of individuals with minor depression.

The potential role of antidepressant medication in preventing the onset of depression in those with cancer is an intriguing area of research which has been investigated in a few studies to date. Musselman and colleagues (2001) demonstrated this effect in patients with melanoma receiving high-dose interferon-alpha who were pretreated with paroxetine. Another RCT of the use of citalopram to prevent depression in patients with head and neck cancer (Lydiatt et al. 2008) revealed significantly less depression after 12 weeks in the treatment group compared with the placebo control group. A further recent RCT by the same group found that prophylactic escitalopram reduced the risk of developing depression by more than 50 % in head and neck cancer patients undergoing first-line cancer treatment (Lydiatt et al. 2013). Although these findings are intriguing, more research is needed to confirm that prophylactic antidepressant medication can prevent depression in high-risk populations of cancer patients.

9.6 Antidepressant Classes

There are several different classes of available antidepressant medications. The following section will briefly outline those which are used in cancer settings, with emphasis on first-line medication classes, such as the selective serotonin reuptake inhibitors [SSRIs, the dual-acting serotonergic/norepinephrine reuptake inhibitors (SNRIs)] and the atypical and tricyclic antidepressants (TCAs) that remain useful options in some cases. The latter's role in the management of depression has declined considerably in recent decades due to the development of better tolerated and safer therapeutic options, though TCAs remain commonly prescribed for their role in the treatment of neuropathic pain in cancer patients. Though monoamine oxidase inhibitors (MAOIs) retain a role in some treatment-resistant depressions, they should be avoided in the oncology setting because of the high risk of potentially lethal drug interactions with other commonly prescribed medications in cancer patients (e.g. opioids). For this reason they are not discussed further in this chapter.

9.6.1 The Selective Serotonin Reuptake Inhibitors

While antidepressants from the different classes have been shown to be equally efficacious, the SSRIs tend to be used first line due to their tolerability and safety profile; this remains true for depressed cancer patients (Caruso et al. 2013). All SSRIs share a similar side effect profile of gastrointestinal disturbance, headache, fatigue or insomnia, sexual dysfunction, and transient increased anxiety after initiation of treatment. However, there are some important differences between each SSRI that may impact on treatment selection. Some SSRIs are potent and dose-related inhibitors of individual or multiple hepatic cytochrome P450 pathways. Owing to its long half-life and strong cytochrome P450 inhibitory effects, fluoxetine is best avoided in the cancer setting, given the risk of interaction with many chemotherapy agents that are metabolised through the cytochrome P450 system. Similarly, paroxetine has prominent P450 inhibitory effects and also significant anticholinergic effects that can be problematic and therefore limit its use in cancer patients. Among the SSRIs, sertraline, citalopram, and escitalopram have the fewest drug–drug interactions and are well tolerated, making them the best first-line treatment options. In addition to relieving symptoms of depression and anxiety, some SSRIs (e.g. citalopram, sertraline, fluoxetine, paroxetine) have also been shown to alleviate hot flash symptoms, which can be a common occurrence related to breast and prostate cancer treatment (Adelson et al. 2005). Several SSRI medications are available in liquid form (e.g. citalopram, fluoxetine) or rapid dissolving formulations (e.g. escitalopram), which are useful options for those cancer patients with dysphagia.

9.6.2 The Serotonin Norepinephrine Reuptake Inhibitors

Venlafaxine, desvenlafaxine, and duloxetine are dual-acting serotonin norepineph-rine reuptake inhibitors (SNRIs). Venlafaxine is effectively an SSRI at lower doses and becomes a dual-acting reuptake inhibitor at doses of 150 mg and higher, whereas duloxetine inhibits both serotonin and norepinephrine reuptake at all therapeutic doses. Desvenlafaxine is the active metabolite of venlafaxine, but is not metabolised by the cytochrome P450 system and thus has a lower potential for drug–drug interactions. SNRIs have been found to have analgesic properties for neuropathic pain and also to be an effective treatment for hot flash symptoms related to tamoxifen use in breast cancer or androgen ablation treatment in prostate cancer. Dose-dependent hypertension may occur in patients taking venlafaxine at high doses, and hepatoxicity has been described as a rare complication of high dose duloxetine. In some countries, the SNRI milnacipran is also available for the treatment of depression. Milnacipran has been shown to be as effective as SSRIs and other SNRIs. Adverse side effects mainly include possible nausea and vomiting, headache, constipation, dizziness, palpitations, heart rate increase, dry mouth, and hypertension.

9.6.3 "Atypical" Antidepressants

Mirtazapine is a noradrenergic and specific serotonergic antidepressant (NaSSA). It exerts anti-anxiety, sleep-inducing, antiemetic and appetite stimulating effects through a combination of histaminic receptor agonism and antagonism of 5HT2 and 5HT3 receptors. Thus, in addition to its antidepressant effect, it can also help to ameliorate somatic cancer-related symptoms such as anorexia, cachexia, and nausea (Riechelmann et al. 2010). Due to its sedative properties, it may also be useful in cases in which prominent insomnia is a feature. Another benefit of mirtazapine is its availability as a rapidly dissolving tablet, making it useful in patients who cannot tolerate oral medications. Side effects include constipation, drowsiness, dry mouth, and, rarely, reversible neutropenia.

Bupropion is a dual norepinephrine and dopamine reuptake inhibitor (NDRI) that is activating in nature and has been shown to improve fatigue and concentration in cancer patients. It tends to be weight neutral, or in some cases to be associated with weight loss, and thus should be used with caution and not as a first-line treatment option in depressed cachectic cancer patients. Common side effects include nausea, dry mouth, constipation, headaches, and insomnia. In some, it may increase agitation and therefore should generally be avoided in those depressed patients who have significant symptoms of anxiety. It increases the seizure threshold (daily doses exceeding 450mg doing so tenfold) and so its use is contraindicated in patients with seizure disorders, intracranial tumours, eating disorders, or alcohol withdrawal.

Trazodone is a serotonin antagonist and reuptake inhibitor (SARI) with an antidepressant and anxiolytic profile. Because of its non-habit-forming action on sleep, it is widely used as medication for sleep disorders. Common side effects include cardiovascular, with the risk of orthostatic hypotension causing dizziness and increasing the risk of falling, particularly in the elderly or fragile patients. Priapism is also a possible rare effect, whereas there are no side effects on sexual function.

Reboxetine is a selective norepinephrine reuptake inhibitor (NRI) used in several countries for the treatment of depression. It is reported to be effective in the treatment of apathy, fatigue, concentration, and anxiety-related symptoms and to restore social functioning. The most common side effects include tachycardia, dry mouth, constipation, headache, drowsiness, dizziness, excessive sweating, and insomnia.

Agomelatine is a new malatonergic antidepressant medication showing an agonist effect on melatonin receptors and an antagonist action on serotonin (5-HT2C) receptors. It has a positive effect on sleep, and it lacks sexual side effects and discontinuation effects shown by some other antidepressants. It is contraindicated in patients with renal or hepatic impairment. Because of the possible increase in the levels of liver enzymes, check-up of liver activity is recommended at the initiation of the treatment and periodically during treatment.

9.6.4 Tricyclic Antidepressants

These are now seldom used first line as antidepressants due to their side effect and safety profile, which can be particularly problematic in the medically ill population. In the elderly or medically frail, TCAs can cause or contribute to the development of acute confusional states, due to central anticholinergic activity, and to a significantly elevated risk of falls, primarily through an orthostatic hypotensive effect. Peripheral anticholinergic effects of TCAs can lead to constipation, urinary retention, blurred vision, and dry mouth, which can be particularly troublesome in some cancer populations depending on tumour site or cancer treatment effects. They are also associated with QT prolongation and thus caution must be used in prescribing TCAs to patients with pre-existing arrhythmias; their use is contraindicated following recent myocardial infarction. Tricyclics retain an important use in the treatment of neuropathic pain, although in doses much lower than those used for depression and therefore with fewer side effects.

9.6.5 Psychostimulants

Psychostimulants (such as methylphenidate and dexamphetamine) may reduce fatigue and promote wakefulness and mood elevation or euphoria, with a rapid onset of action of hours to days rather than weeks. Such effects, which are distinct from that of relieving depression, nevertheless make them a useful treatment option to consider in patients with advanced disease, for whom the quick onset of action is a distinct advantage and the potential problem of dependence or tolerance less relevant. Psychostimulants can also reduce anorexia, improve attention and concentration, counteract opiate-induced sedation, and improve pain. However, evidence of their efficacy in alleviating depression is mixed, with most positive results coming from single-arm studies, rather than from randomised controlled trials (Kerr et al. 2012). The most common adverse effects of psychostimulants are insomnia and agitation, although their prolonged use at high doses may, rarely, be associated with the development of a paranoid psychosis. Due to their ability to stimulate the cardiovascular system, caution is advised when considering their use in patients with hypertension or arrhythmias.

Modafinil, a wakefulness-promoting agent, does not affect the release of dopamine or noradrenaline, but instead likely works through histamine release and agonism of the noradrenaline receptors. It seems to lack the tolerance or dependence effects seen with other stimulants, but also lacks their euphoric effects. There is some evidence from research in other patient populations to support its use as an adjunct in treatment-resistant depression, though data from cancer patients are lacking and there is no evidence that monotherapy with this agent is useful in treating depressed patients (Table 9.4).

9.7   Potential Drug–Drug Interactions Involving Antidepressant Medications

It is vital to consider potential drug interactions when considering the prescription of psychotropics in cancer patients. Given that polypharmacy is common in this population, and that the number and type of drugs which a patient is prescribed may be altered on multiple occasions during the cancer experience (e.g. based on treatment phase, failure of response, side effects of treatment, or complications), it is important to select a medication that is the least likely to have significant pharmacokinetic or pharmacodynamic interactions and to rely on its lowest effective dose. Drug interactions between antidepressants and chemotherapeutic agents may compromise the effectiveness of chemotherapy or increase toxicity of treatment, adversely affecting well-being and survival.

Tamoxifen has been the most extensively studied antineoplastic (AN) agent for drug interactions with antidepressants. It is converted to its active metabolite (endoxifen) by the CYP 2D6 isoenzyme, and several studies have shown that antidepressant drugs that have strong 2D6 inhibition can reduce the conversion of tamoxifen to endoxifen (Desmarais and Looper 2009), though there have been mixed findings regarding the clinical relevance of this interaction (Breitbart 2011). Recent meta-analyses indicate that while CYP 2D6 inhibitors may reduce endoxifen levels, there does not appear to be an impact on recurrence rates or survival (Lash et al. 2011). However, until further research resolves this debate, it may be prudent to avoid potent CYP 2D6 inhibitors, such as fluoxetine and paroxetine, when other options are available.

The effectiveness of cyclophosphamide may be reduced by the concomitant use of either CYP 2B6 inhibitors (e.g. paroxetine, fluoxetine, sertraline, bupropion) or 2C19 inhibitors (e.g. TCAs or sertraline, fluoxetine, fluvoxamine), while higher levels of its active drug (and thus potential toxicity) may be precipitated by 3A4 inhibitors (i.e. fluoxetine, sertraline, paroxetine, fluvoxamine). Procarbazine effectiveness may also be lowered through 2B6 inhibitors and, to a lesser extent, CYP 1A inhibition (e.g. fluvoxamine). Sunitinib is metabolised by CYP 3A4 to its active metabolite, and the therapeutic effect of it may be impaired by 3A4 inhibitors. The taxanes (docetaxel and paclitaxel) are also metabolised by CYP 3A4, and inhibitors of this isoenzyme may increase their plasma concentrations leading to toxicity. The same occurs with the other ANs in the antimicrotubules category (vinblastine, vincristine, vindesine, vinorelbine), corticosteroids, etoposide, irinotecan, sorafenib, imatinib, and dasatinib whose concurrent use with CYP 3A4 inhibitors can increase toxicity, and with CYP 3A4 inducers reduce efficacy. The concomitant use of irinotecan and SSRIs has also been associated with rhabdomyolysis (Richards et al. 2003). Common antineoplastic agents for which there is no current evidence of hepatic cytochrome P450 involvement include temozolamide,

Table 9.4 Specific considerations of common antidepressant medications in the cancer setting

Antidepressant	Minimum effective dose	Most common side effects	Considerations
SSRIs:		All SSRIs:	
Escitalopram	10 mg/day	Nausea, dyspepsia, diarrhoea, sweating, anxiety, insomnia, headache	Good first-line choices
Citalopram	20 mg/day		Minimal P450 effects
			Possible QT prolongation at high doses. Drops/dissolvable formulations are options
Sertraline	50 mg/day	As above	Discontinuation side effects more common
Paroxetine	20 mg/day	Most anticholinergic and sedating SSRI	Strong hepatic enzyme inhibitor; discontinuation symptoms more common
Fluoxetine	20 mg/day	Stimulating	Longest half-life; strong hepatic enzyme inhibitor
SNRIs:			
Venlafaxine	75 mg/day	Nausea, headache, somnolence, insomnia, sweating, dizziness, anxiety, constipation	Additional use for neuropathic pain and hot flash symptoms; discontinuation symptoms common (venlafaxine); may cause elevations in BP at high doses
Desvenlafaxine	50 mg/day		
Duloxetine	60 mg/day		
Atypical Antidepressants:			
Mirtazapine (NaSSA)	15 mg/day	Sedating, weight gain dry mouth	Also available in orodispersible tablet; anti-nausea properties
Bupropion (NDRI)	150 mg/day	Weight neutral or loss, anxiety, seizure risk	Activating; caution in cachectic patients; smoking cessation aid
Reboxetine (NRI)	4 mg/day	Insomnia, sweating, dizziness, tachycardia	Activating; caution in co-morbid cardiac disease
Agomelatine	25 mg/day	Nausea, dizziness, somnolence, insomnia, headache	Changes in liver enzyme activity (esp AST, ALT) merit LFT monitoring. May improve sleep and generally very well tolerated
Tricyclic Antidepressants (e.g. amitriptyline)	Unclear, but at least 75 mg/day	Sedating, orthostatic hypotension, anticholinergic effects	Main use in cancer patients is in neuropathic pain
Psychostimulants			
Methylphenidate	Unclear: Range of 5–60 mg/day	Insomnia, anxiety, tachycardia, hypertension, tremor, confusion	Rapid onset of action; activating; may reduce fatigue and improve concentration Caution in cardiac disease
Dexamphetamine			
Modafinil	100–200 mg/day	Similar profile but less common	Less dependence/tolerance effects.

5-flourouracil, gemcitabine, cisplatin, carboplatin, oxaliplatin, doxorubicin, duanorubicin, melphalan, chlorambucil, and busulfan (Miguel and Albuquerque 2011).

Though there is a lack of research on the impact of antidepressant medications on other antineoplastic agents, knowledge of the individual pharmacokinetics of these medications suggests that interactions may exist that could confer either reduced anticancer efficacy or increased toxicity (Miguel and Albuquerque 2011). The clinician should be alert to the possibility of such effects and seek to avoid any potential negative effects through careful choice of antidepressant.

9.8 Summary

The assessment and treatment of depression in cancer patients are an important clinical activity, given the high prevalence of depression in all phases of the disease. Pharmacotherapy is an important component of care for depressed cancer patients, especially in those with moderate to severe depression. In spite of the limited volume and methodology of reported randomised controlled trials specific for depression in cancer patients, the efficacy of antidepressants can be considered to be robust, based on evidence derived from other medical and general psychiatric populations. However, the use of antidepressants is not without risks, some potentially serious, and clinically significant interactions of these drugs may occur with other commonly prescribed medications in the cancer setting. Physicians working in the oncology setting should screen for depression, conduct diagnostic assessments, and institute appropriate treatment. Attention to the treatment of depression and to the potentially adverse effect of drug interactions associated with antidepressant medication are necessary to ensure safe and high quality patient care. Further research is needed regarding the interactions between antidepressant medication and chemotherapeutic agents, to assess their clinical significance, and on the efficacy of antidepressants across different cancer types and cancer settings.

References

Adelson KB, Loprinzi CL, Hershman DL. Treatment of hot flushes in breast and prostate cancer. Expert Opin Pharmacother. 2005;6(7):1095–106.

American Psychiatric Association (APA). Diagnostic and statistical manual of mental disorders. 5th ed. Arlington, VA: American Psychiatric Publishing; 2013.

American Psychiatric Association (APA). Practice guideline for the treatment of patients with major depressive disorder. 3rd ed; 2010. doi: 10.1176/appi.books.9780890423387.654001

Anderson IM, Ferrier IN, Baldwin RC, Cowen PJ, Howard L, Lewis G, Matthews K, McAllister-Williams RH, Peveler RC, Scott J, Tylee A. Evidence-based guidelines for treating depressive disorders with antidepressants: a revision of the 2000 British Association for Psychopharmacology guidelines. J Psychopharmacol. 2008;22(4):343–96.

Barbui C, Cipriani A, Patel V, Barbui C, Cipriani A, Patel V, Ayuso-Mateos JL, van Ommeren M. Efficacy of antidepressants and benzodiazepines in minor depression: systematic review and meta-analysis. Br J Psychiatry. 2011;198(1):11–6. sup. 1.

Baumeister H. Inappropriate prescriptions of antidepressant drugs in patients with subthreshold to minor depression: time for the evidence to become practice. J Affect Disord. 2012;139(3):240–3.

Blier P, Tremblay P. Physiologic mechanisms underlying the antidepressant discontinuation syndrome. J Clin Psychiatry. 2006;67 Suppl 4:8–13.

Boyer EW, Shannon M. The serotonin syndrome. N Engl J Med. 2005;352:1112–20 [Erratum in: N Engl J Med 2007 Jun 7; 356(23):2437. N Engl J Med 2009 Oct 22; 361(17):1714].

Breitbart W. Do antidepressants reduce the effectiveness of tamoxifen? Psychooncology. 2011;20 (1):1–4.

Caruso R, Grassi L, Nanni MG, Riba M. Psychopharmacology in psycho-oncology. Curr Psychiatry Rep. 2013;15(9):393.

Chochinov HM, Wilson KG, Enns M, Lander S. Depression, hopelessness, and suicidal ideation. Psychosomatics. 1998;39(4):366–70.

Colleoni M, Mandala M, Peruzzotti G, Robertson C, Bredart A, Goldhirsch A. Depression and degree of acceptance of adjuvant cytotoxic drugs. Lancet. 2000;356(9238):1326–7.

Coupland C, Dhiman P, Morriss R, Arthur A, Barton B, Hippisley-Cox J. Antidepressant use and risk of adverse outcomes in older people: population based cohort study. BMJ. 2011;343: d4551.

Desmarais JE, Looper KJ. Interactions between tamoxifen and antidepressants via cytochrome P450 2D6. J Clin Psychiatry. 2009;70(12):1688–97.

Driessen E, Cuijpers P, Hollon SD, Dekker JJ. Does pretreatment severity moderate the efficacy of psychological treatment of adult outpatient depression? A meta-analysis. J Consult Clin Psychol. 2010;78(5):668–80.

Egger C, Muehlbacher M, Nickel M, Geretsegger C, Stuppaeck C. A review on hyponatremia associated with SSRIs, reboxetine and venlafaxine. Int J Psychiatry Clin Pract. 2006;10(1):17–26.

Fitzgerald P, Lo C, Li M, Gagliese L, Zimmermann C, Rodin G. The relationship between depression and physical symptom burden in advanced cancer. BMJ Support Palliat Care. Published Online First: 13 August 2013. doi: 10.1136/bmjspcare-2012-000380

Fournier JC, DeRubeis RJ, Hollon SD, Dimidjian S, Amsterdam JD, Shelton RC, Fawcett J. Antidepressant drug effects and depression severity: a patient-level meta-analysis. JAMA. 2010;303(1):47–53.

Grassi L, Indelli M, Marzola M, Maestri A, Santini A, Piva E, Boccalon M. Depressive symptoms and quality of life in home-care-assisted cancer patients. J Pain Symptom Manage. 1996;12 (5):300–7.

Hegerl U, Schonknecht P, Mergl R. Are antidepressants useful in the treatment of minor depression: a critical update of the current literature. Curr Opin Psychiatry. 2012;25(1):1–6.

Hopko DR, Bell JL, Armento ME, Robertson SM, Hunt MK, Wolf NJ, Mullane C. The phenomenology and screening of clinical depression in cancer patients. J Psychosoc Oncol. 2008;26 (1):31–51.

Iovieno N, Tedeschini E, Ameral VE, Rigatelli M, Papakostas GI. Antidepressants for major depressive disorder in patients with a co-morbid axis III disorder: a metaanalysis of patient characteristics and placebo response rates in randomized controlled trials. Int Clin Psychopharmacol. 2011;26(2):69–74.

Isacsson G, Rich CL, Jureidini J, Raven M. The increased use of antidepressants has contributed to the worldwide reduction in suicide rates. Br J Psychiatry. 2010;196(6):429–33.

Kerr CW, Drake J, Milch RA, Brazeau DA, Skretny JA, Brazeau GA, Donnelly JP. Effects of methylphenidate on fatigue and depression: a randomized, double-blind, placebo-controlled trial. J Pain Symptom Manage. 2012;43(1):68–77.

Laoutidis ZG, Mathiak K. Antidepressants in the treatment of depression/depressive symptoms in cancer patients: a systematic review and meta-analysis. BMC Psychiatry. 2013;13:140. doi:10. 1186/1471-244X-13-140.

Lash TL, Cronin-Fenton D, Ahern TP, Rosenberg CL, Lunetta KL, Silliman RA, Garne JP, Sørensen HT, Hellberg Y, Christensen M, Pedersen L, Hamilton-Dutoit S. CYP2D6 inhibition and breast cancer recurrence in a population-based study in. Denmark J Natl Cancer Inst. 2011;103(6):489–500.

Li M, Fitzgerald P, Rodin G. Evidence-based treatment of depression in patients with cancer. J Clin Oncol. 2012;30(11):1187–96.

Looper KJ. Potential medical and surgical complications of serotonergic antidepressant medications. Psychosomatics. 2007;48(1):1–9.

Lydiatt WM, Denman D, McNeilly DP, Puumula SE, Burke WJ. A randomized, placebo-controlled trial of citalopram for the prevention of major depression during treatment for head and neck cancer. Arch Otolaryngol Head Neck Surg. 2008;134(5):528–35.

Lydiatt WM, Bessette D, Schmid KK, Sayles H, Burke WJ. Prevention of depression with escitalopram in patients undergoing treatment for head and neck cancer: randomized, double-blind, placebo-controlled clinical trial. JAMA Otolaryngol Head Neck Surg. 2013;139(7):678–86.

Massie MJ. Prevalence of depression in patients with cancer. J Natl Cancer Inst Monogr. 2004;32:57–71.

Miguel C, Albuquerque E. Drug interaction in psycho-oncology: antidepressants and antineoplastics. Pharmacology. 2011;88(5–6):333–9.

Mitchell AJ. Screening for cancer-related distress: when is implementation successful and when is it unsuccessful? Acta Oncol. 2013;52(2):216–24.

Mitchell AJ, Meader N, Symonds P. Diagnostic validity of the hospital anxiety and depression scale (HADS) in cancer and palliative settings: a meta-analysis. J Affect Disord. 2010;126 (3):335–48.

Mitchell AJ, Chan M, Bhatti H, Halton M, Grassi L, Johansen C, Meader N. Prevalence of depression, anxiety, and adjustment disorder in oncological, haematological, and palliative-care settings: a meta-analysis of 94 interview-based studies. Lancet Oncol. 2011;12(2):160–74.

Mitchell AJ, Meader N, Davies E, Clover K, Carter GL, Loscalzo MJ, Linden W, Grassi L, Johansen C, Carlson LE, Zabora J. Meta-analysis of screening and case finding tools for depression in cancer: evidence based recommendations for clinical practice on behalf of the depression in cancer care consensus group. J Affect Disord. 2012;140(2):149–60.

Musselman DL, Lawson DH, Gumnick JF, Manatunga AK, Penna S, Goodkin RS, Greiner K, Nemeroff CB, Miller AH. Paroxetine for the prevention of depression induced by high-dose interferon alfa. N Engl J Med. 2001;344:961–6.

National Institute for Health and Care Excellence (NICE). Depression: the treatment and management of depression in adults. NICE Clinical Guideline 90; 2009. http://guidance.nice.org.uk/cg90

Okamura M, Akizuki N, Nakano T, Shimizu K, Ito T, Akechi T, Uchitomi Y. Clinical experience of the use of a pharmacological treatment algorithm for major depressive disorder in patients with advanced cancer. Psychooncology. 2008;17(2):154–60.

Rayner L, Price A, Evans A, Valsraj K, Hotopf M, Higginson IJ. Antidepressants for the treatment of depression in palliative care: systematic review and meta-analysis. Palliat Med. 2011;25 (1):36–51.

Richards S, Umbreit JN, Fanucchi MP, Giblin J, Khuri F. Selective serotonin reuptake inhibitor-induced rhabdomyolysis associated with irinotecan. South Med J. 2003;96(10):1031–3.

Riechelmann RP, Burman D, Tannock IF, Rodin G, Zimmermann C. Phase II trial of mirtazapine for cancer-related cachexia and anorexia. Am J Hosp Palliat Care. 2010;27(2):106–10.

Rodin G, Zimmermann C, Rydall A, Jones J, Shepherd FA, Moore M, Fruh M, Donner A, Gagliese L. The desire for hastened death in patients with metastatic cancer. J Pain Symptom Manage. 2007;33(6):661–75.

Rowe SK, Rapaport MH. Classification and treatment of sub-threshold depression. Curr Opin Psychiatry. 2006;19(1):9–13.

Schneeweiss S, Patrick AR, Solomon DH, Mehta J, Dormuth C, Miller M, Lee JC, Wang PS. Variation in the risk of suicide attempts and completed suicides by antidepressant agents in adults: a propensity score-adjusted analysis of 9 years' data. Arch Gen Psychiatry. 2010;67 (5):497–506.

Stone M, Laughren T, Jones ML, Levenson M, Holland PC, Hughes A, Hammad TA, Temple R, Rochester G. Risk of suicidality in clinical trials of antidepressants in adults: analysis of proprietary data submitted to US food and drug administration. BMJ. 2009;339:b2880.

Taylor S, Harley C, Campbell LJ, Bingham L, Podmore EJ, Newsham AC, Selby PJ, Brown JM, Velikova G. Discussion of emotional and social impact of cancer during outpatient oncology consultations. Psychooncology. 2011a;20(3):242–51.

Taylor D, Meader N, Bird V, Pilling S, Creed F, Goldberg D, Pharmacology Subgroup of the National Institute for Health and Clinical Excellence Guideline Development Group for Depression in Chronic Physical Health Problems. Pharmacological interventions for people with depression and chronic physical health problems: systematic review and meta-analyses of safety and efficacy. Br J Psychiatry. 2011b;198(3):179–88.

Thekkumpurath P, Walker J, Butcher I, Hodges L, Kleiboer A, O'Connor M, Wall L, Murray G, Kroenke K, Sharpe M. Screening for major depression in cancer outpatients: the diagnostic accuracy of the 9-item patient health questionnaire. Cancer. 2011;117(1):218–27.

Treatment of Somatoform Disorders and Other Somatic Symptom Conditions (Pain, Fatigue, Hot Flashes, and Pruritus)

10

Santosh K. Chaturvedi, Valentina Ieraci, and Riccardo Torta

Abstract

This chapter summarizes the role of pharmacological treatment of somatoform disorders and other somatic symptom conditions like cancer pain, cancer-related fatigue, hot flashes, pruritus, anorexia and weight loss, and nausea and vomiting. This chapter highlights the importance of sensitive exploration of somatic symptoms and appropriate intervention. In addition it gives an account of the biological and neurotransmitter mechanisms underlying the action of psychotropic medications on these somatic symptoms. In clinical situations, the psychotropic medications need to be started early and in low doses. The dose should be increased gradually with caution towards the physical side effects on medications. The medications need to be given for a relatively short period of time. When the somatic symptoms are a part of another disorder, like anxiety or depressive disorder, the somatic symptoms remit with the improvement in the underlying disorder. Common side effects, the likelihood of serious adverse events, the route of administration, and the possible drug–drug interactions are all factors that should be considered when selecting a medication, given the fact that most cancer patients are taking many other medications. Relief of somatic symptoms in cancer patients can usually be achieved and is worth the effort as these symptoms may impair the overall quality of life.

S.K. Chaturvedi (✉)
Psychiatric Rehabilitation Services, National Institute of Mental Health and Neurosciences, Bangalore, India
e-mail: skchatur@yahoo.com

V. Ieraci • R. Torta
Department of Neuroscience, University of Turin, Turin, Italy
e-mail: valentina.ieraci@unito.it; riccardo.torta@unito.it

L. Grassi and M. Riba (eds.), *Psychopharmacology in Oncology and Palliative Care*,
DOI 10.1007/978-3-642-40134-3_10, © Springer-Verlag Berlin Heidelberg 2014

10.1 Introduction

Somatoform disorders and somatic symptoms in cancer have attracted clinical and research interest over the last two or three decades. In a way, clinicians found it difficult to conceptualize the occurrence of physical symptoms in a medical disorder occurring due to psychological or emotional factors. In medical disorders, the clinical features are always represented by physical symptoms that are different depending on the different body system involved. But physical or somatic symptoms do not actually occur only in medical diseases but also in psychiatric disorders, in which symptoms are not exclusively represented by emotional, psychological, or cognitive ones. Consequently, when physical symptoms occur in people with a medical disease, such symptoms are believed to be due to the underlying medical disease or its treatment (Chaturvedi et al. 2006). Nevertheless, in a sample of 560 consecutive outpatients, with a major depressive episode, "unexplained" somatic symptoms (i.e., somatic symptoms that are not related to a concomitant physical illness or its treatment) were reported in 84 % of patients (Perugi et al. 2011). Thus, it is possible that emotional disorders, particularly depressive disorders, may manifest with somatic symptoms also in medical diseases, including cancer. It is known that depressive disorder is a systemic disease with several somatic cluster manifestations (Torta and Munari 2010). The term *somatization* refers to patients with emotional problems that express their personal and social distress through bodily complaints and medical help-seeking (Grassi et al. 2013); usually such complaint occurs in the absence of any identifiable organic cause. Understandably, the identification of somatoform disorders is even more difficult when a medical disease is present, because it can be extremely difficult to differentiate somatoform symptoms from those caused by the organic disease. The clinical situation is more complex when a physical symptom, for example, pain or fatigue, demonstrates emotional and physical components, simultaneously.

High levels of somatization have been found in several medical conditions, such as otological (Bakir et al. 2013; Genç et al. 2013), dermatologic (Hassel et al. 2011), gastroenterological (Lee et al. 2012); neurological (Lee et al. 2011; Siri et al. 2010); and endocrinal pathologies (Sonino et al. 2007). Similar data are also demonstrated for patients with cancer (Chaturvedi and Maguire 1998) and cardiological diseases (Laederach-Hofmann et al. 2008). On the other hand, the medical approach to the patients is mainly focused on the physical rather than the psychosocial dimensions: for example, in cancer patients, symptoms such as nausea, vomiting, fatigue, and pain are almost exclusively ascribed to cancer and cancer treatments, and the likelihood that these symptoms are related to possible psychological factors remains low (Grassi et al. 2013).

A poor understanding and distinguishing these somatic symptoms, when present in patients with medical diseases, may result to increase the frequency of requests for medical consultations, unnecessary diagnostic investigations, length of hospitalization (and related costs), non-adherence to treatments, and also wrong therapeutic approaches. These factors negatively affect the clinical outcomes and,

Table 10.1 Factors
related to somatization in
cancer

- Abnormal illness behavior
- Attribution styles
- Somatosensory amplification
- Alexithymia
- Pain catastrophizing
- Psychiatric disorders like anxiety, depression

consequently, the health-related quality of life (Hungin et al. 2009; Shaw and Creed 1991; Thistle et al. 2011; Trafton et al. 2011).

10.1.1 Factors Related to Somatic Presentations

A somatic presentation of an emotional disorder depends on several factors such as personality and other difficulties to express emotional disturbances, cultural and medical context, and so forth. Some factors related to somatization, and particularly with pain, are given in Table 10.1.

Abnormal illness behavior refers how individuals monitor their body and experience and evaluate and respond to their state of health; an abnormal behavior indicates a maladaptive pattern characterized by hypochondriacal disposal, disease conviction with refusal of medical opinion, dysphoria, and friction in interpersonal relationships (Pilowsky 1994). Several studies confirm the relevance of this dimension in cancer patients (Grassi et al. 1989; Grassi and Rosti 1996).

A 41-year-old lady treated for breast cancer with total mastectomy, chemotherapy, and radiation treatment was declared as disease free by her medical team. After a year of the treatment, she started reporting tiredness. The investigations did not reveal any signs of anemia or a medical reason for this tiredness. She would visit the doctors frequently and could not be reassured. She feared if the treatment was incomplete. There were mild depressive features following these symptoms. Preoccupation with her health and body was excessive. A cognitive behavioral approach held her to a certain extent. Sertraline 25 mg was given, which proved to be helpful to some more extent. The features were suggestive of health anxiety and abnormal illness behavior.

Attribution style (Pompili et al. 1990) concerns how individuals process their symptoms: relating them to environmental events (normalizing attributional style), rather than to a psychological status (psychological attributional style) or to a physical background only (somatic attributional style). This last style is predictive of the number of obscure somatic complaints, particularly pain, which patients report to the doctor. Attribution styles, and consequent illness behavior, are also determined by the culture and organization of the health service itself (Cheatle et al. 2012).

Somatosensory amplification is the tendency to experience somatic sensations as intense, noxious, and disturbing. It is linked to bodily hypervigilance, to focusing on weak and infrequent sensations, and considering most visceral and somatic sensations as abnormal (Sarkisian et al. 2007), and it can exacerbate the experience of somatic sensations, particularly in older patients (Torta and Munari 2010).

Alexithymia refers to a condition where individuals are unable to verbally describe their emotional problems, but mainly express them somatically. Alexithymic patients demonstrate higher levels of depressed mood and pain when evaluated in chronic pain conditions (Castelli et al. 2012, 2013; De Vries et al. 2012; Saariaho et al. 2013). Of notable interest is the concept of "secondary alexithymia" which refers to patients with a chronic disease, such as cancer or chronic pain, who focus on the somatic background of the illness and develop an alexithymic style in social relationships (Duddu et al. 2006). Moreover, alexithymic patients show amplified activity in areas considered to be involved in physical sensation, and also an increase in hormonal arousal responses during visceral pain, associated with greater activity of the insula, anterior cingulate cortex, and midbrain (Kano and Fukudo 2013).

Pain catastrophizing is the tendency to ruminate on pain sensations, to feel helpless about pain and to magnify beliefs and feelings toward the painful situation. Catastrophizing is a strong predictor of negative pain-related outcomes, such as clinical pain intensity, and physical disability (Campbell et al. 2012; Pulvers and Hood 2013).

Psychiatric Disorders Anxiety and depressive disorders are commonly observed in cancer patients, and emotional changes of these disorders can influence pain or somatic perception, which may result in heightened experiences of pain and other somatic symptoms, such as fatigue, pruritus, and hot flushes. Somatization is therefore a multisomatoform disorder, characterized by medically unexplained, functional, or psychosomatic symptoms. But similar symptoms (such as hyperalgesia, fatigue, autonomic symptoms, sexual disorders, sleep disorders) are also present in the somatic depressive cluster (Torta and Munari 2010). In cancer patients, experiences of somatic symptoms, due to the disease itself, may be exaggerated because of emotional factors or somatization (Chaturvedi et al. 2006). Moreover, somatic symptoms in cancer patients may be related to a psychiatric disorder (and be independent of cancer) or to the chemotherapy and/or radiation therapy, that may contribute both to mood depression and also cause somatic symptoms.

10.1.2 Diagnosis of Somatic Symptoms Disorders

One of the most relevant problems concerning somatization is the difficulty to make the clinical diagnosis by the usual diagnostic systems, such as the DSM and the ICD. It is possible that the recent reconceptualization of somatiziation and somatoform disorders in the DSM5 category of Somatic Symptom Disorder (SSD) will be of some help in oncology settings. SSD in fact, on the one hand, deletes the term "medically unexplained symptoms," which creates clear problem when dealing with patients with a real medical illness, such as cancer, and, on the other, focuses attention not only on the somatic symptoms themselves but also on the implications on the individual's emotions, thinking, and behavior (Dimsdale et al. 2013). However, several revisions and changes of the classical psychiatric nosological criteria have been proposed over time (Fava and Wise 2007; Kroenke et al. 2007; Sirri et al. 2011), including the most recent DSM 5 (Sirri and Fava 2013). In brief, the proposals suggest a more etiological approach, the use of dimensions rather than categories, changes in the threshold definitions, and issues of reliability, validity, and utility (Grassi et al. 2013).

In the field of diagnostic research, an interesting instrument is represented by Diagnostic Criteria for Psychosomatic Research (DCPR) (Fava et al. 1995; Porcelli and Todarello 2012). The DCPR consists of 12 dimensions grouped into five clusters (i.e., abnormal illness behavior, somatization, irritability, demoralization and alexithymia), and it is extremely helpful in identifying psychosocial dimensions, including somatization, that are difficult to recognize by using standard nosology (Fava et al. 2012).

The use of DCPR in cancer patients demonstrates that 38.1 % were positive for at least one DCPR cluster, with particular reference to AIB (e.g., health anxiety), demoralization, and alexithymia, and that these dimensions were related to higher levels of cancer-related worries and to a poorer quality of life (Grassi et al. 2004). DCPR was also able to diagnose psychological construct such as health anxiety (Grassi et al. 2005).

Thus, somatization in cancer settings can magnify the disability resulting from illness in itself, interfere with adherence to treatments, determine healthcare overutilization, and contribute to poorer outcome and quality of life (Grassi et al. 2013). Hence, treatment of somatic symptoms and somatoform disorders in cancer needs to take into account the above discussion about the intricate and complex phenomena.

10.2 Pharmacological Treatment of Somatoform Disorders in Cancer

Pharmacological interventions should be used carefully and monitored regularly for the treatment of somatoform disorders in oncology. This medical management can play an important role in the treatment of cancer patients suffering from somatic symptoms and syndromes. There are not many studies on the occurrence of somatic symptoms or somatoform disorders in palliative care and hence not much is known by way of evidence-based interventions.

The management of somatoform disorders in cancer requires a combination of psychosocial and pharmacological methods. Low-dose antidepressants are effective though one has to be careful of the drug side effects, as the physical side effects may be further misinterpreted as worsening of disease or new somatic symptoms. The somatoform disorders also need to be managed by behavioral and/or psychosocial methods besides antidepressant medications (Chaturvedi and Uchitomi 2012).

Case Vignette

A 32-year-old gentleman was treated for non-Hodgkins lymphoma successfully. During a follow-up visit, he reported fine tremors of both hands. There was no family history of essential tremor. Neurologists rules out any neurological cause for these. There were no features of autonomic anxiety or depression. Sleep and appetite were normal. The tremors were distressing to the person and causing health worry. He wondered if it was a sign of his disease recurring. He was counseled about the nature of the symptom and given relaxation exercises. He found these strategies useful and reduced his health worries.

Both psychiatric and cancer symptoms should be assessed as cancer patients may be more likely to using medications, if they find benefit in both of these aspects. Many a times the patient will experience improvement in some symptoms quickly like anxiety or sleep disturbance. A good compliance with medication gives additional benefits within few weeks such as improvement in depressive symptoms.

These somatic symptoms are often common causes for medical consultation, but their treatment is complicated by lack of boundary, conceptual clarity, and overemphasis on psychosocial causation and effectiveness of psychological treatments. Actually, most patients with somatoform symptoms are managed by primary care physicians and only severe or chronic cases need specialist treatment: these patients are usually treated with antidepressants, but an effective management of somatoform symptoms is based on fostering a treatment adherence, through a psycho-education and an adequate information about symptoms and their pathogenesis (Gupta et al. 2007; van-Schreiber et al. 2000). In other words, primary care physicians have to maintain a dual role, both on monitoring the patient's physical status and paying attention to psychosocial stress factors that strongly impact on the patient's somatic condition (Gupta et al. 2007).

Several problems that can interfere with such therapeutic management of somatic symptoms are given in Table 10.2.

The difficulty of a correct management of somatization in cancer patients arise also from the fact that somatic symptoms in cancer patients, for example, pain and fatigue, have both organic and psychological components concomitantly (Torta and Ieraci 2013a). Therefore, in order to understand the rationale for the use of psychotropic drugs, and particularly antidepressants, for the treatment of somatic symptoms, it is important to consider certain factors.

Table 10.2 Problems interfering with therapeutic management of somatic symptoms

- The presence of comorbid medical conditions
- Patients' poor awareness
- Poor acceptance of the concept of somatization
- His/her requests for diagnostic investigations
- Frequent "doctor shopping"
- Abnormal illness behavior

First at all, depressive disorder has to be considered as a systemic disease that involves not only peculiar circuits of the central nervous systems, but concerns the total body. In this way, emotional and somatic symptoms overlap and, in each patient, several clinical features, such as pain, fatigue, and sexual disorders, have a double and concomitant psychological and somatic component. Other pathogenic biological hypotheses for depression, complementary to the neurotransmitter-related hypothesis, must also be considered. In any case, the neurotransmitter-related hypothesis of depression must be considered as a widespread somatic pathology, because serotonin (5HT), norepinephrine (NE), and dopamine (DA) are systemic transmitters and not only transmitters within the brain. Therefore, the activity of an antidepressant, that increases the availability of a transmitter, concerns all the body, with a widespread somatic response.

In the hormonal hypothesis of mood depression, several circuits are involved: the hypothalamus-pituitary-adrenocortical axis (HPA), the hypothalamus-pituitary-gonadic axis (HPG), and the hypothalamus-pituitary-thyroid axis (HPA). The hyper-activation of HPA axis, during mood depression, chronic stress, and anxiety, implies an increased release of the hypothalamic factor CRF (Cortisol Releasing Factor) that together with ACTH, cortisol, and vasopressin activates behavior and autonomic responses. Within these circuits, antidepressants reduce the excessive CRF response and the downstream cortisolemic and autonomic alterations. Concerning HPG axis, an important relationship exists between estrogen levels and mood, as confirmed by depression during menopause, after delivery, and, in several cancer patients, after the use of antiestrogen drugs; antidepressants are able to increase the estrogen level produced within brain, thereby regulating the emotional responses related to these hormones, as also confirmed by their effectiveness in improving the phenomenon of hot flashes due to surgical or pharmacological estrogenic depletion (Biglia et al. 2005).

Moreover, the chronic release of glucocorticoids and glutamate, due to the prolonged HPA activation and the increase of proinflammatory cytokines, can induce hippocampal neuronal death and, consequently, shrinkage of this area, as found in several neuroimaging studies of depression and other psychiatric pathologies that may be associated with chronic stress (Anacker et al. 2010). With regard to the neurotrophic hypothesis of depression, antidepressants exert a protective activity on hippocampal neurons, through an increase of the antidepressant-induced production of neurotrophic factors, such as BDNF and NGF (Russo-Neustadt and Chen 2005; Hashimoto 2010). In oncology, such neurogenic effects facilitated by antidepressants can also be useful to counteract the neuronal damage induced by some chemotherapies, thus reducing the neuropathic, cognitive, emotional, and biological consequences during chemotherapies (Durand et al. 2012).

Of major importance, for the use of antidepressants in oncology, is the immunological hypothesis of depression, stating that chronic stress induces a "neuroinflammation" through an increased release of pro-inflammatory cytokines. Particularly at the Central Nervous System (CNS) level, the activation of microglia causes several responses, including, on one hand, an increase of pro-inflammatory cytokines, a reduction of glutamate reuptake, and an increase of glutamate release (increasing excitoxicity) and on the other hand, an induction of IDO, an enzyme that can divert tryptophan from the pathway of serotonin production (causing depression) to the pathway of kinurenines (Krishnadas and Cavanagh 2012; McCarthy et al. 2012; Torta and Ieraci 2013a). The cytokine increase is responsible of a frequent cluster of symptoms (so-called *sickness behavior*), present in oncologic patients (that is characterized by hyperpathy, fatigue, apathy, hyporexia, increased sleep, libido reduction), and it is due to the same pathogenetic background both in inflammation and mood depression. The role of antidepressants in this pathogenetic key is well demonstrated by the fact that they induce an increase of anti-inflammatory cytokines that counteracts the depressant activity of pro-inflammatory ones. This statement is largely confirmed by the protective activity exerted by antidepressants against depression induced by interferon (Capuron et al. 2004). Thus, antidepressants can improve, through these wide activities on hormones and immune system, both the somatic and the psychological component of several symptoms of somatization, particularly pain and fatigue.

Anderson et al. (2013) used the term "physio-somatic" to describe these symptoms resulting from inflammation, immune response, alterations in the tryptophan/kynurenine pathway, and that are present in mood disorder, chronic fatigue syndrome, fibromyalgia, or somatization, suggesting the presence of an emerging organic explanation.

On the other hand, the psychodynamic, and particularly the psychoanalytical, pathogenic interpretation of the somatizing process is clearly expressed by the Paris psychoanalytical school. Two forms of the somatizing process can be recognized: *somatizing through regression*, that typically occurs among subjects whose psychic functioning is organized on a neurotic–normal mode, and the *somatizing process through drive unbinding*, that usually ends in progressive and serious illness such as autoimmune diseases or cancer. All these cases are characterized by a dimension of narcissistic loss that must be correlated to a state of drive unbinding, with a consequent alteration of the subject's psychosomatic equilibrium (Aisenstein and Smadja 2010).

In clinical practice all classes of psychotropics, and particularly antidepressants, are used to treat somatic symptom disorder. Five principal groups of such drugs used are given in Table 10.3.

These psychotropic drugs have been systematically studied in this context and are proved as effective against somatoform and related disorders (Somashekar et al. 2013). SSRIs seem to be more effective against hypochondriasis and body

Table 10.3 Psychotropics used in treatment of somatic symptom disorders	• Tricyclic antidepressants (TCA)
	• Selective serotonin reuptake inhibitors (SSRI)
	• Serotonin and noradrenalin reuptake inhibitors (SNRI)
	• Atypical antipsychotics
	• Herbal medications

dysmorphic disorder (BDD), and SNRIs appear to be more effective than other antidepressants when pain is the predominant symptom. Nevertheless, many unanswered questions concern dosing, duration of treatment, sustainability of improvement in the long term, and differential response to different class drugs (Somashekar et al. 2013).

Psychological interventions for somatization in cancer patients should be aimed at reducing symptoms and improving functioning, by exploring patients' suffering not only in a biological context but also in a psychosocial perspective. Cognitive behavioral therapy (CBT) aims at facilitating patients' identification of their incorrect beliefs about their symptoms and bodily functioning as well as identification of related dysfunctional, avoidable behaviors (Gupta et al. 2007).

However, pharmacological and psychological studies are lacking in the treatment of somatization disorders concerning cancer patients. Frequently, somatic symptoms in cancer patients differ from those observed in psychiatric illness in their context, presentation, severity, duration, and illness behavior. First of all, it is of great importance that clinicians clarify the nature of somatic symptoms and, if no evidence exists of illness progression or recurrence, reassure patients and use techniques facilitating emotional expression (Chaturvedi and Maguire 1998).

To our knowledge there are no controlled trials assessing psychopharmacologic treatment for somatization in cancer patients. Two studies indicated an improvement in somatic symptoms, depression, and anxiety scores secondary to the use of antidepressants (Chaturvedi and Maguire 1998; Chaturvedi et al. 1993). The advantageous use of antidepressants medication in this context is helpful both in treating the somatic component of pain and fatigue (vide infra) and in improving the emotional component associated to the possible superimposed somatoform disorder or in treating the frequent comorbid conditions such as anxiety, depression, and chronic stress. For example, medications that enhance both serotonin and norepinephrine reuptake inhibition, such as duloxetine, venlafaxine, and milnacipran work, in a cancer patient with an emotional exacerbation of pain related to illness or with a somatization that get worse with the true somatic pain, acting on all components, somatic and psychological ones.

Cognitive behavioral therapy, relaxation, and educational approaches may decrease anxiety and tension. The role of counseling is of paramount importance in explaining the nature of somatic symptoms in cancer patients and reassuring them that these symptoms are not indicative of progression of disease, relapse or recurrence, or failure to respond to treatment. Efforts are needed to be made to reduce the somatic concern and preoccupation by distraction and engagement in other recreational activities (Allen and Woolfolk 2010; Chaturvedi et al. 2006; Janca et al. 2006).

Pharmacological, psychotherapeutic, and educational interventions in patients with somatization and cancer must be integrated, and frequently enlarged to the familiar context, in order to face contemporary the biological and psychosocial components of such disorders.

10.3 Pharmacological Treatment of Pain and Chronic Pain in Cancer

More than a third of patients undergoing therapy for cancer and 60–90 % of those with advanced malignancy report significant pain (Foley 2000, 2011). Major depression is commonly present in patients with chronic pain, and the presence of painful symptoms is highly predictive of subsequent major depression (Torta and Munari 2010). Thus, pain intensity depends both on the extent of tissue damage and on the patient's psychological state (Baines 1989) that interferes also in the cancer pain relief (Chaturvedi and Maguire 1998; Torta and Ieraci 2013). The emotional components, in particular, may play a consistent role in the experience of cancer pain, due to its underlying correlation to illness progression or treatment effects, the sense of hopelessness, and the fear that pain can represent a sign of impending death may increase pain (Chaturvedi et al. 2006; Fishbain et al. 2009; Genç and Tan 2011). This relationship has been shown to be reciprocal in that increasing pain intensity leads to greater psychological distress, while pain relief is associated with decreases in distress (Castelli et al. 2013). Somatizing patients, moreover, can show poorer outcomes in pain management, as somatization appears to be a predictor of non-adherence to pharmacologic prescriptions (over- or under-use) (Trafton et al. 2011). Both biological and psychological factors contribute to pain perception. Several psychological factors can modulate pain, such as emotional disorders, prolonged mood depression, chronic anxiety and/or stress, or type of temperament and coping styles, all of which interfere with the individual functioning levels (Torta and Ieraci 2013).

Therapeutic approaches to pain are multifaceted because they have to deal with the complex pain pathogenesis involving biological, psychological, cognitive, and social factors. Consequently, the choice of pain treatment for a patient has to face different pain components (physical, emotional, cognitive, and relational): in this way, pharmacological and non-pharmacological interventions are frequently integrated.

Analgesics, antidepressants, and anticonvulsants frequently have to be utilized to obtain complete remission of pain, particularly when it is comorbid with emotional aspects such as chronic stress, anxiety, and mood depression. Moreover, when the emotional, cognitive, or social pain component is relevant in a given patient, non-pharmacological interventions, such as a psycho-educational or psycho-therapeutic project, must also be associated with the analgesic prescription. In the presence of emotional disorders associated with pain (anxiety, mood depression, chronic stress), the first class of choice among the adjuvants are antidepressants (ADs). ADs are drugs with a broad spectrum of clinical activities, acting on mood depression, anxiety, chronic stress, and pain.

ADs relieve pain through several different mechanisms, and the pain relief is obtained through the same pharmacological mechanisms involved in mood depression (Torta and Munari 2010).

- Neurotransmitter activity, particularly on 5HT and NE, is strictly involved in the fast and direct pain mitigating effect, which is mainly linked to the inhibition of rapid reuptake, with a consequent almost immediate increase of neurotransmitters at the synaptic level. This direct action appears in the first hours after administration of antidepressants and can also be present with low dosages. Such clinical response is not related to the AD's effect on mood.
- The indirect antidepressant pain mitigating effect, on the other hand, appears later, with improvement of the depressed mood after 3–4 weeks of treatment at full dosages. This activity, related to an increase of the threshold for pain (which is reduced by mood depression), is achieved when ADs normalize mood through complex mechanisms (receptor downregulation, HPA normalization, etc.) involved in the slow antidepressant's activity (Torta and Ieraci 2013a).
- Reduction of cytokine pro-inflammatory activity: high cytokine levels actually correlate with mood depression, cognitive dysfunction, pain, and stress levels, as confirmed also by neuroimaging studies (Baudino et al. 2012). ADs counteract the pro-inflammatory activity of cytokines by several mechanisms: reducing CRH activation (and consequently the secondary HPA response to hyperproduction of cytokines), normalizing IDO induction (and secondary tryptophan depletion with reduced 5HT availability), and contributing to the production of anti-inflammatory cytokines (Torta and Ieraci 2013).

An important consequence, coming by the fact that analgesics and antidepressants both act on the structures regulating mood and pain, is that clinicians have carefully to consider the interactions between antidepressants and analgesics. When associated with serotonergic antidepressants (such as SSRIs or SNRIs), several opioids (fentanyl, oxycodone, methadone, etc.) can, in predisposed patients, favor the appearance of a serotonergic syndrome. Actually, through a reduction of GABAergic inhibition, opioids induce an increase of 5HT release, which, when associated with an increased availability of serotonin produced by SSRIs or SNRIs, can cause a serotonergic syndrome (Gnanadesigan et al. 2005). In this way the choice of an antidepressant for an oncologic patient is complex (Torta and Ieraci 2013) and has to face mainly dimensional clinical characteristics of depression, such as the particular symptomatological clusters of each patient (pain, anhedonia, anxiety, inhibition, somatic and cognitive symptoms, etc.).

The wide use of TCAs in patients with pain, particularly neuropathic, is due to their effectiveness. Nevertheless, TCAs induce a large number of side effects, mainly related to their blockade of several kinds of receptors. For this reason, the dosage of TCAs in patients with pain is usually low and inadequate for real antidepressant activity, even if necessary. In spite of a large body of literature concerning the use of TCAs on pain, up-to-date studies on neuropathic oncology pain are lacking. In the few studies available, TCAs are used with low doses, utilizing their sedative and intrinsic analgesic activity, without the synergistic antidepressant effect that is essential to normalize the pain threshold (Torta and Munari 2010).

SSRIs are also effective in several pain syndromes, both experimentally and clinically, because they work on the opioid systems. In several studies on neuropathic pain, SSRIs were less effective than TCAs but better tolerated, particularly in long-term treatments (Gharibian et al. 2013).

As an alternative to the less well-tolerated TCAs (Attal et al. 2010), the dual-acting antidepressants (venlafaxine, duloxetine, and milnacipram) are recommended within the guidelines for the use of antidepressants in neuropathic pain, because of their favorable balance between effectiveness and safety. Venlafaxine (75 mg/day) reduces uncontrolled pain and concomitantly acts on its cognitive and emotional aspects, encouraging better adjustment by the patient to the disease. Duloxetine also demonstrates contextual activity on pain and mood in oncology patients (Torta et al. 2011). In summary, in the presence of uncontrolled pain, particularly if neurogenic, SNRIs should be preferred to SSRIs, because of their double activity on 5HT and NE, and to TCAs, because of their safety concerning side effects.

10.3.1 Psychological Interventions for Pain

Cognitive and emotional components of pain widely justify the psychotherapeutic approach to pain perception. Psychotherapies differ with regard to their approach, perspectives, and goals. CBT, for instance, focuses on the patient's belief system related to problematic behaviors and is often used to modify cognitive strategies and reduce excessive problematic pain-associated behaviors, thus reducing pain perception. In this way, Kashikar-Zuck et al. (2013) recently confirmed CBT effectiveness in pain coping, catastrophizing, and coping efficacy, also in children and adolescents with juvenile fibromyalgia.

In a dynamically oriented therapy, on the other hand, the therapist focuses on integrating and interpreting the material brought forth by the patient in order for the patient to gain insight into its origin and to readjust behavioral recurring patterns. These therapies are designed to bring about fundamental emotional and cognitive changes and address relationship difficulties.

The pain components related to cognition and social aspects are sensitive to interventions that include patient education, and aerobic or other physical exercise, often integrated in a CBT. These non-pharmacological treatments, in particular exercise and CBT (cognitive-behavior therapy), have yielded effect sizes and cost–benefit ratios comparable to medications, particularly in the fibromyalgia context (Prinsloo et al. 2014). The most efficacious non-pharmacological approaches seem to be those with a focus on changing unhelpful beliefs/attitudes and activities associated with the illness. Other non-pharmacological interventions may benefit specific individuals (e.g., massage, nutritional approaches), but to date do not demonstrate sufficient evidence from randomized controlled trials to establish their efficacy (Casale et al. 2008). Noteworthy is the fact that exercise leads to changes in serum BDNF levels: this association highlights the importance of exercise in FMS and other chronic pain conditions (De Silva et al. 2010).

To conclude, an important bridge linking pharmacological and psychological treatment is the fact that both the pharmacodynamic and pharmacokinetic properties and the emotional aspects of the patient contribute to the effectiveness of a given drug. This consideration is strictly related to the placebo paradigm and mainly involves the patient's expectations concerning a given treatment.

10.4   Pharmacological Management of Cancer-Related Fatigue

Cancer-related fatigue (CRF) is a subjective sensation that is extremely more severe than the feeling of being tired, and it is characterized by being pervasive and not relieved by rest (Cella et al. 2002; Stone and Minton 2008; NCCN 2009). CRF is related to the disease in itself, increases its prevalence with advancing disease, and can also be a side effect of oncologic treatments (surgery, chemotherapy, and radiotherapy). Moreover, CRF can also affect disease-free survivors, and its presence represents an adjunctive cost in cancer management (Carlotto et al. 2013). Cancer-related fatigue (CRF) is present during all phases of the disease trajectory, with prevalence rates that range from 40 % to 100 %, during active treatments, and about 30 % in posttreatment survivors (Prue et al. 2006; Howell et al. 2013).

10.4.1 Pathophysiology of Cancer-Related Fatigue

The pathophysiology of cancer-related fatigue is poorly understood, but surely multifactorial, arising from a complex interplay of physical factors (such as the cancer in itself or its treatment, long lasting pain, etc.) and psychological (as mood disorder, chronic stress, insomnia), environmental (poor nutrition, deconditioning, support), physiological, and biological factors (such as an increase of inflammatory cytokines) (Barsevick et al. 2001; Howell et al. 2013) (Fig. 10.1).

A close relationship exists between fatigue severity and psychological distress in cancer patients, as also reported in patients with other chronic illnesses (Stone and Minton 2008): actually mechanisms that link stress and fatigue are mainly mediated by the HPA system and particularly through the increased release of proinflammatory cytokines due to the HPA hyper-activation during chronic stress (Torta and Ieraci 2013a). A quantitative, systematic review has reported a consistent correlation between interleukin 6 (IL-6), interleukin 1 receptor antibody (IL-1ra), neopterin, and CRF (Schubert et al. 2007). Moreover, the majority of cancer symptoms, including fatigue, are associated with inflammation (Laird et al. 2013).

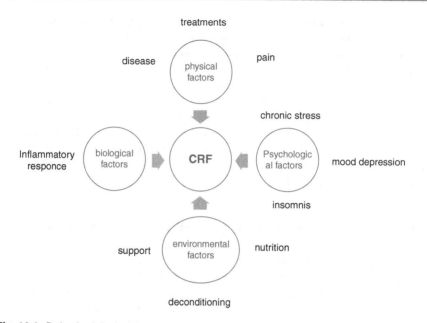

treatments

disease | physical factors | pain

chronic stress

Inflammatory responce | biological factors | CRF | Psychologic al factors | mood depression

insomnis

support | environmental factors | nutrition

deconditioning

Fig. 10.1 Pathophysiological factors involved in CRF

The NCCN Guideline (2009) recommends a complete evaluation with an in-depth fatigue history, including a review of clinical status and medications and a physical exam. Parameters that have to be taken into consideration are summarized in Table 10.4.

10.4.2 Management of Cancer-Related Fatigue

Treatment depends on the patient's overall situation and her/his different priorities, largely dependent on the stage of disease.

Nonpharmacologic interventions improving fatigue are mainly represented by physical therapy, such as enhanced physical activity (Kummer et al. 2013) or exercise, cognitive approaches, such CBT or psycho-educational ones, and psychosocial interventions (NCCN 2009).

Exercise

Exercise is an useful intervention that is supported by RCT data (Mitchell et al. 2007; Cuesta-Vargas et al. 2014), and it is mainly proposed as exercise programs based at home, concerning patients on treatment or disease-free survivors, while few data are disposable for palliative care population (Oldervoll et al. 2006). Moreover, a recent review of six studies revealed a statistically significant effect of exercise interventions in reducing general fatigue in children and adolescents with cancer (Chang et al. 2013).

Table 10.4 Parameters of assessment for cancer-related fatigue

Pattern of fatigue	Onset, duration, changes over time, relation to treatments
Patient description of fatigue	Clinical interview
Fatigue intensity evaluation	ESAS, FACT-F, FQ, DICRFS
Comorbid factors	Disease status, treatments, sleep, current medications, stressors, nutrition
Fatigue and daily living	Interferences on work, social life, cognitive performance
Contributing factors	Anemia, emotional disorders, pain, sedating medications, inflammation, sleep disturbances, inactivity, inadequate nutrition
Physical examination	Signs of anemia, vitamin deficiencies, muscle wasting

ESAS Edmonton Symptom Assessment System, *FACT-F* Functional Assessment of Cancer Therapy-Fatigue, *FQ* Fatigue Questionnaire, *DICRFS* Diagnostic Interview for Cancer-Related Fatigue Syndrome

Cognitive Behavioral Therapy

A meta-analysis carried out by Jacobsen et al. (2007) identified a heterogeneous group of interventions that included CBT, supportive and expressive therapies, and psycho-education. Overall, the authors reported a small but significant positive effect for psychological interventions when compared to controls. More recent studies also support the effectiveness of an educational intervention during chemotherapy (Ream et al. 2006), mainly through a reduction in the distress but with no change in CRF severity.

CBT is focused on the reframing of negative thinking patterns that can influence the perception of problems and, subsequently, behavior. Negative attributions are reported in patients with CRF, and warped perceptions about fatigue can represent a potential contributor to the fatigue in itself (Seigel et al. 2012; Pertl et al. 2012). The effectiveness of CBT on CRF is still debated, with recent favorable (Goedendorp et al. 2012) and previous critical (Mitchell et al. 2007) reports.

Psycho-education

Psycho-educational strategies include scheduling high-priority tasks during the patient's best time of day, avoiding unimportant activities, so that the patient will have more energy available for other activities. The goal of energy conservation is to balance rest and activities so that prioritized activities are more likely to be achieved (Howell et al. 2013). Results coming from a recent review suggest that also yoga interventions may be beneficial for reducing cancer-related fatigue in women with breast cancer, even if such conclusions should be interpreted with caution because of methodological bias across studies (Sadja and Mills 2013).

Acupuncture, Acupressure, Moxibustion

A systematic review and meta-analysis of acupuncture and moxibustion for CRF was performed by He and colleagues: in a total of seven studies involving 804 participants, real acupuncture improved fatigue level of 36 % versus 19 %

with acupressure and 0.6 % with sham acupuncture. Data on moxibustion are positive but few high quality RCTs are disposable (He et al. 2013).

Pharmacological Interventions in CRF

These were evaluated by guidelines (NCCN 2009) and by a Cochrane review (Minton et al. 2008). Six different classes of drugs were identified: hematopoietic growth factors, psychostimulants, bisphosphonates, anti-TNF-a antibodies, antidepressants, and steroids.

All interventions were considered of limited effectiveness, with the exception of methylphenidate that the National Cancer Institute, in the light of the limited documented experience (Fleishman et al. 2005; Bruera et al. 2006; Hardy 2009), suggests to consider only in the treatment of severe fatigue (Anderson et al. 2013). Some preliminary data support using modafinil in cancer-related fatigue with less concern about tolerance or dependence (Breitbart and Alici-Evcimen 2007).

Erythropoietin and darbepoetin were reported to be effective for CRF in patients who were anemic as a result of chemotherapy (Minton et al. 2008). A recent study reported that dexamethasone is more effective than placebo in improving CRF and quality of life in patients with advanced cancer (Yennurajalingam et al. 2013).

Antidepressant studies have shown mixed results. The NCCN guideline also did not recommend the use of antidepressants to reduce fatigue; however, underlying clinical depression, a contributing factor in CRF, should still be treated according to best practices. Paroxetine seems to show benefit for fatigue primarily when it is a symptom of clinical depression (Breitbart and Alici-Evcimen 2007). A possible explanation is that cancer-related fatigue does not involve a reduction in brain 5-HT levels (Morrow et al. 2003). But also recently Heras et al. (2013) confirmed that paroxetine is effective for the treatment of depression during chemotherapy, but has no benefit for the treatment of fatigue. Bupropion, a norepinephrine/dopamine reuptake inhibitor, may have psychostimulant-like effects and therefore may be more beneficial for treating fatigue (Schönfeldt-Lecuona et al. 2006), but without data concerning CFS.

Some open studies have reported the effectiveness and safety of phytotherapeutic drugs such as oral Withania somnifera (ashwagandha) (Biswal et al. 2013) and American ginseng against CRF (Barton et al. 2013).

10.5   Treatment of Other Somatic Symptoms in Cancer Care

The choice of medication should be dictated by side effects profile and potential drug–drug interactions of the medications. There are limited numbers of clinical trials evaluating antidepressant efficacy in cancer patients; however, this is an area in need of further study (Torta and Munari 2010).

10.5.1 Hot Flashes

Hot flashes are common among individuals with cancer, more in women, and at times in men. Hot flashes have a complex pathophysiology. Hot flashes are experienced as sudden and transient episodes of heat emerging out of the body, sweating, palpitations, and anxiety. Hot flashes are reported by up to 86 % in menopausal women without cancer, 51–81 % in women with breast cancer, 69–76 % in men with prostate cancer, and 85–90 % in patients with carcinoid syndrome (Fisher et al. 2013). Other cancer patients who may report hot flashes due to tumor secretion include those with medullary thyroid cancer, pancreatic cancer, or renal cell carcinoma. Hot flashes can interfere with adherence to lifesaving therapies such as estrogen- or testosterone-reducing or ablative therapies that are used to prevent or treat cancer (Fisher et al. 2013). Despite the lack of a full understanding of hot flash etiology, clinical trials testing different hot flash treatment options continue. A wide variety of options have been recommended by experts in the field and/or researched for treating hot flashes in populations with and without cancer. Pharmaceutical therapies include antidepressants, anticonvulsants, antiadrenergics, anticholinergics, progestins, and tibolone (Fisher et al. 2013).

Management of hot flashes in breast cancer survivors can be done using bupropion, venlafaxine, fluoxetine, and paroxetine. Some of these medications are still being studied. It is important to consider caution regarding specific medications for women taking tamoxifen (Thekdi et al. 2012). Antidepressants including venlafaxine and paroxetine, gabapentin, and clonidine have been recommended for treatment of hot flashes in young women being treated for breast cancer. Many RCTs have been conducted on the effectiveness of these medications (Rosenberg and Partridge 2013). In contrast, there has not been strong evidence that natural supplements, including Vitamin E, phyto-estrogens, and black cohosh, are better compared to placebos (Rada et al. 2010).

Four antidepressants (venlafaxine, paroxetine, sertraline, and fluoxetine), representing both selective serotonin reuptake inhibitors and serotonin/norepinephrine reuptake inhibitors, were anecdotally and independently noted to decrease hot flashes in clinical practice in the late 1980s. Along with pilot trials involving some of these agents, a number of placebo-controlled, double-blinded, randomized clinical trials were performed (Loprinzi et al. 2006). A pooled analysis, based on individual patient data, on all known published placebo-controlled trials demonstrated that significant reductions of hot flashes were seen with paroxetine and venlafaxine, as compared with fluoxetine and sertraline. Additional RCTs have demonstrated that venlafaxine and citalopram also significantly reduced hot flashes more than does placebo, to a similar degree as seen with venlafaxine and paroxetine. Gabapentin and pregabalin are other agents that have been shown to decrease hot flashes substantially more than placebos (Loprinzi et al. 2006).

10.5.2 Pruritus

Pruritus is a distressing symptom associated with cholestasis, renal failure, and malignancies. When associated with malignancy it may be one of the most bothersome symptoms in advanced cancer. Its control is difficult to achieve and is a challenge to palliative medicine specialists. The pathogenesis is complex and is not fully understood although there is evidence of involvement of a number of mediators from which treatment options are developing.

In cancer patients pruritus may be directly related to the cancer, indirectly related (e.g., cholestasis) or associated with treatment. It is not always possible to treat the underlying cause of the pruritus in these patients or desirable to stop treatments that may contribute and in these cases we must address the pruritus itself (Lidstone and Thorns 2001). The evidence base is not extensive, but some high quality studies exist.

Itching is a common symptom in cancer patients and is usually managed by local applicants of anti-itching agents. A systematic review and meta-analysis of the literature were conducted for targeted therapies (Ensslin et al. 2013). The incidences of all-grade and high-grade pruritus were 17.4 % and 1.4 %, respectively. There is a significant risk of developing pruritus in patients receiving targeted therapies. To prevent suboptimal dosing and decreased quality of life, patients should be counseled and treated against this untoward symptom.

Low-dose anti-anxiety medications may help specially when itching is interfering with sleep or causing irritations to the patients. Mainly antihistaminics have been used to treat Pruritus. The opioid antagonists, the serotonin receptor blocker ondansetron, and the selective serotonin reuptake inhibitor (SSRI) paroxetine are playing an increasingly important role in the management of pruritus. Antihistaminics frequently are not helpful with cholestatic pruritus, pruritus associated with renal failure, or paraneoplastic pruritus. Selective serotonin reuptake inhibitors (SSRIs) are helpful in the itch associated with myeloproliferative disorders. Paroxetine relieves paraneoplastic, opioid, and cholestatic pruritus. Opioid antagonists (i.e., parenteral naloxone or oral naltrexone) can relieve cholestatic pruritus. Ondansetron relieves cholestatic, opioid, and renal failure-associated pruritus. Ondansetron is expensive and SSRIs, although less expensive, are associated with significant drug–drug interactions and adverse drug effects. Opioid antagonists will reverse analgesia and are contraindicated in hepatic failure. Mirtazapine, an H_1, $5HT_2$, and $5HT_3$ receptor blocker, may be an effective alternative treatment for pruritus arising from cancer, cholestasis, and renal failure. Davis et al. (2003) reported four cases to illustrate its potential therapeutic role.

Zylicz et al. (1998) described five patients suffering from pruritus of different etiologies who responded rapidly to administration of paroxetine, a serotonin reuptake inhibitor, in a dose-dependent manner. Two patients experienced transient but severe nausea and vomiting. Paroxetine's antipruritic effect may be explained by rapid downregulation of the 5-HTs receptors, which may have an important role in the generation of pruritus and pain.

10.5.3 Anorexia and Weight Loss

Weight loss and anorexia in the terminally ill patient are complex problems that can arise due to a number of causes. Medical factors are observed for the anorexia and cachexia associated with terminal illness. Psychiatric and psychological factors, like anxiety, depression, and conditioned food aversions, may also play a role in the etiology of anorexia and weight loss.

Psychopharmacologic interventions with antidepressants and anxiolytics are indicated, when poor appetite is a symptom of underlying depression or anxiety. Behavioral interventions are commonly used to treat a variety of eating disorders in cancer patients including conditioned anorexia and swallowing difficulties. Conditioned difficulties with eating, swallowing, and nausea have been managed successfully with systematic desensitization. Hypnosis has been utilized in children with cancer, resulting in improved appetite and weight gain.

10.5.4 Nausea and Vomiting

Approximately, 50 % of patients with advanced cancer experience anticipatory nausea and vomiting (ANV) during the course of their illness. Antiemetic drugs are the mainstay of managing chemotherapy induced nausea and vomiting in patients with advanced disease. Rapid onset, short-acting benzodiazepines are helpful in controlling ANV once it has developed. Alprazolam has been shown to be clinically effective in reducing ANV in low divided doses, given for 1 to 2 days prior to chemotherapy (Razavi et al. 1993; Ruzsa et al. 2013). In many centers other benzodiazepines are preferred. Conditioned nausea and vomiting are often quite responsive to relaxation training, guided imagery, video game distraction (in children), and other behavioral techniques.

10.6   Effectiveness of Treatment of Somatoform Disorders

The effectiveness of the pharmacological agents in somatoform disorders is not very evident. There are not many randomized control trials. However, there are case reports indicating effectiveness of medications.

The area of somatization and somatoform disorders in cancer patients, how these clinical aspects can worsen the patients' quality of life, and the treatments strategies have been, for a long time, neglected, and no conclusive evidence on effectiveness of interventions are available. Chaturvedi and Maguire (1998), evaluating the nature and frequency of somatic symptoms in cancer patients, found that the most common somatic symptoms (such as pain and fatigue) were often associated with depressive or anxiety disorders: the use of psychotropic medications and counselling for emotional symptoms produced, after 4–6 months, not only an improvement of anxiety and depression scores, but also a significant reduction of somatic symptoms. On the other hand, symptoms of somatization, in patients with active cancer, can complicate the course of disease, for example, by increasing the burden of physical component of pain (Zimmerman et al. 1996; Torta and Munari 2010) and fatigue (Anderson et al. 2013; Martin et al. 2007). Moreover, persistent somatization symptoms in survivors of childhood cancer increase the risk of health-related unemployment status, when compared to survivors with a normal health status (Kirchhoff et al. 2011).

The efficacy of treatment for somatoform disorders was reviewed by Kroenke et al. of 34 randomized controlled trials involving 3,922 patients. Two-thirds of the studies involved somatization disorder and its variants. Cognitive behavior therapy was effective in most studies (11 of 13), as were antidepressants in a small number (4 of 5) (Kroenke 2007).

Conclusions

Patients need to be encouraged to accept medications for the treatment of psychiatric symptoms. This is one of the most challenging tasks for a clinician. Stigma related to psychiatric and psychological symptoms such as depression and anxiety is quite high in most countries and cultures. Awareness of the underlying stigma and shame that patients may feel about accepting help in the form of medications will serve the clinician well (Thekdi et al. 2012).

The availability of new drugs, with less side-effects and safer pharmacological profiles, has been a major advance in this field. Interestingly, several drugs have also been found to be helpful for the adjuvant treatment of cancer-related symptoms, such as pain, hot flashes, pruritus, nausea and vomiting, fatigue, and cognitive impairment, making psychopharmacology an important tool for the improvement of cancer patients' quality of life (Caruso et al. 2013). Clinicians need to share their experiences about use of psychotropic in cancer patients, and more clinical trials will help clinicians to use safer and effective medications to reduce distress and improve quality of life of cancer patients. The management of somatic symptom conditions are a big challenge in cancer patients and need more stringent studies, as well as empirical evidence, to help clinicians care for their cancer patients.

References

Aisenstein M, Smadja C. Conceptual framework from the Paris psychosomatic school: a clinical psychoanalytic approach to oncology. Int J Psychoanal. 2010;91:621–40.

Allen LA, Woolfolk RL. Cognitive behavioral therapy for somatoform disorders. Psychiatr Clin North Am. 2010;33:579–93.

Anacker C, Zunszain PA, Carvgalho LA, et al. The glucocorticoid receptor: pivot of depression and of antidepressant treatment? Psychoneuroendocrinology. 2010;36:415–25.

Anderson G, Berk M, Maes M. Biological phenotypes underpin the physio-somatic symptoms of somatization, depression, and chronic fatigue syndrome. Acta Psychiatr Scand. 2013;129 (2):83–97. doi:10.1111/acps.12182.

Attal N, Cruccu G, Baron R, European Federation of Neurological Societies, et al. EFNS guidelines on the pharmacological treatment of neuropathic pain: 2010 revision. Eur J Neurol. 2010;17:1113–88.

Baines M. Pain relief in active patients with cancer: analgesic drugs are the foundation of management. Br Med J. 1989;298:36–8.

Bakir S, Kinis V, Bez Y, et al. Mental health and quality of life in patients with chronic otitis media. Eur Arch Otorhinolaryngol. 2013;270:521–6.

Barsevick AM, Whitmer K, Walker L. In their own words: using the common sense model to analyze patient descriptions of cancer-related fatigue. Oncol Nurs Forum. 2001;28:1363–9.

Barton DL, Liu H, Loprinzi CL, et al. Wisconsin Ginseng (Panax quinquefolius) to improve cancer-related fatigue: a randomized, double-blind trial, N07C2. J Natl Cancer Inst. 2013;105:1230–8.

Baudino B, Geminiani GC, Torta R, et al. The chemotherapy long-term effect on cognitive functions and brain metabolism in lymphoma patients. Q J Nucl Med Mol Imaging. 2012;56:12–28.

Biglia N, Torta R, Roagna R, et al. Evaluation of low-dose venlafaxine hydrochloride for the therapy of hot flushes in breast cancer survivors. Maturitas. 2005;52:78–85.

Biswal BM, Sulaiman SA, Ismail HC, et al. Effect of Withania somnifera (Ashwagandha) on the development of chemotherapy-induced fatigue and quality of life in breast cancer patients. Integr Cancer Ther. 2013;12:312–22.

Breitbart W, Alici-Evcimen Y. Update on psychotropic medications for cancer-related fatigue. J Natl Compr Canc Netw. 2007;5:1081–91.

Bruera E, Valero V, Driver L, et al. Patient-controlled methylphenidate for cancer fatigue: a double-blind, randomized, placebo-controlled trial. J Clin Oncol. 2006;24:2073–8.

Campbell CM, McCauley L, Bounds SC, et al. Changes in pain catastrophizing predict later changes in fibromyalgia clinical and experimental pain report: cross-lagged panel analyses of dispositional and situational catastrophizing. Arthritis Res Ther. 2012;14(5):R231.

Capuron L, Ravaud A, Miller AH, et al. Baseline mood and psychosocial characteristics of patients developing depressive symptoms during interleukin-2 and/or interferon-alpha cancer therapy. Brain Behav Immun. 2004;18:205–13.

Carlotto A, Hogsett VL, Maiorini EM, et al. The economic burden of toxicities associated with cancer treatment: review of the literature and analysis of nausea and vomiting, diarrhoea, oral mucositis and fatigue. Pharmacoeconomics. 2013;31:753–66.

Caruso R, Grassi L, Nanni MG, Riba M. Psychopharmacology in psycho-oncology. Curr Psychiatry Rep. 2013;15(9):393.

Casale R, Cazzola M, Torta R, et al. Non-pharmacological treatments in fibromyalgia. Reumatismo. 2008;60 Suppl 1:59–69.

Castelli L, Tesio V, Torta R, et al. Alexithymia and psychological distress in fibromyalgia: prevalence and relation with quality of life. Clin Exp Rheumatol. 2012;30(6 Suppl 74):70–7.

Castelli L, De Santis F, Torta R, et al. Alexithymia, anger and psychological distress in patients with myofascial pain: a case–control study. Front Psychol. 2013;4(490):1–8.

Cella D, Lai JS, Chang CH, et al. Fatigue in cancer patients compared with fatigue in the general United States population. Cancer. 2002;94:528–38.

Chang CW, Mu PF, Chen YC, et al. Systematic review and meta-analysis of nonpharmacological interventions for fatigue in children and adolescents with cancer. Worldviews Evid Based Nurs. 2013;10(4):208–17.

Chaturvedi S, Maguire GP. Persistent somatization in cancer: A controlled follow-up study. J Psychosom Res. 1998;45:249–56.

Chaturvedi SK, Uchitomi Y. Psychosocial and psychiatric disorders. In: Grassi L, Riba M, editors. Clinical psycho oncology. Chichester, UK: Wiley Publications; 2012. p. 55–70.

Chaturvedi SK, Hopwood P, Maguire P. Nonorganic somatic symptoms in cancer. Eur J Cancer. 1993;29:1006–8.

Chaturvedi SK, Maguire G, Somashekar BS. Somatization in cancer. Int Rev Psychiatry. 2006;18:49–54.

Cheatle MD, Brady JP, Ruland T, et al. How does subjective experience of pain relate to psychopathology among psychiatric patients? Gen Hosp Psychiatry. 2012;34:534–40.

Cuesta-Vargas AI, Buchan J, Arroyo-Morales M. A multimodal physiotherapy programme plus deep water running for improving cancer-related fatigue and quality of life in breast cancer survivors. Eur J Cancer Care (Engl). 2014;23(1):15–21.

Davis MP, Franssen JL, Walsh D, et al. Mirtazapine for Pruritus. J Pain Symptom Manage. 2003;25:288–91.

De Silva V, El-Metwally A, Ernst E, et al. Arthritis Research Campaign working group on complementary and alternative medicines. Evidence for the efficacy of complementary and alternative medicines in the management of fibromyalgia: a systematic review. Rheumatology (Oxford). 2010;49:1063–8.

De Vries AM, Forni V, Voellinger R, et al. Alexithymia in cancer patients: review of the literature. Psychother Psychosom. 2012;81:79–86.

Dimsdale JE, Creed F, Escobar J, Sharpe M, Wulsin L, Barsky A, Lee S, Irwin MR, Levenson J. Somatic symptom disorder: an important change in DSM. J Psychosom Res. 2013;75 (3):223–8.

Duddu V, Isaac MK, Chaturvedi SK. Somatization, somatosensory amplification, attribution styles and illness behaviour: a review. Int Rev Psychiatry. 2006;18:25–33.

Durand JP, Deplanque G, Montheil V, et al. Efficacy of venlafaxine for the prevention and relief of oxaliplatin-induced acute neurotoxicity: results of EFFOX, a randomized, double-blind, placebo-controlled phase III trial. Ann Oncol. 2012;23:200–5.

Ensslin CJ, Rosen AC, Wu S, et al. Pruritus in patients treated with targeted cancer therapies. Systematic review and meta-analysis. J Am Acad Dermatol. 2013;69(5):708–20.

Fava GA, Wise TN. Issues for DSM-V: psychological factors affecting either identified or feared medical conditions: a solution for somatoform disorders. Am J Psychiatry. 2007;164:1002–3.

Fava GA, Freyberger HJ, Wise TN. Diagnostic criteria for use in psychosomatic research. Psychother Psychosom. 1995;63:1–8.

Fava GA, Guidi J, Sonino N, et al. A cluster analysis derived classification of psychological distress and illness behavior in the medically ill. Psychol Med. 2012;42:401–7.

Fishbain DA, Bruns D, Disorbio JM, et al. Risk for five forms of suicidality in acute pain patients and chronic pain patients vs pain-free community controls. Pain Med. 2009;10:1095–105.

Fisher WI, Johnson AK, Elkins GR, et al. Risk factors, pathophysiology, and treatment of hot flashes in cancer. CA Cancer J Clin. 2013;63:167–92.

Fleishman S, Lower E, Zeldis J, et al. A phase 2 randomized, placebo-controlled trial of the safety and efficacy of dexmethylphenidate (d-MPH) as a treatment for fatigue and "chemobrain in adult cancer patients. Br Cancer Res Treat. 2005;94:S214.

Foley KM. Controlling cancer pain. Hosp Pract. 2000;15(35):101–8.

Foley KM. How well is cancer pain treated? Palliat Med. 2011;25:398–401.

Genç F, Tan M. Symptoms of patients with lung cancer undergoing chemotherapy and coping strategies. Cancer Nurs. 2011;34:503–9.

Genç GA, Muluk NB, Belgin E. The effects of tinnitus and/or hearing loss on the Symptom Checklist-90-Revised test. Auris Nasus Larynx. 2013;40:154–61.

Gharibian D, Polzin JK, Rho JP. Compliance and persistence of antidepressants versus anticonvulsants in patients with neuropathic pain during the first year of therapy. Clin J Pain. 2013;29:377–81.

Gnanadesigan N, Espinoza RT, Smith R, et al. Interactions of seriotonergic antidepressants and opioid analgesic: is serotonin syndrome going undetected? J Am Med Dir Assoc. 2005;6:265–9.

Goedendorp MM, Andrykowski MA, Donovan KA, et al. Prolonged impact of chemotherapy on fatigue in breast cancer survivors: a longitudinal comparison with radiotherapy treated breast cancer survivors and noncancer controls. Cancer. 2012;118:3833–41.

Grassi L, Rosti G. Psychosocial morbidity and adjustment to illness among long-term cancer survivors. A six-year follow-up study. Psychosomatics. 1996;37:523–32.

Grassi L, Rosti G, Albieri G, et al. Depression and abnormal illness behaviour in cancer patients. Gen Hosp Psychiatry. 1989;11:404–11.

Grassi L, Rossi E, Sabato S, et al. Diagnostic criteria for psychosomatic research and psychosocial variables in breast cancer patients. Psychosomatics. 2004;45:483–91.

Grassi L, Sabato S, Rossi E, et al. Use of the diagnostic criteria for psychosomatic research in oncology. Psychother Psychosom. 2005;74:100–7.

Grassi L, Caruso R, Nanni MG. Somatization and somatic symptom presentation in cancer: a neglected area. Int Rev Psychiatry. 2013;25:41–51.

Gupta D, Mishra S, Bhatnagar S. Somatization disorder, a cause of difficult pain: a case report. Am J Hosp Palliat Care. 2007;24:219–23.

Hardy SE. Methylphenidate for the treatment of depressive symptoms, including fatigue and apathy, in medically ill older adults and terminally ill adults. Am J Geriatr Pharmacother. 2009;7:34–59.

Hashimoto K. Brain-derived neurotrophic factor as a biomarker for mood disorders: an historical overview and future directions. Psychiatry Clin Neurosci. 2010;64:341–57.

Hassel JC, Danner D, Hassel AJ. Psychosomatic or allergic symptoms? High levels for somatization in patients with drug intolerance. J Dermatol. 2011;38:959–65.

He XR, Wang Q, Li PP. Acupuncture and moxibustion for cancer-related fatigue: a systematic review and meta-analysis. Asian Pac J Cancer Prev. 2013;14:3067–74.

Heras P, Kritikos K, Hatzopoulos A, et al. The role of paroxetine in fatigue and depression of patients under chemotherapeutic treatment. Am J Ther. 2013;20:254–6.

Howell D, Keller-Olaman S, Oliver TK, et al. A pan-Canadian practice guideline and algorithm: screening, assessment, and supportive care of adults with cancer-related fatigue. Curr Oncol. 2013;20:e233–46.

Hungin AP, Hill C, Raghunath A. A systematic review: frequency and reasons for consultation for gastro-oesophageal reflux disease and dyspepsia. Aliment Pharmacol Ther. 2009;30:331–42.

Jacobsen PB, Donovan KA, Vadaparampil ST, et al. Systematic review and meta-analysis of psychological and activity-based interventions for cancer-related fatigue. Health Psychol. 2007;26:660–7.

Janca A, Isaac M, Ventouras J. Towards better understanding and management of somatoform disorders. Int Rev Psychiatry. 2006;18:5–12.

Kano M, Fukudo S. The alexithymic brain: the neural pathways linking alexithymia to physical disorders. Biopsychosoc Med. 2013;9(7):1–6.

Kashikar-Zuck S, Sil S, Lynch-Jordan AM, et al. Changes in pain coping, catastrophizing, and coping efficacy after cognitive-behavioral therapy in children and adolescents with juvenile fibromyalgia. J Pain. 2013;14:492–501.

Kirchhoff AC, Krull KR, Leisenring W, et al. Physical, mental, and neurocognitive status and employment outcomes in the childhood cancer survivor study cohort. Cancer Epidemiol Biomarkers Prev. 2011;20:1838–49.

Krishnadas R, Cavanagh J. Depression: an inflammatory illness? J Neurol Neurosurg Psychiatry. 2012;83:495–502.

Kroenke K. Efficacy of treatment for somatoform disorders: a review of randomized controlled trials. Psychosom Med. 2007;69:881–8.

Kroenke K, Sharpe M, Sykes R. Revising the classification of somatoform disorders: Key questions and preliminary recommendations. Psychosomatics. 2007;48:277–85.

Kummer F, Catuogno S, Perseus JM, et al. Relationship between cancer-related fatigue and physical activity in inpatient cancer rehabilitation. Anticancer Res. 2013;33:3415–22.

Laederach-Hofmann K, Rüddel H, Mussgay L. Pathological baroreceptor sensitivity in patients suffering from somatization disorders: do they correlate with symptoms? Biol Psychol. 2008;79:243–9.

Laird BJ, McMillan DC, Fayers P, et al. The systemic inflammatory response and its relationship to pain and other symptoms in advanced cancer. Oncologist. 2013;18:1050–5.

Lee JJ, Song HS, Park SP, et al. Psychiatric symptoms and quality of life in patients with drug-refractory epilepsy receiving adjunctive levetiracetam therapy. J Clin Neurol. 2011;7:128–36.

Lee SP, Lee KN, Lee OY, et al. The relationship between existence of typical symptoms and psychological factors in patients with erosive esophagitis. J Neurogastroenterol Motil. 2012;18:284–90.

Lidstone V, Thorns A. Pruritus in cancer patients. Cancer Treat Rev. 2001;27:305–12.

Loprinzi CL, Levitt R, Barton D, et al. Phase III comparison of depomedroxyprogesterone acetate to venlafaxine for managing hot flashes: North Central Cancer Treatment Group Trial N99C7. J Clin Oncol. 2006;24:1409–14.

Martin A, Chalder T, Rief W, et al. The relationship between chronic fatigue and somatization syndrome: a general population survey. J Psychosom Res. 2007;63:147–56.

McCarthy DJ, Alexander R, Smith MA, et al. Glutamate-based depression GBD. Med Hypotheses. 2012;78:675–81.

Minton O, Stone P, Richardson A, et al. Drug therapy for the management of cancer related fatigue. Cochrane Database Syst Rev. 2008;23(1), CD006704.

Mitchell SA, Beck SL, Hood LE, et al. Putting evidence into practice: evidence-based interventions for fatigue during and following cancer and its treatment. Clin J Oncol Nurs. 2007;11:99–113.

Morrow GR, Hickok JT, Roscoe JA, et al. Differential effects of paroxetine on fatigue and depression: a randomized, double-blind trial from the University of Rochester Cancer Center Community Clinical Oncology Program. J Clin Oncol. 2003;15(21):4635–41.

National Comprehensive Cancer Network NCCN Clinical Practice Guidelines in Oncology: Cancer-Related Fatigue. Ver. 2.2009. Fort Washington, PA: NCCN; 2009.

Oldervoll LM, Loge JH, Paltiel H, et al. The effect of a physical exercise program in palliative care: a phase II study. J Pain Symptom Manage. 2006;31:421–30.

Pertl MM, Hevey D, Donohoe G, et al. Assessing patients' beliefs about their cancer-related fatigue: validation of an adapted version of the Illness Perception Questionnaire. J Clin Psychol Med Settings. 2012;19:293–307.

Perugi G, Canonico PL, Torta R, et al. Unexplained somatic symptoms during major depression: prevalence and clinical impact in a national sample of Italian psychiatric outpatients. Psychopathology. 2011;44:116–24.

Pilowsky I. Abnormal illness behaviour: A 25th anniversary review. Aust N Z J Psychiatry. 1994;28:566–73.

Pompili M, Innamorati M, Serafini G, et al. Chronic low back pain, depression, and attributional style. Clin J Pain. 1990;6:114–7.

Porcelli P, Todarello O. Psychological factors in medical disorders assessed with the diagnostic criteria for psychosomatic research. Adv Psychosom Med. 2012;32:108–17.

Prinsloo S, Gabel S, Lyle R, et al. Neuromodulation of cancer pain. Integr Cancer Ther. 2014;13 (1):30–7.

Prue G, Rankin J, Allen J, et al. Cancer-related fatigue: a critical appraisal. Eur J Cancer. 2006;42:846–63.

Pulvers K, Hood A. The role of positive traits and pain catastrophizing in pain perception. Curr Pain Headache Rep. 2013;17:330.

Rada G, Capurro D, Pantoja T, et al. Non-hormonal interventions for hot flushes in women with a history of breast cancer. Cochrane Database Syst Rev. 2010;9, CD004923.

Razavi D, Delvaux N, Farvacques C, De Brier F, Van Heer C, Kaufman L, Derde MP, Beauduin M, Piccart M. Prevention of adjustment disorders and anticipatory nausea secondary to adjuvant chemotherapy: a double-blind, placebo-controlled study assessing the usefulness of alprazolam. J Clin Oncol. 1993;11(7):1384–90.

Ream E, Richardson A, Alexander-Dann C. Supportive intervention for fatigue in patients undergoing chemotherapy: a randomized controlled trial. J Pain Symptom Manage. 2006;31:148–61.

Rosenberg SM, Partridge AH. Premature menopause in young breast cancer: effects on quality of life and treatment interventions. J Thorac Dis. 2013;5 Suppl 1:S55–61.

Russo-Neustadt AA, Chen MJ. Brain-derived neurotrophic factor and antidepressant activity. Curr Pharm Des. 2005;11:1495–510.

Ruzsa A, Lelovics Z, Hegedűs K. The influence of patients' gender and education level on the incidence of chemotherapy-induced anticipatory nausea and vomiting] [Hungarian]. Orv Hetil. 2013;154(21):820–4.

Saariaho AS, Saariaho TH, Mattila AK, et al. Alexithymia and depression in a chronic pain patient sample. Gen Hosp Psychiatry. 2013;35:239–45.

Sadja J, Mills PJ. Effects of yoga interventions on fatigue in cancer patients and survivors: a systematic review of randomized controlled trials. Explore (NY). 2013;9:232–43.

Sarkisian CA, Prohaska TR, Davis C, et al. Pilot test of an attribution retraining intervention to raise walking levels in sedentary older adults. J Am Geriatr Soc. 2007;55:1842–6.

Schönfeldt-Lecuona C, Connemann BJ, Wolf RC, et al. Bupropion augmentation in the treatment of chronic fatigue syndrome with coexistent major depression episode. Pharmacopsychiatry. 2006;39:152–4.

Schubert C, Hong S, Natarajan L, et al. The association between fatigue and inflammatory marker levels in cancer patients: a quantitative review. Brain Behav Immun. 2007;21:413–27.

Seigel K, Lekas HM, Maheshwari D. Causal attributions for fatigue by older adults with advanced cancer. J Pain Symptom Manage. 2012;44:52–63.

Shaw J, Creed F. The cost of somatization. J Psychosom Res. 1991;35(2–3):307–12.

Siri C, Cilia R, Antonini A, et al. Psychiatric symptoms in Parkinson ' s disease assessed with the SCL-90R self-reported questionnaire. Neurol Sci. 2010;31:35–40.

Sirri L, Fava GA. Diagnostic criteria for psychosomatic research and somatic symptom disorders. Int Rev Psychiatry. 2013;25(1):19–30.

Sirri L, Fava GA, Wise TN. Psychiatric classification in the setting of medical disease: Comparing the clinical value of different proposals. J Psychosom Res. 2011;70:493–5.

Somashekar B, Jainer A, Wuntakal B. Psychopharmacotherapy of somatic symptoms disorders. Int Rev Psychiatry. 2013;25:107–15.

Sonino N, Tomba E, Fava GA. Psychosocial approach to endocrine disease. Adv Psychosom Med. 2007;28:21–33.

Stone PC, Minton O. Cancer-related fatigue. Eur J Cancer. 2008;44:1097–104.

Thekdi SM, Irurrazaval ME, Dunn LB. Psychopharmacological interventions. In: Grassi L, Riba M, editors. Clinical psycho oncology. Chichester, UK: Wiley Publications; 2012. p. 109–26.

Thistle JL, Longstreth GF, Zinsmeister AR, et al. Factors that predict relief from upper abdominal pain after cholecystectomy. Clin Gastroenterol Hepatol. 2011;9:891–6.

Torta RG, Ieraci V. Pharmacological management of depression in patients with cancer: practical considerations. Drugs. 2013;73:1131–45.

Torta RG, Ieraci V. Depressive disorders and pain: A joint model of diagnosis and treatment. J Pain Relief. 2013;S2:003. doi:10.4172/2167-0846.S2-003.

Torta RG, Munari J. Symptom cluster: depression and pain. Surg Oncol. 2010;19:155–9.

Torta R, Leombruni P, Borio R, et al. Duloxetine for the treatment of mood disorder in cancer patients: a 12 week casecontrol clinical trial. Hum Psychopharmacol. 2011;26:291–9.

Trafton JA, Cucciare MA, Lewis E, et al. Somatization is associated with non-adherence to opioid prescriptions. J Pain. 2011;12:573–80.

van-Schreiber D, Tabas G, Kolb NR. Somatizing patients: Part II. Practical management. Am Fam Physician. 2000;61:1423–32.

Yennurajalingam S, Frisbee-Hume S, Bruera E, et al. Reduction of cancer-related fatigue with dexamethasone: a double-blind, randomized, placebo-controlled trial in patients with advanced cancer. J Clin Oncol. 2013;31:3076–82.

Zimmerman L, Story KT, Gaston-Johansson F, et al. Psychological variables and cancer pain. Cancer Nurs. 1996;19:44–53.

Zylicz Z, Smits C, Krajnik MJ. Paroxetine for pruritus in advanced cancer. J Pain Symptom Manage. 1998;16:121–4.

Bipolar Disorder in the Cancer Patient

11

Daniel L. Hertz, Vicki L. Ellingrod, and Melvin G. McInnis

Abstract

The diagnosis of any cancer is typically accompanied with instabilities of general health, disposition, and mood. Once the urgency of the cancer is addressed, additional health concerns, comorbidities, and conditions may be compromised and attention must be paid to these details in the context of the cancer. Mood disorders, including major depression and bipolar disorder, as well as distressful reactions are common and often ignored due to an inherent expectation of a sadness and distress associated with such a life-threatening disease. However, pathological mood swings are eminently treatable, and the management of mood disorders is particularly gratifying to the individual with cancer and rewarding for the practitioner. Adherence to treatment and improvements to quality of life are immediate, and enhancements in survivorship emerge over time. Bipolar disorder represents a particular challenge for the oncology team as gyrations of mood may jeopardize every aspect of management. This chapter discusses clinical strategies for the bipolar patient and includes the mood stabilizing and antipsychotic medications, emphasizing the need for regular monitoring of clinical mood symptoms, medication levels when possible, and physical health to gauge progress. Periods of unstable moods should be anticipated in the individual with concomitant cancer and specifically

D.L. Hertz
University of Michigan College of Pharmacy, Ann Arbor, MI, USA
e-mail: dlhertz@med.umich.edu

V.L. Ellingrod
John Gideon Serle Professor of Clinical and Translational Pharmacy, University of Michigan College of Pharmacy and School of Medicine, Ann Arbor, MI, USA
e-mail: vellingr@med.umich.edu

M.G. McInnis (✉)
Thomas B and Nancy Upjohn Woodworth Professor of Bipolar Disorder and Depression, Professor of Psychiatry, University of Michigan School of Medicine, Ann Arbor, MI, USA
e-mail: mmcinnis@med.umich.edu

L. Grassi and M. Riba (eds.), *Psychopharmacology in Oncology and Palliative Care*,   189
DOI 10.1007/978-3-642-40134-3_11, © Springer-Verlag Berlin Heidelberg 2014

in the patient with bipolar disorder. Negotiating care involves clinical judgment at an interface of medicine wherein limited knowledge of pharmacological interactions is a major challenge; there are no clinical trials of mood management in the cancer patient with bipolar disorder. This chapter discusses the treatments of bipolar disorder and unstable moods in cancer.

11.1   Overview of Major Depressive Disorder and Bipolar Disorder

Within the United States, approximately 15–20 % of the population will experience a Major Depressive Disorder (MDD) (Kessler et al. 2003), and approximately 5 % will be diagnosed with Bipolar Affective Disorder (BPAD) or one of its subtypes (Merikangas et al. 2007). BPAD is a cyclic, severe, chronic psychiatric disorder requiring both nonpharmacologic and pharmacologic management. In general for those with depression, the occurrence of this mental illness is often debilitating and may involve mood alterations, sleep disturbances, weight changes, energy loss, decreased concentration, suicidal ideation, feelings of worthlessness, psychomotor agitation or depression, and/or an inability to experience pleasure (AP Association et al. 2000). For those with BPAD, all of these symptoms can be seen while the patient is undergoing a depressive episode; however, they also experience periods of mania characterized by increased energy, an elevated or expansive mood, irritability, hostility, decreased need for sleep, and an increase in goal-directed activity (AP Association et al. 2000).

11.2   Managing MDD and BPAD in the Cancer Patient

Although non-pharmacologic treatments for both MDD and BPAD exist and may be useful in management of these illnesses or as an adjunct to medications, the mainstay of treatment consists of antidepressants for the depressive symptoms and a mood stabilizer for the periods of mania. The goal of therapy is to achieve remission of acute symptoms followed by a prevention of further episodes while maintaining optimal functioning.

The management of mood disorders in the cancer patient is confounded by the compromised physical health that often accompanies cancer and its treatments. There are few, if any, clinical studies that directly evaluate mood management strategies in the cancer patient and are unlikely to be forthcoming as each individual treated for cancer has features that are unique according to the primary cancer and its treatments and sequelae. The previous medical, psychiatric, and personal history of the individual will figure prominently in formulating a treatment plan. The clinician treating a mood disorder in a cancer patient will have a wide range of pharmacological and social interventions available. Below we discuss pharmacological treatments. A general consideration is that management of mood disorders in the cancer patient is similar to treatments in general mood disorders clinic. However, as in any medically compromised patient, we must be guided by the clinical condition of the individual, adjusting doses and monitoring side effects, toxicity, and efficacy of the interventions. Knowledge of the medications used in all treatments and their interactions is essential in effective management.

The first-line pharmacological treatment for MDD is the antidepressants such as the selective serotonin reuptake inhibitors (SSRIs) (escitalopram, citalopram, fluoxetine, fluvoxamine, paroxetine, and sertraline) (Mann 2005). When used at therapeutic doses, the response rates to these medications are approximately 60 % (Anonymous 2000). Most importantly when used for the treatment of depression, the risk of relapse is significantly reduced if these medications are used acutely for a minimum of 8 weeks, followed by a 6–9-month continuation phase, and then a 12- or more month maintenance phase for those who are at high risk (Anonymous 2000).

For the treatment of bipolar disorder, the treatment of mania consists of two primary considerations: an acute phase aimed at the treatment of the acute manic symptoms followed by a maintenance phase that is aimed at preventing recurrence. For the acute phase, an urgent assessment should be performed, usually within the emergency room to rule out any physical conditions that may be contributing to the current manic symptoms. The assessment will be guided by the clinical concerns and may include biochemistry and/or neuroimaging. First onset of symptoms or changes in the symptom patterns in the context of medical disease are indicators for detailed medical evaluation. Immediate management of acute symptoms is indicated with an antipsychotic and/or mood stabilizing agent. There are currently three mood stabilizing medications (valproate, lithium, and carbamazepine) and six antipsychotics (risperidone, olanzapine, quetiapine, aripirazole, chlorpromazine, and ziprasidone) that have been FDA approved for acute mania. The acute phase can be less than 1 month or as long as several months in duration. However, a significant number of individuals may continue with unstable fluctuations in mood, particularly if there are concomitant unstable medical conditions such as cancer. The pharmacological management strategy for each individual patient is governed by the emerging symptom pattern; frequently, in the acute phase a combination strategy of an antipsychotic and mood stabilizer is employed. Once the individual is stable (free from or with minimal symptoms) a monotherapy approach with the mood stabilizer is suggested for the maintenance phase. There are many patients with bipolar disorder for whom depression is a major clinical problem. Lamotrigine and quetiapine are FDA approved for the prevention of recurring depression in BPAD (Suppes et al. 2005); however, management with an antidepressant may be needed. This often presents a substantial challenge as the management of depression using an antidepressant in a patient with BPAD may bring about antidepressant-induced mania or "switching" in which the antidepressant quickly induces a mania state that may require treatment. Patients with BPAD treated with an antidepressant should also be treated with a mood stabilizing medication or antipsychotic or monitored very closely for emerging mood instability in order to minimize the risk of antidepressant-induced manias. Guidelines and algorithms have been reviewed and published for further guidance in BPAD management (Suppes et al. 2005; Yatham et al. 2013; Perlis 2005).

The choice of BPAD management will be guided by the presenting clinical features of the patient combined with the knowledge of the pharmacology and pharmacokinetics of the medications. The complex medical condition found in patients with cancers calls for the expert involvement of the pharmacy team to review the medication history of responses, the current ongoing treatment, and the plans and needs for future pharmacotherapies in order to account for the possible drug–drug interactions and side effects that may arise. Significant and life-threatening medical complications may be inadvertently introduced in a complex metabolically challenged cancer patient that in another setting, such as a college mental health clinic, would be of minimal concern. Management of bipolar in the cancer setting is clearly challenged by overlapping pharmacological side effect profiles. In the brief descriptions of the common options used to manage BPAD, it is evident that the management of BPAD in the medically compromised or cancer patient benefits from a team-based approach that accommodates the concerns and recommendations of the multiple disciplines.

11.3 Lithium

Despite very little data regarding its mechanism of action, lithium is the mainstay of treatment for bipolar disorder. Pharmacokinetically, lithium is very different from the other mood stabilizers in that it is completely eliminated by the kidneys. Due to this, regular monitoring of serum creatinine and lithium levels is required and in patients with unstable renal function, or the potential for unstable renal function, lithium needs to be used with caution and monitored closely. In the complex medical patient, a beginning dose of 150 mg daily is recommended followed by an increase of 150 mg every 3 days as tolerated. Blood levels will generally stabilize after 3–4 days of a constant dose. The target blood level in the classic BPAD patient is in the 0.7 mEq/L vicinity; however, many patients appear to do well at lower levels while others need more. Monitoring is best done with a 12 h trough assessment; however, if there is concern about a toxic state, an immediate level is indicated. It is to be appreciated that the lithium blood levels are guidelines and that in complex medical conditions, the stability of the patient is an important guiding factor. As the level of lithium increases so does the risk of toxicity and levels beyond 1.2 mEq/L should be avoided. For maintenance therapy some work supports the use of lower levels and recommends that a level closer to 0.6 mEq/L is adequate (Anonymous 2000; Hopkins and Gelenberg 2000). Medical monitoring of lithium includes baseline thyroid function, renal function, and an ECG. When lithium therapy is being established in the medically compromised patient, twice weekly lithium levels are recommended, and once stable this level may be checked at monthly intervals. Monitoring frequency is subsequently guided by the clinical presentation, when medically stable, interval monitoring of up to 3–6 months is acceptable. Any significant change in the medical condition of the individual is an

Table 11.1 Lithium side effects and potential signs of toxicity

Common side effects seen with lithium use
• Fine tremor
• Dry mouth
• Altered taste sensation
• Increased thirst
• Increased frequency of urination
• Mild nausea
• Weight gain
Potential signs and symptoms of lithium toxicity
• Vomiting or diarrhea
• Coarse tremor (larger movements, especially of hands)
• Muscle weakness
• General lack of coordination, including ataxia
• Slurred speech
• Blurred vision
• Lethargy
• Confusion
• Seizures

BMJ 2010;341:c6258

indication for increased monitoring of lithium. Use of lithium in patients with unstable renal status or renal insufficiency is often avoided, but it is acceptable with proper monitoring of lithium levels and engagement of the nephrology service. Patient education regarding the side effects of lithium (listed in Table 11.1) is part of the treatment, as occurrence of these side effects are common and may occur in the medically compromised patient even within the accepted therapeutic range.

11.4   Anticonvulsants

These mediations were originally approved by the FDA as anticonvulsants; however given that these medications pharmacologically affect GABA neurotransmission, their role in the treatment of BPAD comes primarily from noted improvement in mood stability amongst patients with epilepsy. Regardless, all of these mediations now currently have FDA approval either for the acute or maintenance treatment of BPAD mania and/or depression.

11.4.1 Valproic Acid, Valproate, or VPA

In general, valproate is considered either a first- or second-line treatment for BPAD and is also very effective in reducing or preventing recurrent manic, depressive, and mixed episodes. There are several dosing strategies for its use, one of which is a loading dose of 20 mg/kg divided over 12 h. Dosing is then adjusted daily by 250–500 mg based on response and tolerability. Alternatively, a cautious approach in the medically compromised patient will include beginning with a low dose of 250 mg/d and increased every 2–3 days as tolerated. Although a strong dose response relationship between valproate levels and mood response has not been critically defined, a suggested therapeutic range between 50–150 mg/ml exists (Allen et al. 2006). This range is often used when making therapeutic decisions in patients who are either not responding to VPA, as those with lower levels may tolerate a higher dose, or are experiencing side effects, as those at higher levels may benefit from a reduced dose. Similar to lithium, use of VPA also necessitates careful monitoring which includes laboratory values along with drug interactions and side effects. Most of the side effects seen with VPA are gastrointestinal in nature and will reduce in severity over the first 2–3 weeks of treatment. For those who are highly sensitive to these gastrointestinal side effects, the use of Depakote, an enteric coated form of divalproic acid, will help reduce the occurrence of these adverse effects. The greatest risk with VPA use is hepatotoxicity and is greatest in young children and those taking more than one medication to prevent seizures. In the medically compromised patient, metabolic monitoring of liver function is clearly indicated on all accounts and should be included in any follow-up therapeutic monitoring or if there is any medical change of clinical concern. For patients who develop acute liver injury, the use of VPA is not necessarily contraindicated but does require close and careful monitoring, generally with the expert consultation from the gastrointestinal service. Patient education regarding the signs and symptoms of liver insufficiency such as new onset tiredness, lack of energy, weakness, stomach pain, loss of appetite, nausea, and vomiting helps in the identification of potential hepatotoxicity; however, these symptoms clearly may overlap with the primary cancer. Other potential side effects from VPA use include pancreatitis, weight gain, alopecia, and thrombocytopenia, as well as common central nervous system (CNS) side effects such as drowsiness, ataxia, and hand tremor. Although VPA has been associated with the thrombocytopenia, its occurrence is rare and routine platelet monitoring is not necessary unless the patient notes frequent bruising. For those in which this does occur, platelet counts may return to normal with continued use or may require treatment discontinuation.

Perhaps the greatest challenge associated with VPA use is its effect on the cytochrome P450 system, as VPA is an inhibitor of CYP3A4 as well as CYP2C9; however, the degree to which VPA inhibits these enzymes has not been fully established. Importantly though, wide variation in the expression of these enzymes, especially CYP3A4, has been reported, thus for some patients drug interactions with VPA may be clinically relevant while for others not. Therefore, prudent monitoring of medication related side effects is necessary whenever medications are either being added to VPA or VPA is being removed from a patient's medication profile.

11.4.2 Carbamazepine

An additional anticonvulsant used for the acute and maintenance treatment of BPAD is carbamazepine (CBZ); however, its use is usually considered a second- or third-line approach. Although effective for the treatment of bipolar disorder, its use is often associated with troublesome side effects such as dizziness, drowsiness, nausea, vomiting, cardiac conduction changes, loss of balance or coordination, as well as some blood dyscrasias. Due to the incidence of these side effects and the relatively narrow therapeutic range that is used to monitor this medication (4–12 mcg/ml), the popularity of carbamazepine use has declined among patients and care providers (McEvoy et al. 2007a). Similar to VPA the therapeutic range that has been suggested for CBZ has not been substantially linked with therapeutic outcomes, but rather is used for making dosing changes based on the occurrence of side effects as well as medication response. For an acute manic episode CBZ can generally be started around 400–600 mg/day in divided doses and taken with meals. This may be increased by 200 mg/day based on clinical response. Blood dyscrasias have been reported with CBZ use; thrombocytopenia and leukopenia have been found to occur most commonly, while aplastic anemia is a rare possibility. For these reasons, monitoring of blood counts is recommended with any clinical concerns in the medically compromised patent, and the use of CBZ is not recommended with other medications that may cause reductions in platelets or leukocytes. Another potential side effect associated with CBZ use is rash which in very rare cases can progress to Stevens–Johnson Syndrome. This risk may be higher in patients of Asian descent and has been linked to certain pharmacogenomic risk factors such as the patient's human leukocyte antigen (HLA) 1502 allele status. Therefore, routine monitoring for this allele is recommended in all patients of Asian descent in which CBZ is being initiated. Other issues associated with CBZ use center around potential drug interactions as CBZ has been found to be an inducer of cytochrome P450 3A4 and 2C19. Therefore, when CBZ is taken in combination with other medications that use these metabolic pathways, reduced blood levels of these substrates may be experienced, possibly resulting in subtherapeutic blood levels and reduced efficacy (McEvoy et al. 2007a). Similar to VPA these drug interactions become extremely important when CBZ is being added on to or removed from existing therapies or when another medication is being initiated in a patient on CBZ.

11.4.3 Lamotrigine

Another commonly used anticonvulsant is lamotrigene which blocks voltage-gated sodium channels and modifies aspartate and glutamate release. The efficacy of lamotrigine in BPAD has been established through randomized controlled trials (Malhi et al. 2003, 2009). It has antidepressant and mood stabilizing effects in BPAD patients and also is considered to have augmenting properties when combined with lithium or valproic acid. For maintenance treatment the usual dosage range of lamotrigine is 50 to 300 mg/day. Trials have shown that doses above this range do not provide any further benefit. A dose titration strategy (25 mg/day for the first 2 weeks, 50 mg/day for weeks 3 and 4, 100 mg/day for week 5 and 200 mg/day for week 6 and on) is employed when starting lamotrigine. Although such a titration strategy does not completely eliminate the risk of Stevens–Johnson Syndrome, it is rare for problems to emerge in such a cautious approach. The occasional skin rash associated with lamotrigine therapy is usually self-limiting; however, in rare instances it may progress to Stevens–Johnson Syndrome; patient education regarding rashes should include advice on maintaining a constancy of use of external soaps and exposures and to seek advice should a rash occur while taking lamotrigine. Drug interactions are possible with lamotrigine as it is metabolized by glucuronidation. Valproic acid, or any substance that inhibits glucuronidation can decreases the clearance of lamotrigne, affecting the metabolisms of lamotrigine. The dose of lamotrigine should be reduced by approximately half when used concomitantly with a significant inhibitor of glucurionidase (McEvoy et al. 2007b).

11.5 Antipsychotics

Another class of medications that is commonly used for the treatment of BPAD are the atypical antipsychotics such as quetiapine, risperidone, and aripipazole. In general these medications work through the regulation of dopamine and serotonin neurotransmission. When used acutely for the treatment of mania, medications in this class act more as a sedative agent, while with continued use they have some direct mood stabilization properties. All three of these medications have been approved by the Food and Drug Administration (FDA) for the acute treatment of mania, while aripiprazole has been approved for both acute and maintenance therapy of BPAD either as monotherapy or as adjunct treatment. These medications are generally well tolerated and effective in the treatment of BPAD; therefore, choice of which agent to use depends on prescriber preference, side effects, and drug interactions. Perhaps the most worrisome side effect seen with these medications is metabolic and relate to an increased risk of cardiovascular disease. Approximately, 40 % of patients who take these medications go on to develop metabolic syndrome which is a constellation of symptoms relating to central adiposity, hypercholesterolemia, hypertension, and glucose dysregulation. Developing a metabolic syndrome places individuals at greater risk for overall cardiovascular disease then having any one specific individual symptom in isolation, e.g., being overweight or just having elevated fasting glucose. Therefore, monitoring guidelines for these metabolic complications have been established which start with baseline monitoring of the above parameters, followed by continued monitoring while the patient is taking the medication (Tohen and Vieta 2009; Marder et al. 2004). Table 11.2 outlines the routine monitoring recommended for atypical antipsychotic use. Although all of these medications fall within the class of atypical antipsychotic, not all of these medications carry the same risk. Of those listed above, aripiprazole seems to be the most metabolically benign; however, routine monitoring is still recommended (Marder et al. 2004).

Each of the atypical antipsychotic medications are extensively metabolized by the liver; they are all substrates for various CYP450 enzymes and carry the potential for drug interactions. In particular, both CYP3A4 and 2D6 are involved in the

Table 11.2 Recommend monitoring for second generation antipsychotics

Monitoring parameter	Baseline	12 week	Annually	Every 5 years
Personal/family history	X		X	
Weight (BMI)[a]	X	X	Obtain quarterly	
Waist circumference	X		X	
Blood pressure	X	X	X	
Fasting plasma glucose	X	X	X	
Fasting lipid panel	X	X		X

Adapted from: Diabetes Care. 2004;27(2):596–601
[a]Additionally obtain weight at weeks 4 and 8

metabolism of aripiprazole. Therefore, if patients are put on medications that induce or inhibit this metabolic enzyme, the metabolism of aripiprazole could be affected. Risperidone is primarily metabolized by CYP2D6 to the active metabolite 9-OH-risperdone as well as being a substrate for the drug efflux transporter, P-glycoprotein. When used with medications that are also 2D6 inhibitors, careful monitoring should occur and if necessary the dosage of ripseridone will need to be adjusted. Alternatively, if risperidone is given with a P-glycoprotein inducer, the dosage of risperione may need to be increased. For quetiapine, its metabolism is primarily mediated through 3A4; therefore, if this medication is to be used with any 3A4 inhibitors or inducers, appropriate modifications to the quetiapine dosage are necessary. Although this can potentially be a serious drug interaction, quetiapine itself does not seem to inhibit or induce any of the cytochrome P450 enzymes and therefore may not cause additional drug interactions.

11.6 Drug Interactions

For the medications listed above, numerous potential drug interactions may occur either due to direct or competitive metabolic inhibition. In the first scenario, either the BPAD medication or the chemotherapeutic agent may directly inhibit the enzyme(s) responsible for drug metabolism. This may result in the inhibition of metabolism resulting in elevated levels of the substrate medication, with no change in serum concentrations for the inhibiting medication. In the second scenario, both the BPAD medication and the chemotherapeutic medication are eliminated through the same isoenzyme resulting in competition that prevents the breakdown of both medications. The end result is an elevation in both medications, albeit the elevation in serum concentrations may not be to the same extent as that seen with direct metabolic inhibition. On the flip side of this are medications that induce the production of the CYP450 enzymes, resulting in reduced serum concentrations of medications whose metabolism is facilitated by these enzymes. Because the induction process takes time for the synthesis of new enzyme formation, these drug interactions may not be seen until about 2 weeks after both medications have been given. This is in contrast to inhibitory drug interactions where the interaction of

Table 11.3 CYP450 enzymes status by medication class for specific medications traditionally used in bipolar affective disorder (adapted from http://medicine.iupui.edu/clinpharm/ddis/)

	CYP1A2	CYP2B6	CYP2C9	CYP2C19	CYP2D6	CYP3A4
Antidepressants						
Amitriptyline	Substrate		Substrate	Substrate	Substrate	Substrate
Clomipramine	Substrate			Substrate	Substrate	Substrate
Atomoxetine					Substrate	Substrate
Despramine					Substrate	Substrate
Imipramine	Substrate			Substrate	Substrate	Substrate
Paroxetine					Substrate Inhibitor	Substrate
Fluoxetine			Substrate	Inhibitor	Substrate Inhibitor	Substrate
Fluvoxamine	Inhibitor		Inhibitor	Inhibitor	Substrate	Substrate Inhibitor
Nortriptyline					Substrate	Substrate
Venlafaxine					Substrate	Substrate
Bupropion		Substrate			Inhibitor	
Citalopram				Substrate		
Duloxetine					Inhibitor	
Sertraline					Inhibitor	
Escitalopram					Inhibitor	
Nefazodone						Inhibitor
Mood stabilizers/antipsychotics						
Haloperidol	Substrate				Substrate	Substrate
Perphenazine					Substrate Inhibitor	Substrate
Risperidone					Substrate	Substrate
Thioridazine					Substrate	Substrate
Aripiprazole						Substrate
Clozapine	Substrate					
Olanzapine	Substrate					
Chlorpromazine					Substrate Inhibitor	
Oxcarbamazepine				Inhibitor		Inducer
Carbamazepine				Inducer		Inducer
Valproate						Inhibitor
Nontraditional medications						
St. Johns Wort						Inducer

metabolism can be seen within hours or days. Table 11.3 is a listing of common medications used in bipolar disorder, followed by their CYPP450 substrate, inhibition, and inducer status. The fourth column in Table 11.4 refers to the drug efflux transporter, P-glycoprotein, which is encoded by the ATP-binding cassette, sub-family B (MDR/TAP), member 1(ABCB1) gene also known as the Multi

Table 11.4 Potential effects of chemotherapy agents on drug metabolism

| Cancer drug | Cytochrome P450 | | | P-Glycoprotein interaction |
	Substrate	Inhibitor	Inducer	
5-Fluorouracil		2C9		
Abiraterone	3A4	2D6		
Camptothecin			1A1, 1A4	Substrate
Cyclophosphamide	2B6, 2C19, 3A4		2B6, 3A4	
Dasatinib	3A4			
Daunorubicin				Substrate
Docetaxel	3A4	3A4	3A4	Substrate
Doxorubicin	3A4	2D6, 3A4		Substrate and inhibitor
Erlotinib	3A4			
Etoposide	3A4	2C8, 3A4		Substrate
Everolimus	2C8, 3A4			Substrate
Ifosfamide	2B6, 3A4	3A4		
Imatinib	3A4	2C9, 2D6, 3A4		Substrate
Irinotecan	2C9, 3A4			Substrate
Lapatinib	3A4	3A4		Substrate
Nilotinib	3A4			Substrate
Nitrosoureas	2C19	2D6		
Paclitaxel	2C8, 3A4	3A4	3A4	Substrate
Procarbazine	3A4			
Sorafenib	3A4			
Sunitinib	3A4			
Tamoxifen	2D6, 1A2, 2C9, 3A4		2B6, 2D6, 3A4	Inhibitor
Teniposide	2C19, 3A4	2C8, 2C9, 3A4	3A4	Substrate
Thiotepa	2B6, 3A4	2B6		
Topotecan	3A4			Substrate
Vinblastine	3A4	2D6, 3A4		Substrate
Vincristine	3A4	2D6		Substrate

Drug Resistance (MDR) gene. While many of the oncologic agents are known to be substrates of P-glycoprotein, the effect of this drug transporter on most of the medications used for the treatment of BPAD is unknown. In theory, drug interactions that may occur through this transporter system would most likely result in a reduction in the elimination of both oncologic and bipolar disorder substrates, resulting in higher blood concentrations. Therefore, the information included in this table may serve as a future reference as we work to understand the role of this drug transporter in mental illness.

11.7   Summary

Management of the oncology patient with BPAD is an interdisciplinary team effort. While generally, treatment of the patient's cancer is the priority, an acute manic or depressive episode will often need to be managed urgently in order to secure compliance with medical care. BPAD treatment in the maintenance phase should be adjusted and modified based on cancer treatment. Close involvement of the oncology team with psychiatry and pharmacy will ensure that the patient gets the best possible management of their bipolar symptoms while minimizing debilitating side effects and drug interactions. The pharmacist is particularly well placed in strategic medication changes, as drug interactions involving oncology and psychiatric medications are common. However, randomized placebo-controlled trial data of interactions with oncology medications are lacking. Drug interactions with oncologic medication are not typically studied during the drug discovery and approval process, due to the unacceptable risks of administering these medications to a non-oncology population. Therefore, potential drug interactions identified before the patient starts therapy are important to discuss so that a decision can be made based on a risk–benefit assessment. The reader is to be advised that there are ongoing attempts to catalogue and describe oncology–psychiatry medicine interactions (http://www.onco-informatics.com/); however, they are as yet underdeveloped and incomplete. Overall, close monitoring and evaluation of a BPAD patient with cancer will maximize success of therapy from both an oncology and psychiatric perspective.

> **Clinical Case**
>
> TR is a 62-year-old male with a long standing history of bipolar affective disorder (BPAD) I. His first episode of mania was at the age of 25; however, prior to this he was first diagnosed with depression starting in his late teens. Over the years, he has been placed on many medications for the treatment of BPAD. His most recent episode was a major depressive episode. His current regimen consists of Valproate 1,500 mg BID and Paroxetine 30 mg QD. He has been stable on this combination for the past two years and reports good medication compliance.
>
> Approximately 6 months ago, TR noticed some abdominal issues (discomfort in the GI/pelvic area) but thought this was due to his Valproate since he experienced these type of symptoms when he was started on this medication; he also noticed that he has had some trouble urinating and decided to seek medical attention. At this time he was diagnosed with prostate cancer and unsuccessfully underwent hormonal therapy. He was recently started on Abiraterone (Zytiga) and currently is experiencing a manic episode. His psychiatrist diagnoses him with antidepressant-induced mania caused by Abiraterone inhibition of CYP2D6 which has resulted in higher paroxetine

(continued)

drug levels. Additionally, his psychiatrist wonders if there is a potential drug interaction between the Abiraterone and his Valproate since Valporate inhibits CYP3A4 which is responsible for the metabolism of Abiraterone. Therefore, what changes should be made to his BPAD treatments?

Suggested Further Reading

• Drug Interactions Table at http://medicine.iupui.edu/clinpharm/ddis/

References

Allen MH, Hirschfeld RM, Wozniak PJ, Baker JD, Bowden CL. Linear relationship of valproate serum concentration to response and optimal serum levels for acute mania. Am J Psychiatry. 2006;163:272–5.

Anonymous. Practice guideline for the treatment of patients with major depressive disorder (revision). Am J Psychiatry. 2000;157:1–45

AP Association, STAT!Ref, Teton Data Systems. Diagnostic and statistical manual of mental disorders. Washington, DC: American Psychiatric Association; 2000.

Hopkins HS, Gelenberg AJ. Serum lithium levels and the outcome of maintenance therapy of bipolar disorder. Bipolar Disord. 2000;2:174–9.

Kessler RC, Berglund P, Demler O, Jin R, Koretz D, Merikangas KR, Rush AJ, Walters EE, Wang PS, National Comorbidity Survey Replication. The epidemiology of major depressive disorder: results from the National Comorbidity Survey Replication (NCS-R). JAMA. 2003; 289:3095–105.

Malhi GS, Mitchell PB, Salim S. Bipolar depression: management options. CNS Drugs. 2003;17: 9–25.

Malhi GS, Adams D, Berk M. Medicating mood with maintenance in mind: bipolar depression pharmacotherapy. Bipolar Disord. 2009;11 Suppl 2:55–76.

Mann JJ. The medical management of depression. N Engl J Med. 2005;353:1819–34.

Marder SR, Essock SM, Miller AL, Buchanan RW, Casey DE, Davis JM, Kane JM, Lieberman JA, Schooler NR, Covell N, Stroup S, Weissman EM, Wirshing DA, Hall CS, Pogach L, Pi-Sunyer X, Bigger Jr JT, Friedman A, Kleinberg D, Yevich SJ, Davis B, Shon S. Physical health monitoring of patients with schizophrenia. Am J Psychiatry. 2004;161:1334–49.

McEvoy GK, Miller J, Snow EK, et al. Carbamazepine. AHFS Drug Information 2007. Bethesda, MD: American Society of Health-System Pharmacists; 2007a. p. 2220–5

McEvoy GK, Miller J, Snow EK, et al. Lamotrigine. AHFS Drug Information 2007. Bethesda, MD: American Society of Health-System Pharmacists; 2007b. p. 2233–9

Merikangas KR, Akiskal HS, Angst J, Greenberg PE, Hirschfeld RM, Petukhova M, Kessler RC. Lifetime and 12-month prevalence of bipolar spectrum disorder in the National Comorbidity Survey replication. Arch Gen Psychiatry. 2007;64:543–52.

Perlis RH. The role of pharmacologic treatment guidelines for bipolar disorder. J Clin Psychiatry. 2005;66 Suppl 3:37–47.

Suppes T, Dennehy EB, Hirschfeld RM, Altshuler LL, Bowden CL, Calabrese JR, Crismon ML, Ketter TA, Sachs GS, Swann AC, Texas Consensus Conference Panel on Medication Treatment of Bipolar Disorder. The Texas implementation of medication algorithms: update to the algorithms for treatment of bipolar I disorder. J Clin Psychiatry. 2005;66:870–86.

Tohen M, Vieta E. Antipsychotic agents in the treatment of bipolar mania. Bipolar Disord. 2009;
  11 Suppl 2:45–54.
Yatham LN, Kennedy SH, Parikh SV, Schaffer A, Beaulieu S, Alda M, O'Donovan C,
  Macqueen G, McIntyre RS, Sharma V, Ravindran A, Young LT, Milev R, Bond DJ,
  Frey BN, Goldstein BI, Lafer B, Birmaher B, Ha K, Nolen WA, Berk M. Canadian Network
  for Mood and Anxiety Treatments (CANMAT) and International Society for Bipolar Disorders
  (ISBD) collaborative update of CANMAT guidelines for the management of patients with
  bipolar disorder: update 2013. Bipolar Disord. 2013;15:1–44.

Treatment of Delirium and Confusional States in Oncology and Palliative Care Settings

12

William S. Breitbart and Yesne Alici

Abstract

Delirium is one of the most common neuropsychiatric complications seen in cancer patients, associated with significant morbidity and mortality. Delirium is frequently under recognized, misdiagnosed, and undertreated among cancer patients and in palliative care settings. Psycho-oncologists should be familiar with early recognition, accurate assessment, and proper management of delirium to prevent adverse outcomes of delirium. There have been a growing number of studies in management and prevention of delirium published over the last decade. Antipsychotics, cholinesterase inhibitors, melatonin, and alpha-2 agonists are the pharmacological management options studied in randomized controlled trials in a variety of patient populations, not all in cancer patients or in the terminally ill. In oncology and palliative care settings, the evidence is most clearly supportive of short-term, low-dose use of antipsychotics for the control of the symptoms of delirium, with close monitoring for possible side effects especially in older patients and patients with multiple medical comorbidities. This chapter presents an overview of the pharmacological management options for delirium in cancer patients and in palliative care settings.

12.1 Introduction

Delirium is one of the most common and often serious neuropsychiatric complications seen in oncology and palliative care settings. Delirium is characterized by an abrupt onset of disturbances of awareness and alertness, attention, cognition, and perception that fluctuate over the course of the day (Breitbart and Alici 2008). In addition to these core symptoms, the clinical features of delirium are numerous

W.S. Breitbart (✉) • Y. Alici
Department of Psychiatry and Behavioral Sciences, Memorial Sloan Kettering Cancer Center, 614 Lexington Avenue, 7th Floor, New York, NY 10022, USA
e-mail: breitbaw@MSKCC.ORG; Aliciy@mskcc.org

L. Grassi and M. Riba (eds.), *Psychopharmacology in Oncology and Palliative Care*,
DOI 10.1007/978-3-642-40134-3_12, © Springer-Verlag Berlin Heidelberg 2014

and include a variety of neuropsychiatric symptoms that are also common to other psychiatric disorders, such as depression, cognitive disturbances, and psychotic symptoms (APA 2013).

Delirium is caused by a significant physiologic disturbance, usually involving multiple medical etiologies among patients with cancer, including infections, major organ failure, and medication adverse effects (Gaudreau et al. 2005; Spiller and Keen 2006). In patients with cancer, delirium can result either from the direct effects of cancer (e.g., metastatic brain lesions) on the central nervous system (CNS) or from indirect CNS effects of the disease or treatments (e.g., medications, electrolyte imbalance, dehydration, major organ failure, infection, vascular complications, paraneoplastic syndromes) (APA 1999; Breitbart and Alici 2008).

Clinically, the diagnostic gold standard for delirium is the clinician's assessment utilizing the Diagnostic and Statistical Manual of Mental Disorders, 5th edition (DSM-V) criteria (APA 2013). Several delirium assessment tools, including the Memorial Delirium Assessment Scale (MDAS) (Breitbart et al. 1997), the Delirium Rating Scale-Revised 98 (DRS-R-98) (Trzepacz et al. 2001), and the Confusion Assessment Method (CAM) (Inouye et al. 1990), have been validated in oncology and palliative care settings and are used to maximize diagnostic precision for clinical and research purposes and to assess delirium severity (Wong et al. 2010). Based on psychomotor behavior, three clinical subtypes of delirium have been described (Stagno et al. 2004). The subtypes include the hyperactive subtype, the hypoactive subtype, and a mixed subtype with alternating features of each (Stagno et al. 2004).

Delirium is a dysfunction of multiple regions of the brain, a global cerebral dysfunction. Several hypotheses have been proposed and studied to explain the pathogenesis of delirium including but not limited to the neurotransmitter hypothesis (e.g., decreased acetylcholine, increased dopamine), oxygen deprivation hypothesis, inflammatory hypothesis, and physiologic stress hypothesis. Most hypotheses are complementary rather than competing. It is likely that two or more of these hypotheses act together leading to syndromes of delirium as opposed to the earlier proposition of a final common pathway (Maldonado 2008).

The diagnostic workup of delirium should include an assessment of potentially reversible causes of delirium. The clinician should obtain a detailed history from family and staff of the patient's baseline mental status and verify the current fluctuating mental status. It is important to inquire about alcohol, or other substance use disorders in hospitalized cancer patients to be able to recognize and treat alcohol or other substance-induced withdrawal delirium appropriately. Medications that could contribute to delirium should be reviewed (Breitbart and Alici 2008). Predisposing risk factors for delirium should be reviewed including old age, physical frailty, multiple medical comorbidities, dementia, admission to the hospital with infection or dehydration, visual impairment, hearing deficits, polypharmacy, renal impairment, and malnutrition (Inouye et al. 2013). A screen of laboratory parameters allows assessment of the possible role of metabolic abnormalities, such as hypercalcemia, and other problems, such as hypoxia or disseminated intravascular coagulation. In some instances, an EEG (to rule out seizures), brain imaging studies (to rule out brain metastases, intracranial bleeding, or ischemia), or lumbar puncture (to rule out leptomeningeal carcinomatosis or meningitis) may be appropriate (Breitbart and Alici 2008).

It is well recognized that delirium is associated with increased morbidity and mortality, increased length of hospitalization, higher healthcare costs, and significant distress in patients, family members, and professional caregivers (Inouye et al. 2013). There has been growing data on the long-term cognitive and behavioral adverse outcomes of delirium mostly based on studies among intensive care unit survivors and older adults (Pandharipande et al. 2013). Delirium is often under recognized or misdiagnosed; even when recognized, it frequently goes untreated or is inappropriately treated. Psycho-oncology clinicians must be able to diagnose delirium accurately, undertake appropriate assessment of etiologies, and understand the risks and benefits of the currently available management options. This chapter presents an overview of the pharmacological management options for delirium in cancer patients and in palliative care settings. Readers should refer to the further readings section for a list of the key references on prevalence, pathophysiology, and assessment of delirium. In Tables 12.1, 12.2, and 12.3 a summary of delirium prevalence, potential etiologies, and clinical features has been provided.

12.2 Treatment of Delirium

The standard approach to treating delirium in cancer patients, even in those with advanced disease, includes a search for underlying causes, correction of those factors, and concurrent management of the symptoms of delirium utilizing both pharmacologic and non-pharmacologic strategies (Breitbart and Alici 2012). Treatment of the symptoms of delirium should be initiated before, or in concert with, a diagnostic assessment of the etiologies to minimize distress to patients, staff, and family members. Modifiable predisposing risk factors (e.g., visual impairment, hearing impairment, malnutrition, dehydration, polypharmacy) should be identified and corrected diligently (Inouye et al. 2013). In the terminally ill patient who develops delirium in the last days of life, the management of delirium is unique, presenting a number of dilemmas, and the desired clinical outcome may be significantly altered by the dying process. The goal of care in the terminally ill may shift to providing comfort through the judicious use of sedatives, even at the expense of alertness.

12.2.1 Pharmacological Interventions in the Treatment of Delirium

Treatment with psychotropic medications is often necessary to control the symptoms of delirium in cancer patients. Antipsychotics, cholinesterase inhibitors, melatonin, and alpha-2 agonists are the main classes of medications studied in the treatment and prevention of delirium, not all in cancer patients or in the terminally ill (Breitbart and Alici 2012). None of the medications have been approved by the

Table 12.1 Prevalence of delirium

Patient population	Prevalence (%)
Cancer and AIDS patients with advanced disease	25–85
Hospitalized cancer patients seen in psychiatric consultation	25
Hematopoietic stem cell transplant patients around the time of transplant	50
Postoperative patients	50
Elderly patients (>70 years) admitted to medical wards	30–50

Adapted from Breitbart and Alici 2014, IPOS Handbook on Palliative Care for the Psycho-Oncology Clinician

Table 12.2 Clinical features of delirium

Disturbance in level of awareness (reduced orientation to the environment)
Disturbances in level of consciousness (alertness or arousal)[a]
Attentional disturbances
Rapidly fluctuating clinical course and abrupt onset of symptoms that present a change from baseline level of functioning
Disorientation
Cognitive disturbances (i.e., Memory impairment, executive dysfunction, apraxia, agnosia, visuospatial dysfunction, and language disturbances)
Increased or decreased psychomotor activity
Disturbances of sleep–wake cycle
Mood symptoms (depression, dysphoria, mood lability, euphoria)
Perceptual disturbances (hallucinations or illusions) or delusions
Disorganized thought process
Incoherent speech
Neurological findings (may include asterixis, myoclonus, tremor, presence of primitive frontal lobe reflexes also known as frontal release signs, changes in muscle tone)

Adapted from Breitbart W., Alici Y. Agitation and Delirium at the End of Life: "We Couldn't Manage Him". JAMA 2008;300:2898–2910
[a]The Diagnostic and Statistical Manual of Mental Disorders 5th edition (DSM-V) diagnostic criteria for delirium specify that the disturbances in attention and cognition do not occur in the context of a severely reduced level of arousal, such as coma

Food and Drug Administration, (FDA), for treatment or prevention of delirium to date.

Antipsychotic Medications

There have been case reports, case series, retrospective chart reviews, open-label trials, randomized controlled comparison trials, and most recently placebo-controlled trials with both typical and atypical antipsychotics in the treatment of delirium. Study populations mostly include postoperative patients, patients in intensive care unit settings, patients in general medical settings, and only a few focus specifically on patients in oncology and palliative care settings. Table 12.4 presents a summary of the open-label and randomized controlled trials with antipsychotics in the treatment of patients with delirium in oncology and palliative

Table 12.3 Potential etiologies of delirium

Metabolic encephalopathy due to major organ failure (e.g., acute kidney injury, acute hepatic failure)
Electrolyte imbalance
Treatment side effects from
Chemotherapeutic agents
Narcotic analgesics
Corticosteroids
Radiation therapy
Exogenous cytokines—interferon, interleukin
Anticholinergics
Antivirals and antibiotics
Other medications and therapeutic modalities
Infections
Hematologic abnormalities
Nutritional deficiencies
Paraneoplastic syndromes: limbic encephalitis
Primary brain tumor
Metastatic spread to CNS
Seizures including nonepileptiform status epilepticus

care settings as well as randomized controlled trials with antipsychotics in the treatment of patients with delirium in other settings.

Despite the growing number of studies with antipsychotics for the treatment of the symptoms of delirium, there are several limitations to the published studies that should be taken into account. Common problems in most delirium trials include small sample size, heterogeneous samples, lack of systematic assessment of side effects, utilizing valid side effect rating scales, lack of differentiation between subtypes of delirium, and the lack of control for as needed use of additional psychotropic agents.

Evidence-based recommendations for the use of antipsychotics in the treatment of patients with delirium in oncology and palliative care settings can be summarized as follows:

- The American Psychiatric Association (APA) practice guidelines published in 1999 recommended the use of antipsychotics as the first-line pharmacologic option in the treatment of symptoms of delirium (APA 1999).
- A 2004 Cochrane review on drug therapy for delirium in the terminally ill (Jackson and Lipman 2004) concluded that haloperidol was the most suitable medication for the treatment of patients with delirium near the end of life, with chlorpromazine being an acceptable alternative. A 2012 update of this Cochrane review of drug therapy for terminally ill delirium patients (Candy et al. 2012) did not find any additional trials that met the inclusion criteria for the review and therefore concluded that the practitioners should follow the current clinical guidelines on delirium treatment.

Table 12.4 Open-label and randomized controlled trials with antipsychotics in the treatment of delirium

	Intervention	Dose and duration, mean (SD)	Results	Comments
Open-label studies in oncology and palliative care settings				
Breitbart et al. (2002)	Open-label trial of olanzapine for 79 hospitalized advanced cancer patients with delirium	The average starting dose was in the 2.5–5 mg range and patients were given up to 20 mg/day of olanzapine	Olanzapine was effective in resolving delirium in 76 % of patients with no incidence of extrapyramidal side effects. The mean MDAS scores declined from 19.85 to 10.78 in 7 days	Sedation was the most common side effect. Age over 70, history of dementia, and hypoactive delirium were found to be significantly associated with poorer response to olanzapine
Kim et al. (2003)	Open-label trial of 12 patients (most with leukemia) with delirium treated with quetiapine	The average dose was 93.75 mg. The mean duration for stabilization was 5.91 days. The quetiapine dose was tapered down about a month after discharge from the hospital	The DRS scores declined from 18.25 to 8.00	None of the patients experienced any parkinsonian side effects; sedation and vivid dreaming were the only reported side effects
Elsayem et al. (2010)	Open-label trial in 24 advanced cancer patients with delirium using subcutaneous olanzapine	Patients received olanzapine 5 mg SC every 8 h for 3 days and continued haloperidol for breakthrough agitation	Efficacy was achieved in nine (37.5 %) patients. Intramuscular olanzapine was well tolerated subcutaneously in the treatment of delirium	No injection site toxicity was observed after 167 injections. Probable side effects were observed in four patients [severe hypotension (blood pressure <90/50 mmHg), paradoxical agitation, diabetes insipidus, and seizure]
Boettger et al. (2011)	Prospective, case-matched control comparison trial of aripiprazole ($n = 21$) vs. haloperidol ($n = 21$) treated cancer patients with delirium	The mean aripiprazole dose was 15.2 mg at study entry and 18.3 mg at the end. The mean haloperidol dose was 4.9 and 5.5 mg, respectively	Over the course of treatment, MDAS scores improved from 18.1 to 8.3 for aripiprazole and 19.9 to 6.8 for haloperidol. The delirium resolution rate was 76.2 % for aripiprazole and 76.2 % for haloperidol	There were no significant differences in treatment results between aripiprazole and haloperidol for cancer patients with either hypoactive or hyperactive subtypes of delirium. However there was a trend for poor response to aripiprazole among patients with hyperactive delirium. Treatment with haloperidol resulted in more extrapyramidal side effects

Crawford et al. (2013)	Prospective trial of haloperidol for treatment of delirium in hospice and palliative care settings (n = 119)	Haloperidol with a mean dose of 2.1 mg/24 h	Of the 119 participants included, the average dose was 2.1 mg per 24 h; 42 of 106 (35.2 %) reported benefit at 48 h	Harm was reported in 14 of 119 (12 %) at 10 days, the most frequent being somnolence (n = 11) and urinary retention (n = 6). Seven participants had their medication ceased due to harms (two for somnolence and two for rigidity). The researchers concluded that one in three participants gained net clinical benefit at 10 days

Randomized controlled trials in oncology and palliative care settings

Breitbart et al. (1996)	Double-blind RCT of terminally ill AIDS patients: 11, haloperidol; 13, chlorpromazine; and 6, lorazepam for treatment of delirium	1.4 (1.2) mg/day haloperidol, 36 (18.4) mg/day chlorpromazine, 4.6 (4.7) mg/day lorazepam Used for up to 6 days	DRS scores significantly improved in haloperidol and chlorpromazine groups (P < 0.05) No significant extrapyramidal symptoms were observed	Lorazepam group was discontinued early due to worsening of delirium symptoms
Hu et al. (2004)	Double-blind RCT of hospitalized patients: 75, olanzapine; 72, intramuscular haloperidol; and 29, oral placebo for the treatment of delirium	4.5 (4) mg/day olanzapine, 7 (2.3) mg/day haloperidol, and placebo Used for 7 days	The improvement in DRS scores were significantly higher in the olanzapine (72 %) and haloperidol (70 %) groups vs. placebo (29.7 %) (P < 0.01). Increased rates of extrapyramidal symptoms observed in the haloperidol group	Comparison of oral olanzapine and oral placebo with intramuscular haloperidol hinders the quality of double-blind study design
Kim et al. (2010)	A randomized, single-blind, comparative clinical trial comparing the effectiveness of risperidone (n = 17) and olanzapine (n = 15) in the treatment of delirium among mostly oncology patients	Study period: 7 days The mean starting doses were 0.6 (0.2) mg/day risperidone and 1.8 (0.6) mg/day olanzapine. The mean doses at last observation were 0.9 (0.6) mg/day risperidone and 2.4 (1.7) mg/day olanzapine	Significant within-group improvements in the DRS-R-98 scores over time were observed in both treatment groups; the response (defined as a 50 % reduction in the DRS-R-98 scores) rates did not differ significantly between the two groups (risperidone group: 64.7 %, olanzapine group: 73.3 %)	The response to risperidone was significantly poorer in patients > or = 70 years of age compared with those aged <70 years. There was no significant difference in the safety profiles, including extrapyramidal symptoms (EPSs), between the two groups

(continued)

Table 12.4 (continued)

Randomized controlled trials in other settings (e.g., postoperative, ICU)

	Intervention	Dose and duration, mean (SD)	Results	Comments
Han and Kim (2004)	Double-blind RCT of hospitalized patients: 12, haloperidol; 12, risperidone for the treatment of delirium	1.7 (0.84) mg/day haloperidol, 1 (0.4) mg/day Risperidone. Used for 7 days	MDAS scores improved significantly in both groups, but no significant difference between groups was observed	Researchers were not able to provide tablets identical in appearance, which might have hindered the double-blind study design. No significant difference in adverse effects observed
Girard et al. (2010)	Placebo-controlled randomized feasibility trial of intensive care unit patients: 35 haloperidol, 30 ziprasidone, 36 placebo for the treatment of delirium	Patients in the haloperidol group received 15.0 mg/day (10.8–17.0 mg/day) and patients in the ziprasidone group received 113.3 mg/day (81.0–140.0 mg/day) for an average of 4 days	There were no differences in the number of days alive without delirium between the three treatment groups. The study did not find any differences in other outcomes such as ventilator-free days, hospital length of stay, or mortality	The study reported no difference in any safety concerns (ie, akathisia, neuroleptic malignant syndrome, extrapyramidal symptoms, QT prolongation, or arrhythmias). The adverse events were similar between the three groups with no serious events
Devlin et al. (2010)	Placebo-controlled randomized pilot trial of intensive care unit patients with delirium who had an as-needed haloperidol order: 18 quetiapine or 18 placebo for the treatment of delirium	Quetiapine 110 mg (88–191 mg) for 102 h (84–168); placebo group for 186 (108–228) $P = 0.04$	Quetiapine add-on was associated with a shorter time to first resolution of delirium [1.0 (inter quartile range [IQR], 0.5–3.0) vs. 4.5 days (IQR, 2.0–7.0; $P = 0.001$)], and a reduced duration of delirium [36 (IQR, 12–87) vs. 120 h (IQR, 60–195; $P = 0.006$)]	The incidence of extrapyramidal symptoms was similar between groups; however more somnolence was observed with quetiapine (22 % vs. 11 %; $P = 0.66$)
Tahir et al. (2010)	Placebo-controlled randomized trial in medical and surgical patients with delirium: 21 patients with quetiapine and 20 patients with placebo	The mean dose of quetiapine was 40 mg on day 4; 25 mg on day 1; 37.5 mg on day 10	The quetiapine group recovered 82.7 % (37.1 %) faster ($P = 0.026$) than the placebo group in terms of DRS-R-98 severity score. However there was no difference in the total DRS-R-98 scores at anytime	The study reported no difference in any safety concerns between medication and placebo arms

| Grover et al. (2011) | A single-blind randomized controlled trial to compare the efficacy and safety of olanzapine ($n = 23$) and risperidone ($n = 21$) vs. haloperidol ($n = 20$) in patients with delirium admitted to medical and surgical wards | A flexible dose regimen (haloperidol −0.25 to 10 mg; risperidone −0.25 to 4 mg; olanzapine −1.25 to 20 mg) was used | There was a significant reduction in DRS-R98 severity scores over the period of 6 days, but there was no difference between the three medication groups | Researchers concluded that risperidone and olanzapine are as efficacious as haloperidol in the treatment of delirium |
| Maneeton et al. (2013) | A 7-day double-blind, randomized controlled trial in medically ill patients with delirium comparing the efficacy and tolerability of quetiapine and haloperidol. Measures used for daily assessment included the Delirium Rating Scale-revised 98 (DRS-R-98) and total sleep time | Fifty-two subjects were randomized to receive 25–100 mg/day of quetiapine ($n = 24$) or 0.5–2.0 mg/day of haloperidol ($n = 28$). Mean (standard deviation) doses of quetiapine and haloperidol were 67.6 (9.7) and 0.8 (0.3) mg/day, respectively | Means (standard deviation) of the DRS-R-98 severity scores were not significantly different between the quetiapine and haloperidol groups (−22.9 [6.9] vs. −21.7 [6.7]; $P = 0.59$). The DRS-R-98 noncognitive and cognitive subscale scores were not significantly different. At end point, the response and remission rates, the total sleep time, and the Modified (nine-item) Simpson–Angus scores were also not significantly different between groups | Hypersomnia was common in the quetiapine-treated patients (33.3 %), but not significantly higher than that in the haloperidol-treated group (21.4 %) |

This table was compiled based on a comprehensive search of PubMed using the search terms "delirium," "treatment," "antipsychotic" from 1960 through November 2013

- A 2007 Cochrane review, comparing the efficacy and the incidence of adverse effects between haloperidol and atypical antipsychotics, concluded that, like haloperidol, selected atypical antipsychotics (risperidone, olanzapine) were effective in managing delirium (Lonergan et al. 2007). Haloperidol doses greater than 4.5 mg/day resulted in increased rates of extrapyramidal symptoms compared with the atypical antipsychotics, but low-dose haloperidol (i.e., less than 3.5 mg/day) was not shown to result in a greater frequency of extrapyramidal adverse effects.
- A recent review of 28 prospective studies of delirium treatment with antipsychotics among hospitalized adults has concluded that 75 % of delirious patients who receive short-term treatment with low-dose antipsychotics experience clinical response. Response rates appeared consistent across different patient groups and treatment settings. Studies did not suggest significant differences in efficacy for haloperidol vs. atypical agents, except for higher rates of extrapyramidal side effects with haloperidol. A reduced response rate with comorbid dementia was questioned based on the reviewed studies; however further studies were suggested to further explore this association. Review of the 28 prospective delirium treatment trials did not indicate major differences in response rates between clinical subtypes of delirium (Meagher et al. 2013).
- Despite the limitations noted above for antipsychotic medication trials in the treatment of delirium, the evidence to date suggests that antipsychotic medications are effective in improving or resolving the symptoms of delirium in oncology and palliative care settings. Most recent evidence supports the recommendations of the American Psychiatric Association guidelines (APA 1999) for the management of delirium in that low-dose haloperidol (i.e., 1–2 mg po every 4 h as needed or 0.25–0.5 mg po every 4 h for the elderly) continues to be the first-line agent for treatment of symptoms of delirium. The recent evidence further supports the 2007 Cochrane review (Lonergan et al. 2007) that atypical antipsychotics (e.g., olanzapine, risperidone) should be considered as an effective alternative to haloperidol, particularly in patients who are sensitive or intolerant to the use of haloperidol.
- The evidence for efficacy in the improvement of the symptoms of delirium exists for the following atypical antipsychotics: olanzapine, risperidone, aripiprazole, quetiapine. None of the antipsychotics were found to be superior when compared to others in the treatment of delirium symptoms. There is evidence suggesting that the subtypes of delirium may have different treatment responses. A randomized controlled trial of haloperidol and chlorpromazine found that both medications were equally effective in hypoactive and hyperactive subtypes of delirium (Breitbart et al. 1996). Two open-label trials showed different treatment responses to different antipsychotics. In an open-label trial the hypoactive subtype was associated with poorer treatment response to olanzapine (Breitbart et al. 2002). Another open-label study suggested that the hypoactive subtype of delirium was associated with better response to treatment with aripiprazole (Boettger et al. 2011).
- There have not been any trials testing the efficacy and safety of newer antipsychotics (e.g., iloperidone, paliperidone, asenapine, or lurasidone) in the treatment of delirium.

Table 12.5 presents a list of the antipsychotic medications and dosages recommended for use in the treatment of delirium.

Important considerations in starting treatment with any antipsychotic for delirium should primarily include the following: risk of extrapyramidal side effects, sedation, anticholinergic side effects, cardiac arrhythmias, and possible drug–drug interactions (Table 12.6). Despite its widespread use especially in postoperative patients and in ICU settings, there is an FDA warning on the risk of QTc prolongation and torsades de pointes with the use of intravenous haloperidol. Therefore monitoring QTc intervals at least daily among medically ill patients receiving intravenous haloperidol has become the standard clinical practice. The FDA has issued a "black box" warning of increased risk of death when antipsychotics are used to treat elderly patients with dementia-related psychoses. Initial warning for atypical antipsychotics was based on a meta-analysis by Schneider et al. (2005) of 17 placebo-controlled trials involving patients with dementia. The risk of death in patients treated with atypical antipsychotic agents was 1.6–1.7 times greater than in those who received placebo. Most deaths were associated with cardiovascular disease or infection. A second retrospective study of nearly 23,000 older patients found higher mortality rates associated with typical than with atypical antipsychotics—whether or not they had dementia (Wang et al. 2005). This finding has led to an extension of the FDA warning to typical antipsychotics. Caution is advised when using antipsychotic medications especially in elderly patients with dementia. A retrospective case–control analysis of 326 elderly hospitalized patients with delirium at an acute care community hospital comparing risk of mortality among patients who received an antipsychotic vs. those who did not showed that of the 111 patients who received an antipsychotic a total of 16 patients died during that hospitalization. The odds ratio of association between antipsychotic use and death was 1.53 (95 % C.I, 0.83–2.80) in univariate and 1.61 (95 % C.I, 0.88–2.96) in multivariate analysis. The researchers concluded that among elderly medical inpatients with delirium, administration of antipsychotics was not associated with a statistically significant increased risk of mortality (Elie et al. 2009). However larger studies are needed to clarify this conclusion (Table 12.5).

It is important to recognize that antipsychotics have complex mechanisms of action, mostly affecting multiple neurotransmitter systems that can lead to unwanted side effects. Therefore the benefits of initiating antipsychotic treatment for delirium should be weighed against risks associated with their use. Additionally, it remains unknown to what extent the treatment effects of antipsychotics can be explained by specific symptoms control vs. an actual treatment of the delirium syndrome. Future research is needed to explore this further and to develop high-quality evidence-based pharmacologic treatment guidelines for delirium.

Psychostimulants

Psychostimulants have been suggested for the treatment of the hypoactive subtype of delirium, alone or in combination with antipsychotics. Studies with psycho-stimulants in treating delirium are limited to case reports and one open-label study

Table 12.5 Antipsychotic medications used in the treatment of delirium in oncology and palliative care settings (Adapted from Breitbart W, Alici Y: Evidence-Based Treatment of Delirium in Patients with Cancer. J Clin Oncol 2012: 30;1206–1214)

Medication	Dose range	Routes of administration	Side effects	Comments
Typical antipsychotics				
Haloperidol	0.25–2 mg every 2–12 h	PO, IV, IM, SC	Extrapyramidal adverse effects can occur at higher doses (such as doses higher than 4 mg/day). Monitor QT interval on EKG	Remains the gold standard therapy for delirium. May add lorazepam (0.25–1 mg every 2–4 h) for agitated patients. Double-blind controlled trials support efficacy in treatment of symptoms of delirium. A pilot placebo-controlled trial suggests no difference in treatment of delirium when compared to placebo
Chlorpromazine	6.25–50 mg every 4–6 h	PO, IV, IM, SC, PR	More sedating and anticholinergic compared with haloperidol. Monitor blood pressure for hypotension. More suitable for use in ICU settings for closer blood pressure monitoring	May be preferred in agitated patients due to its sedative effect. Double-blind controlled trials support efficacy in treatment of symptoms of delirium No placebo-controlled trials
Atypical antipsychotics				
Olanzapine	2.5–5 mg every 12–24 h	PO[a], IM	Sedation is the main dose-limiting adverse effect in short-term use	Older age, preexisting dementia, and hypoactive subtype of delirium have been associated with poor response. Double-blind comparison trials with haloperidol and risperidone support efficacy in the treatment of delirium. A pilot placebo-controlled prevention trial suggested worsening in delirium severity. A placebo-controlled study is supportive of efficacy in reducing delirium severity and duration
Risperidone	0.125–1 mg every 12–24 h	PO[a]	Extrapyramidal adverse effects can occur with doses >6 mg/day (or in lower doses among patients at high risk). Orthostatic hypotension	Double-blind comparison trials support efficacy in the treatment of delirium. No placebo-controlled trials

(continued)

Table 12.5 (continued)

Medication	Dose range	Routes of administration	Side effects	Comments
Quetiapine	6.25–100 mg every 12–24 h	PO	Sedation, orthostatic hypotension	Sedating effects may be helpful in patients with sleep–wake cycle disturbance. Pilot placebo-controlled trials suggest efficacy in treatment of delirium. However most studies allowed for concomitant use of haloperidol which makes the results difficult to interpret
Ziprasidone	10–40 mg every 12–24 h	PO, IM	Monitor QT interval on EKG	Placebo-controlled, double-blind trial suggests no difference in the treatment of delirium when compared to placebo
Aripiprazole	2–30 mg every 24 h	PO[a], IM	Monitor for akathisia	Evidence is limited. A prospective open-label trial suggests comparable efficacy to haloperidol. There is some evidence to suggest its efficacy in hypoactive subtype of delirium. No placebo-controlled trials

[a]Risperidone, olanzapine, and aripiprazole are available in orally disintegrating tablets

that are supportive of its use in terminally ill cancer patients with no significant adverse events (Breitbart and Alici 2012). However, in the absence of further evidence psychostimulants cannot be recommended for the treatment of patients with delirium in oncology and palliative care settings. The risks of precipitating agitation and exacerbating psychotic symptoms should be carefully evaluated when psychostimulants are considered in the treatment of hypoactive subtype of delirium.

Cholinesterase Inhibitors

Impaired cholinergic function has been implicated as one of the neurochemical imbalances in the neuropathogenesis of delirium (Maldonado 2008). Despite case reports of beneficial effects of donepezil and rivastigmine, a 2008 Cochrane review concluded that there is currently no evidence from controlled trials supporting use of cholinesterase inhibitors in the treatment of delirium (Overshott et al. 2008). A small, double-blind, placebo-controlled trial with the use of rivastigmine in the treatment of delirium patients in general hospital settings failed to show any differences in the duration of delirium between rivastigmine and placebo groups (Overshott et al. 2010). A European multicenter double-blind study in intensive

Table 12.6 Recommendations on monitoring patients with delirium for antipsychotic side effects in oncology and palliative care settings[a] (Adapted from Breitbart W, Alici Y: Evidence-Based Treatment of Delirium in Patients with Cancer. J Clin Oncol 2012: 30;1206–1214)

EKG—baseline, and with every dose increase [consider daily monitoring if on high doses (e.g., haloperidol > 5–10 mg daily), patients with underlying unstable cardiac disease, patients with electrolyte disturbances, patients on other QT prolonging medications[b], medically frail, older patients; patients with unstable cardiac diseases or those on intravenous antipsychotics may require continuous monitoring in consultation with cardiology]

Fasting lipid profile—baseline and every 3 months

Fasting blood glucose—baseline and weekly

Body Mass Index—baseline and weekly

Extrapyramidal side effects (including parkinsonism, dystonia, akathisia, neuroleptic malignant syndrome)—baseline and daily

Blood pressure, pulse-baseline, and at least daily (high-risk patients should be monitored more closely, continuous monitoring may be required in medically unstable patients; orthostatic measurements should be considered with antipsychotics with alpha-1 antagonist effects such as chlorpromazine, risperidone)

[a]Recommendations are based on the Consensus Development Conference on antipsychotic drugs and obesity and diabetes (American Diabetes Association 2004)

[b]The risk of QT prolongation is directly correlated with higher antipsychotic doses, with parenteral formulations (e.g., intravenous haloperidol) of antipsychotics, and with certain medications (e.g., ziprasidone, thioridazine). In individual patients an absolute QTc interval of >500 ms or an increase of 60 ms (or more than 20 %) from baseline is regarded as indicating an increased risk of torsades des pointes. Discontinuation of the antipsychotic and a consultation with cardiology should be considered especially if there is continued need for the use of antipsychotics

care units comparing rivastigmine and placebo for the treatment of delirium was stopped prematurely due to increased mortality in the rivastigmine group (Van Eijk et al. 2010). No common cause of mortality could be identified among patients who died while on rivastigmine.

The use of cholinesterase inhibitors in delirium has not been studied in oncology and palliative care settings. Based on the existing evidence from general hospital and intensive care unit settings, cholinesterase inhibitors could not be recommended in treatment of delirium.

12.2.2 Pharmacologic Interventions in Prevention of Delirium

Several researchers studied both pharmacologic and non-pharmacologic interventions in the prevention of delirium among older patient populations, particularly in surgical and ICU settings. However, there have been no delirium prevention trials with any of the pharmacologic agents in oncology settings to date. Antipsychotics, cholinesterase inhibitors, melatonin, and dexmedetomidine have been studied in the prevention of delirium in randomized controlled delirium prevention studies conducted in different settings (Breitbart and Alici 2012). A 2007 Cochrane review of delirium prevention studies in different patient populations concluded that the evidence on effectiveness of interventions to prevent

Table 12.7 Summary of non-pharmacologic interventions used in the prevention and treatment of delirium (Inouye et al. 2013)

Review of medication list to avoid polypharmacy
Control of pain
Promoting good sleep pattern and sleep hygiene
Monitoring closely for dehydration and fluid-electrolyte disturbances
Monitoring nutrition
Monitoring for sensory deficits, provide visual and hearing aids
Avoiding immobility, encouraging early mobilization (minimizing the use of immobilizing catheters, intravenous lines, and physical restraints)[a]
Monitoring bowel and bladder functioning
Reorienting the patient frequently
Placing an orientation board, clock, or familiar objects in patient rooms
Encouraging cognitively stimulating activities

[a]Physical restraints should be avoided both in patients who are at risk for developing delirium and in those with delirium. The use of physical restraints has been identified as an independent risk factor for delirium persistence at the time of hospital discharge. Restraint-free care should be the standard of care for prevention and treatment of delirium in oncology and palliative care settings

delirium was sparse; therefore no recommendations could be made regarding the use of pharmacologic interventions for prevention of delirium (Siddiqi et al. 2007).

The findings of the delirium prevention studies conducted in general postoperative and ICU settings can be summarized as follows:

– Antipsychotics: A randomized controlled prevention trial with low-dose haloperidol was not found to be effective in reducing delirium incidence; however, it was shown to decrease delirium severity and duration (Kalisvaart et al. 2005). A delirium prevention trial with olanzapine among postoperative patients was suggestive of decrease in delirium incidence with the prophylactic use of olanzapine; however, increase in the severity and duration of delirium with olanzapine in this study raised concerns (Larsen et al. 2010). The positive results (decrease in delirium incidence) of a prevention trial with risperidone were found to be imprecise in a deliberate review of delirium trials (Prakanrattana and Prapaitrakool 2007). A trial of 457 postoperative patients admitted to ICUs in Beijing did show a reduction in the incidence of delirium using prophylactic, low-dose haloperidol (0.5 mg bolus followed by 0.1 mg/h for 12 h) compared with placebo. Only 35 patients (15.3 %) in the haloperidol group and 53 (23.2 %) patients in the placebo group developed delirium (Wang et al. 2012). A recent, double-blind, placebo-controlled, randomized trial in a general adult ICU, to establish whether early treatment with haloperidol would decrease the duration of delirium or coma, showed that patients in the haloperidol group spent the same number of days alive, without delirium, and without coma as did patients in the placebo group (median 5 days vs. 6 days; $P = 0.53$). The most common adverse events were oversedation (11 patients in the haloperidol group vs. 6 patients in the placebo group) and QTc prolongation (7 patients in the haloperidol group and 6 patients in the placebo group). No serious adverse events were noted. Patients received haloperidol 2.5 mg IV q8h ($n = 71$) and placebo ($n = 70$) for a maximum of 14 days. The importance of this study is the finding that haloperidol can be safely used in this population of patients (Page et al. 2013)

- Cholinesterase inhibitors: Cholinesterase inhibitors were not found to be effective in reducing delirium incidence or severity based on the evidence from three different placebo-controlled prevention trials with donepezil, and rivastigmine.
- Melatonin: Melatonin has been suggested to play a role in the treatment of delirium through direct antioxidant and anti-inflammatory activity, in addition to its effects on the sleep–wake cycle. A small randomized, double-blind placebo-controlled study suggested that low-dose melatonin (0.5 mg/night) administered nightly to elderly patients admitted to acute care represents a potential protective agent against development of delirium (Al-Aama et al. 2011).
- Alpha-2 agonists: Dexmedetomidine is a selective $\alpha(2)$-adrenergic receptor agonist that is indicated in the USA for the sedation of mechanically ventilated adult patients in intensive care settings and in non-intubated adult patients prior to and/or during surgical and other procedures. Clinical trials with dexmedetomidine have shown mixed results for the prevention and treatment of delirium in the intensive care unit setting. A recent meta-analysis of randomized controlled trials involving the use of dexmedetomidine in ICU patients has shown that the incidence of delirium was significantly reduced in comparison with propofol based on three studies including a total of 658 patients (relative risk 0.40; confidence interval 0.22–0.74) (Xia et al. 2013). The potential use of dexmedetomidine in the palliative care population has been considered for the prevention and treatment of delirium, and enhancing analgesia. However there have not been any studies with dexmedetomidine in palliative care settings to the best of our knowledge.

In summary, none of the pharmacologic agents were studied specifically in oncology and palliative care settings for prevention of delirium; therefore no recommendations could be made regarding use of these medications in the prevention of delirium in these settings.

12.2.3 Non-pharmacologic Management of Delirium in Cancer Patients

There have been several non-pharmacologic intervention trials in the treatment and prevention of delirium among older patients in general medical and surgical settings. A list of non-pharmacologic interventions is included in Table 12.7. Although these interventions were not found to have any beneficial effects on mortality or health-related quality of life when compared with usual care there is evidence that they result in faster improvement of delirium and slower deterioration in cognition especially among older patients with delirium in general hospital settings (Inouye et al. 2013). Prevention trials yielded more encouraging results in reducing delirium incidence and decreasing delirium duration and severity in geriatric patient population. The study effect sizes suggested statistically significant reductions in delirium incidence of about one-third reduction with multicomponent interventions (Inouye et al. 2013).

The applicability of a multicomponent intervention, to prevent delirium in cancer patients in palliative care settings, has been studied (Gagnon et al. 2012). A cohort of 1,516 patients was followed from admission to death at seven palliative care centers. In two of these centers, routine care included a delirium preventive intervention targeting physicians (written notice on selective delirium risk factors and inquest on intended medication changes), patients, and their family (orientation to time and place, information about early delirium symptoms). Delirium frequency and severity were compared between patients at the intervention ($N = 674$) and usual care ($N = 842$) centers based on thrice-daily symptom assessments with the Confusion Rating Scale. The overall rate of adherence to the intervention was 89.7 %. The incidence of delirium was 49.1 % in the intervention group, compared with 43.9 % in the usual care group [odds ratio (OR) 1.23, $P = 0.045$]. When confounding variables were controlled for, no difference was observed between the intervention and the usual care groups in delirium incidence (OR 0.94, $P = 0.66$), delirium severity (1.83 vs. 1.92; $P = 0.07$), total days in delirium (4.57 vs. 3.57 days; $P = 0.63$), or duration of first delirium episode (2.9 vs. 2.1 days; $P = 0.96$). Researchers concluded that a simple multicomponent preventive intervention was ineffective in reducing delirium incidence or severity among cancer patients receiving end-of-life care. It would be important to study these interventions in the treatment of delirium and among cancer patients in non-palliative care settings.

In summary, non-pharmacologic prevention and treatment strategies are supported by the evidence-based literature in general hospital settings especially among older patients (National Institute for Health and Clinical Excellence, 2010). Although they have not shown to be effective in preventing delirium in palliative care settings, they may have a role in controlling delirium symptoms in oncology and palliative care settings. The use of non-pharmacologic interventions to prevent and treat delirium is recommended when feasible. There are no known risks associated with the use of non-pharmacologic interventions in delirium patients. They may also play a role in reducing delirium-induced distress among patients, families, and caregivers.

Conclusion

Psycho-oncology clinicians commonly encounter delirium as a major complication of cancer and its treatments, particularly among hospitalized cancer patients. Proper assessment, diagnosis, and management of delirium are essential in improving quality of life and minimizing morbidity in cancer patients. The current evidence supports the use of pharmacologic agents in the control of symptoms of delirium, with the best evidence, demonstrating efficacy for short-term, low-dose use of antipsychotics in oncology and palliative care settings. Current evidence does not support the use of psychostimulants or cholinesterase inhibitors for the treatment or prevention of delirium. Psycho-oncology clinicians should make every effort to minimize the well-documented patient, family, and caregiver distress associated with delirium in these settings. The prophylactic use of antipsychotics, alpha-2 agonists, and melatonin in the prevention of delirium is one of the more interesting new frontiers of delirium management, and the evidence to date suggests some promise for olanzapine, risperidone, and mela-tonin in non-oncology settings. The use of alpha-2 agonists in the prevention of delirium has shown mixed results in ICU settings. Larger, well-designed, pla-cebo-controlled trials are required for any prophylactic drug recommendations to be made among cancer patients and the terminally ill.

Clinical Case

Ms. Jones is an 82-year-old retired high school teacher with a history of postpartum depression, a 3-year-long history of gradual cognitive decline primarily affecting short-term memory and ability to manage finances, and a past medical history of hypertension, right bundle branch block, hyper-cholesterolemia, osteoarthritis, and diffuse large B cell lymphoma diagnosed about a year ago. Ms. Jones has recently completed tenth cycle of her chemotherapy with RCHOP and has tolerated the treatment well so far. Ms. Jones was brought into the Emergency Room by the police after having been found in front of her apartment building in her nightgown in an agitated state. During triage she was noted to be hyperpneic with a heart rate of 110bPM and a blood pressure of 80/51 mmHg. She was hypoalert, agitated, and inattentive throughout the assessment, asking an attorney to be present throughout her assessment so that the people in white coats do not arrest her. The psycho-oncology service was consulted to assess patient for severe agitation and to rule out psychotic depression based on patient's history of postpartum depression.

In this everyday clinical scenario the role of the psycho-oncologist can be summarized as follows:

1. Primum non nocere: "First do no harm."
2. Educate the ER staff that the patient's presentation is consistent with delirium until proven otherwise. Assessment and management of delirium take precedence over any other psychiatric diagnoses that the patient has or had in the past.
3. Start treatment of symptoms of delirium with pharmacologic and non-pharmacologic measures. Given patient's age, underlying cognitive deficits, and vascular comorbidities use of antipsychotics should be limited to low dose and short duration to control symptoms of delirium that represent a danger to self or others. EKG should be obtained if and when possible. It should be noted that patients with right bundle branch block might present with a prolonged QTc secondary to prolonged ventricular depolarization. Do not be alarmed! A consultation with cardiology or

(continued)

assessment of the JT interval would help clinicians determine the actual risk of torsade des pointes.

4. Concurrent with the treatment start assessment of underlying etiologies for delirium including but not limited to obtaining labs for complete blood count, electrolytes, renal and hepatic functioning; consider brain imaging, arterial blood gases, and urinalysis with culture.

5. Review medication list for possible drug–drug interactions.

6. Obtain collateral information from the family and other caregivers to determine the course of events, possible missed or doubled doses of medications, alcohol use, use of benzodiazepines or barbiturates, and history of recent falls. The psycho-oncologist should educate the family on diagnosis and management of delirium.

7. Given underlying cognitive deficits, a possible diagnosis of underlying dementia, or mild cognitive impairment, the psycho-oncologist should educate the staff that the patient is at high risk for increased delirium duration and severity, for worsening cognitive decline, and increased morbidity and mortality.

▶ **Key Points (Breitbart and Alici 2014)**

1. Current evidence is supportive of short-term use of low-dose antipsychotics in the treatment of symptoms of delirium (i.e., agitation, sleep–wake cycle disturbances, delusions, hallucinations) with close monitoring for possible side effects especially in elderly patients with multiple medical comorbidities.

2. The longest clinical and research experience and safety/efficacy data are available for haloperidol. Therefore low-dose haloperidol is still considered the gold standard in treatment of delirium. There is growing evidence for the efficacy of atypical antipsychotics in the management of delirium as well.

3. The choice of antipsychotic medication for the treatment of delirium should be based on the clinical presentation of the patient and the side-effect profile and routes of availability of each antipsychotic drug, as none of the antipsychotics were found to be superior to others in comparison trials.

4. A more cautious approach may be appropriate for patients with a hypoalert or hypoactive presentation of delirium, or those who are having frankly pleasant or comforting hallucinations in using antipsychotic medications. It should be noted, however, that a hypoalert or "hypoactive" delirium may very quickly and unexpectedly elevate to an agitated or "hyperactive" delirium that can threaten the serenity and safety of the patient, family and staff.

5. Current evidence is not supportive of the use of antipsychotics for the prevention of delirium in oncology and palliative care settings.

6. It is strongly recommended to implement non-pharmacologic interventions in the routine care of patients who are either at risk for delirium and for patients

with established delirium, based on the evidence from non-oncology settings. There are no known risks associated with the use of non-pharmacologic interventions.

7. There is no evidence to support the use of cholinesterase inhibitors in treatment or prevention of delirium in oncology and palliative care settings.

8. The use of psychostimulants in the treatment of hypoactive subtype of delirium in terminally ill patients has been considered. In the absence of randomized controlled trials psychostimulants cannot currently be recommended in the treatment of patients with delirium in oncology and palliative care settings.

9. There has been some evidence to suggest use of low-dose melatonin for elderly patients admitted to acute care as a potential protective agent against development of delirium. The applicability of these findings to oncology settings should further be explored with well-designed studies.

10. The evidence supporting the use of intravenous dexmedetomidine for the prevention of delirium has been mixed and is limited to patients in intensive care settings only; there is currently no evidence to support its use in oncology and palliative care settings as a treatment for delirium.

11. In terminally ill patients:

    (a) The clinician must consult with the family (and the patient, when lucid) to elicit their concerns and wishes for care during the dying process. The clinician should describe the optimal achievable goals of therapy as they currently exist.

    (b) If sedation becomes necessary, family members should be informed that the goal of sedation is to provide comfort and symptom control, and not to hasten death. They should also be advised that sedation may result in a premature sense of loss.

    (c) Ultimately, the clinician must always keep in mind the goals of care and communicate these goals to the staff, patients, and family members while preserving and respecting the dignity and values of that individual and family.

Suggested Further Reading

- Meagher DJ, Moran M, Raju B, Gibbons D, Donnelly S, Saunders J, Trzepacz PT. Motor symptoms in 100 patients with delirium versus control subjects: comparison of subtyping methods. Psychosomatics. 2008;49(4):300–8. PMID: 18621935.

- Breitbart W, Gibson C, Tremblay A. The delirium experience: delirium recall and delirium-related distress in hospitalized patients with cancer, their spouses/caregivers, and their nurses. Psychosomatics. 2002b;43(3):183–94.

- Boettger S, Breitbart W. Phenomenology of the subtypes of delirium: phenomenological differences between hyperactive and hypoactive delirium. Palliat Support Care. 2011;9:129–35.

- Boettger S, Passik S, Breitbart W. Delirium superimposed on dementia versus delirium in the absence of dementia: phenomenological differences. Palliat Support Care. 2009;7(4):495–500.
- Bruera E, Bush SH, Willey J, et al. Impact of delirium and recall on the level of distress in patients with advanced cancer and their family caregivers. Cancer. 2009;115(9):2004–12.
- Buss MK, Vanderwerker LC, Inouye SK, Zhang B, Block SD, Prigerson HG. Associations between caregiver-perceived delirium in patients with cancer and generalized anxiety in their caregivers. J Palliat Med. 2007;10(5):1083–92.
- Fann JR, Roth-Roemer S, Burington BE, et al. Delirium in patients undergoing hematopoietic stem cell transplantation. Cancer. 2002;95:1971–81.
- Fang CK, Chen HW, Liu SI, Lin CJ, Tsai LY, Lai YL. Prevalence, detection and treatment of delirium in terminal cancer inpatients: a prospective survey. Jpn J Clin Oncol. 2008;38(1):56–63.
- Gagnon P, Charbonneau C, Allard P, Soulard C, Dumont S, Fillion L. Delirium in advanced cancer: a psychoeducational intervention for family caregivers. J Palliat Care. 2002;18(4):253–61.
- Lawlor P, Gagnon B, Mancini I, et al. The occurrence, causes and outcomes of delirium in advanced cancer patients: a prospective study. Arch Intern Med. 2002;160:786–94.
- Leonard M, Raju B, Conroy M, et al. Reversibility of delirium in terminally ill patients and predictors of mortality. Palliat Med. 2008;22(7):848–54.
- Leonard M, Donnelly S, Conroy M, Trzepacz P, Meagher DJ. Phenomenological and neuropsychological profile across motor variants of delirium in a palliative-care unit. J Neuropsychiatry Clin Neurosci. 2011;23(2):180–8.
- Meagher DJ, O'Hanlon D, O'Mahony E, Casey PR, Trzepacz PT. Relationship between symptoms and motoric subtype of delirium. J Neuropsychiatry Clin Neurosci. 2000;12(1):51–6.
- Morita T, Tei Y, Tsunoda J, Inoue S, Chihara S. Underlying pathologies and their associations with clinical features in terminal delirium of cancer patients. J Pain Symptom Manage. 2001;22(6):997–1006.
- Morita T, Tei Y, Inouye S. Impaired communication capacity and agitated delirium in the final week of terminally ill cancer patients: prevalence and identification of research focus. J Pain Symptom Manage. 2003;26:827–34.
- Morita T, et al. Family-perceived distress from delirium-related symptoms of terminally ill cancer patients. Psychosomatics. 2004;45(2):107–13.
- Stagno D, Gibson C, Breitbart W. The delirium subtypes: a review of prevalence, phenomenology, pathophysiology, and treatment response. Palliat Support Care. 2004b;2(2):171–9.
- Gagnon B, et al. The impact of delirium on the circadian distribution of breakthrough analgesia in advanced cancer patients. J Pain Symptom Manage. 2001; 22(4):826–33.
- Trzepacz PT. Is there a final common neural pathway in delirium? Focus on acetylcholine and dopamine. Semin Clin Neuropsychiatry. 2000;5(2):132–48.

- Lawlor P, Nekolaichuck C, Gagnon B, et al. Clinical utility, factor analysis and further validation of the Memorial Delirium Assessment Scale (MDAS). Cancer. 2000;88:2859–67.
- Ryan K, Leonard M, Guerin S, et al. Validation of the confusion assessment method in the palliative care setting. Palliat Med. 2009;23:40–55.
- Gagnon B, Low G, Schreier G. Methylpheni- date hydrochloride improves cognitive function in patients with advanced cancer and hypoactive delirium: a prospective clinical study. J Psychiatry Neurosci. 2005;30:100–7.
- Keen JC, Brown D. Psychostimulants and delirium in patients receiving palliative care. Palliat Support Care. 2004;2:199–202.
- Morita T, Otani H, Tsunoda J, et al. Successful palliation of hypoactive delirium due to multi-organ failure by oral methylphenidate. Support Care Cancer. 2000;8:134–7.
- Kiely DK, Jones RN, Bergmann MA, Marcantonio ER. Association between psychomotor activity delirium subtypes and mortality among newly admitted postacute facility patients. J Gerontol A Biol Sci Med Sci. 2007;62(2):174–9.
- Agar M, Currow D, Plummer J, et al. Changes in anticholinergic load from regular prescribed medications in palliative care as death approaches. Palliat Med. 2009;23(3):257–65.
- Boettger S, Breitbart W. Atypical antipsychotics in the management of delirium: a review of the empirical literature. Palliat Support Care. 2005;3(3):227–37.
- Flaherty JH. The evaluation and management of delirium among older persons. Med Clin North Am. 2011;95(3):555–77. xi.
- Harrigan EP, Miceli JJ, Anziano R, et al. A randomized evaluation of the effects of six antipsychotic agents on QTc, in the absence and presence of metabolic inhibition. J Clin Psychopharmacol. 2004;24(1):62–9.
- Haddad PM, Anderson IM. Antipsychotic-related QTc prolongation, torsade de pointes and sudden death. Drugs. 2002;62(11):1649–71.
- Liptzin B, Laki A, Garb JL, Fingeroth R, Krushell R. Donepezil in the prevention and treatment of post-surgical delirium. Am J Geriatr Psychiatry. 2005; 13(12):1100–6.
- Sampson EL, Raven PR, Ndhlovu PN, et al. A randomized, double-blind, placebo controlled trial of donepezil hydrochloride (Aricept) for reducing the incidence of postoperative delirium after elective total hip replacement. Int J Geriatr Psychiatry. 2007;22(4):343–9.
- Inouye SK, Bogardus Jr ST, Charpentier PA, et al. A multicomponent intervention to prevent delirium in hospitalized older patients. N Engl J Med. 1999; 340(9):669–766.
- Marcantonio ER, Flacker JM, Wright RJ, Resnick NM. Reducing delirium after hip fracture: a randomized trial. J Am Geriatr Soc. 2001;49(5):516–22.
- Gamberini M, Bolliger D, Lurati Buse GA, Burkhart CS, Grapow M, Gagneux A, Filipovic M, Seeberger MD, Pargger H, Siegemund M, Carrel T, Seiler WO, Berres M, Strebel SP, Monsch AU, Steiner LA. Rivastigmine for the prevention of postoperative delirium in elderly patients undergoing elective cardiac surgery—a randomized controlled trial. Crit Care Med. 2009;37(5):1762–8.

- Prommer E. Review article: dexmedetomidine: does it have potential in palliative medicine? Am J Hosp Palliat Care. 2011;28(4):276–83.
- Cole MG, Primeau FJ, Bailey RF, et al. Systematic intervention for elderly in patients with delirium: a randomized trial. CMAJ. 1994;151(7):965–70.
- Cole MG, McCusker J, Bellavance F, et al. Systematic detection and multidisciplinary care of delirium in older medical inpatients: a randomized trial. CMAJ. 2002;167(7):753–9.
- Pitkälä KH, Laurila JV, Strandberg TE, Tilvis RS. Multicomponent geriatric intervention for elderly inpatients with delirium: a randomized, controlled trial. J Gerontol A Biol Sci Med Sci. 2006;61(2):176–81.
- Flaherty JH, Steele DK, Chibnall JT, et al. An ACE unit with a delirium room may improve function and equalize length of stay among older delirious medical inpatients. J Gerontol A Biol Sci Med Sci. 2010;65(12):1387–92.
- Pitkala KH, Laurila JV, Strandberg TE, Kautiainen H, Sintonen H, Tilvis RS. Multicomponent geriatric intervention for elderly inpatients with delirium: effects on costs and health-related quality of life. J Gerontol A Biol Sci Med Sci. 2008;63(1):56–61.
- Milisen K, Lemiengre J, Braes T, Foreman MD. Multicomponent intervention strategies for managing delirium in hospitalized older people: systematic review. J Adv Nurs. 2005;52(1):79–90.
- Inouye SK, Zhang Y, Jones RN, Kiely DK, Yang F, Marcantonio ER. Risk factors for delirium at discharge: development and validation of a predictive model. Arch Intern Med. 2007;167(13):1406–13.
- Ventafridda V, Ripamonti C, DeConno F, Tamburini M, Cassileth BR. Symptom prevalence and control during cancer patients' last days of life. J Palliat Care. 1990;6(3):7–11.
- Fainsinger RL, Waller A, Bercovici M, et al. A multicentre international study of sedation for uncontrolled symptoms in terminally ill patients. Palliat Med. 2000;14(4):257–65.
- Rietjens JA, van Zuylen L, van Veluw H, van der Wijk L, van der Heide A, van der Rijt CC. Palliative sedation in a specialized unit for acute palliative care in a cancer hospital: comparing patients dying with and without palliative sedation. J Pain Symptom Manage. 2008;36(3):228–34.
- Mercadante S, DeConno F, Ripamonti C. Propofol in terminal care. J Pain Symptom Manage. 1995;10(8):639–42.
- Lo B, Rubenfeld G. Palliative sedation in dying patients: "we turn to it when everything else hasn't worked". JAMA. 2005;294(14):1810–6.
- Sykes N, Thorns A. Sedative use in the last week of life and the implications for end-of-life decision making. Arch Intern Med. 2003;163(3):341–4.
- Morita T, Chinone Y, Ikenaga M, et al. Efficacy and safety of palliative sedation therapy: a multicenter, prospective, observational study conducted on specialized palliative care units in Japan. J Pain Symptom Manage. 2005; 30(4):320–8.

References

Al-Aama T, Brymer C, Gutmanis I, Woolmore-Goodwin SM, Esbaugh J, Dasgupta M. Melatonin decreases delirium in elderly patients: a randomized, placebo-controlled trial. Int J Geriatr Psychiatry. 2011;26(7):687–94.

American Diabetes Association, American Psychiatric Association, American Association of Clinical Endocrinologists, North American Association for the Study of Obesity. Consensus development conference on antipsychotic drugs and obesity and diabetes. Diabetes Care. 2004; 27:596–601.

American Psychiatric Association. Practice guidelines for the treatment of patients with delirium. Am J Psychiatry. 1999;156:S1–20.

American Psychiatric Association. Diagnostic and statistical manual of mental disorders. 5th ed. Washington, DC: American Psychiatric Association, Published online in March 2013.

Boettger S, Friedlander M, Breitbart W, Passik S. Aripiprazole and haloperidol in the treatment of delirium. Aust N Z J Psychiatry. 2011;45(6):477–82.

Breitbart W, Alici Y. IPOS handbook on palliative care for the psycho-oncology clinician. New York: Oxford publishing; 2014.

Breitbart W, Alici Y. Agitation and delirium at the end of life: "we couldn't manage him". JAMA. 2008;300:2898–910.

Breitbart W, Alici Y. Evidence-based treatment of delirium in patients with cancer. J Clin Oncol. 2012;30:1206–14.

Breitbart W, Marotta R, Platt M, et al. A double-blind trial of haloperidol, chlorpromazine, and lorazepam in the treatment of delirium in hospitalized AIDS patients. Am J Psychiatry. 1996; 153(2):231–7.

Breitbart W, Rosenfeld B, Roth A. The memorial delirium assessment scale. J Pain Symptom Manage. 1997;13:128–37.

Breitbart W, Tremblay A, Gibson C. An open trial of olanzapine for the treatment of delirium in hospitalized cancer patients. Psychosomatics. 2002;43(3):175–82.

Candy B, Jackson KC, Jones L, Leurent B, Tookman A, King M. Drug therapy for delirium in terminally ill adult patients. Cochrane Database Syst Rev. 2012;11, CD004770. doi:10.1002/14651858.CD004770.pub2.

Crawford GB, Agar MM, Quinn SJ, Phillips J, Litster C, Michael N, Doogue M, Rowett D, Currow DC. Pharmacovigilance in hospice/palliative care: net effect of haloperidol for delirium. J Palliat Med. 2013;16:1335–41.

Devlin JW, Roberts RJ, Fong JJ, et al. Efficacy and safety of quetiapine in critically ill patients with delirium: a prospective, multicenter, randomized, double-blind, placebo controlled pilot study. Crit Care Med. 2010;38(2):419–27.

Elie M, Boss K, Cole MG, et al. A retrospective, exploratory, secondary analysis of the association between antipsychotic use and mortality in elderly patients with delirium. Int Psychogeriatr. 2009;21(3):588–92.

Elsayem A, Bush SH, Munsell MF, Curry 3rd E, Calderon BB, Paraskevopoulos T, Fadul N, Bruera E. Subcutaneous olanzapine for hyperactive or mixed delirium in patients with advanced cancer: a preliminary study. J Pain Symptom Manage. 2010;40(5):774–82.

Gagnon P, Allard P, Gagnon B, Mérette C, Tardif F. Delirium prevention in terminal cancer: assessment of a multicomponent intervention. Psychooncology. 2012;21:187–94.

Gaudreau JD, Gagnon P, et al. Psychoactive medications and risk of delirium in hospitalized cancer patients. J Clin Oncol. 2005;23(27):6712–8.

Girard TD, Pandharipande PP, Carson SS, et al. Feasibility, efficacy, and safety of antipsychotics for intensive care unit delirium: the MIND randomized, placebo-controlled trial. Crit Care Med. 2010;38(2):428–37.

Grover S, Kumar V, Chakrabarti S. Comparative efficacy study of haloperidol, olanzapine and risperidone in delirium. J Psychosom Res. 2011;71(4):277–81.

Han CS, Kim Y. A double-blind trial of risperidone and haloperidol for the treatment of delirium. Psychosomatics. 2004;45(4):297–301.

Hu H, Deng W, Yang H. A prospective random control study comparison of olanzapine and haloperidol in senile delirium. Chongqing Med J. 2004;8:1234–7.

Inouye B, Vandyck C, Alessi C. Clarifying confusion: the confusion assessment method, a new method for the detection of delirium. Ann Intern Med. 1990;113:941–8.

Inouye SK, Westendorp RGJ, Saczynski JS. Delirium in elderly people. Lancet. 2013;383:911–22.

Jackson KC, Lipman AG. Drug therapy for delirium in terminally ill patients. Cochrane Database Syst Rev. 2004;2, CD004770.

Kalisvaart KJ, de Jonghe JF, Bogaards MJ, et al. Haloperidol prophylaxis for elderly hip-surgery patients at risk for delirium: a randomized placebo-controlled study. J Am Geriatr Soc. 2005; 53(10):1658–66.

Kim KY, Bader G, Kotlyar V, Gropper D. Treatment of delirium in older adults with quetiapine. J Geriatr Psychiatry Neurol. 2003;16(1):29–31.

Kim SW, Yoo JA, Lee SY, et al. Risperidone versus olanzapine for the treatment of delirium. Hum Psychopharmacol. 2010;25(4):298–302.

Larsen KA, Kelly SE, Stern TA, Bode Jr RH, Price LL, Hunter DJ, Gulczynski D, Bierbaum BE, Sweeney GA, Hoikala KA, Cotter JJ, Potter AW. Administration of olanzapine to prevent postoperative delirium in elderly joint-replacement patients: a randomized, controlled trial. Psychosomatics. 2010;51(5):409–18.

Lonergan E, Britton AM, Luxenberg J, Wyller T. Antipsychotics for delirium. Cochrane Database Syst Rev. 2007;2, CD005594.

Maldonado JR. Pathoetiological model of delirium: A comprehensive understanding of the neurobiology of delirium and an evidence-based approach to prevention and treatment. Crit Care Clin. 2008;24:789–856.

Maneeton B, Maneeton N, Srisurapanont M, Chittawatanarat K. Quetiapine versus haloperidol in the treatment of delirium: a double-blind, randomized, controlled trial. Drug Des Devel Ther. 2013;7:657–67. doi:10.2147/DDDT.S45575. Print 2013.

Meagher D, McLoughlin L, Leonard M, et al. What do we really know about the treatment of delirium with antipsychotics? Ten key issues for delirium pharmacotherapy. Am J Geriatric Psychiatry. 2013;21:1223–38.

National Institute for Health and Clinical Excellence. Delirium: diagnosis, prevention and management (clinical guideline 103). Published July 2010. Accessed at http://www.nice.org.uk/nicemedia/live/13060/49909/49909.pdf. 17 Sept 2011.

Overshott R, Karim S, Burns A. Cholinesterase inhibitors for delirium. Cochrane Database Syst Rev. 2008;1, CD005317.

Overshott R, Vernon M, Morris J, Burns A. Rivastigmine in the treatment of delirium in older people: a pilot study. Int Psychogeriatr. 2010;22(5):812–8.

Page V, Ely W, Gates S, et al. Effect of intravenous haloperidol on the duration of delirium and coma in critically ill patients (Hope-ICU): a randomized, double-blind, placebo-controlled trial. Lancet Respir Med. 2013;1:515–53.

Pandharipande PP, Girard TD, Jackson JC, et al. Long-term cognitive impairment after critical illness. N Engl J Med. 2013;369:1306–16.

Prakanrattana U, Prapaitrakool S. Efficacy of risperidone for prevention of postoperative delirium in cardiac surgery. Anaesth Intensive Care. 2007;35(5):714–9.

Schneider LS, Dagerman KS, Insel P. Risk of death with atypical antipsychotic drug treatment for dementia: meta-analysis of randomized placebo-controlled trials. JAMA. 2005;294(15): 1934–43.

Siddiqi N, Stockdale R, Britton AM, Holmes J. Interventions for preventing delirium in hospitalised patients. Cochrane Database Syst Rev. 2007;2, CD005563.

Spiller JA, Keen JC. Hypoactive delirium: assessing the extent of the problem for inpatient specialist palliative care. Palliat Med. 2006;20(1):17–23.

Stagno D, Gibson C, Breitbart W. The delirium subtypes: a review of prevalence, phenomenology, pathophysiology, and treatment response. Palliat Support Care. 2004;2(2):171–9.

Tahir TA, Eeles E, Karapareddy V, et al. A randomized controlled trial of quetiapine versus placebo in the treatment of delirium. J Psychosom Res. 2010;69(5):485–90.

Trzepacz PT, Mittal D, Torres R, Kanary K, Norton J, Jimerson N. Validation of the delirium rating scale-revised-98: comparison with the delirium rating scale and the cognitive test for delirium. J Neuropsychiatry Clin Neurosci. 2001;13(2):229–42.

Van Eijk MM, Roes KC, Honing ML, et al. Effect of rivastigmine as an adjunct to usual care with haloperidol on duration of delirium and mortality in critically ill patients: a multicentre, double-blind, placebo-controlled randomised trial. Lancet. 2010;376:1829–37.

Wang PS, Schneeweiss S, Avorn J, et al. Risk of death in elderly users of conventional vs atypical antipsychotic medications. N Engl J Med. 2005;353(22):2335–41.

Wang W, Li HL, Wand DX, et al. Haloperidol prophylaxis decreases delirium incidence in elderly patients after noncardiac surgery: a randomized controlled trial. Crit Care Med. 2012;40: 731–9.

Wong CL, Holroyd-Leduc J, Simel DL, Straus SE. Does this patient have delirium?: value of bedside instruments. JAMA. 2010;304(7):779–86.

Xia ZQ, Chen SQ, Yao X, Xie CB, Wen SH, Liu KX. Clinical benefits of dexmedetomidine versus propofol in adult intensive care unit patients: a meta-analysis of randomized clinical trials. J Surg Res. 2013;185:833–43. doi:10.1016/j.jss.2013.06.062. pii: S0022-4804(13)00685-9.

Pharmacological Treatment of Psychotic Disorders

13

Jong-Heun Kim and Chun-Kai Fang

Abstract

Treatment of psychotic disorders in cancer patients represents a challenge for clinicians. Psychotic symptoms (e.g., delusions, perceptual disorders), unusual behavior or inappropriate affect, and low adherence may be a problem for healthcare teams in oncology and palliative care. Pharmacotherapy is the key of management of psychotic disorders, along with psychosocial therapies. Antipsychotic agents (APs) (first-generation or typical or conventional APs; atypical APs), benzodiazepines, or possibly certain anticonvulsants are used to manage psychotic disorders in cancer and palliative care settings. Attention to side effects of APs, including extra-pyramidal symptoms (e.g., acute dystonia, akathisia, parkinsonism-like symptoms, and tardive dyskinesia), possible antimuscarinic symptoms (e.g., xerostomia, tachycardia, peristalsis impairment, urinary retention), neuroleptic malignant syndrome, and others, is necessary. Also possible cardiologic side effects (e.g., increase QTc length) should be monitored. Drug–drug interaction, given the possible overlapping of metabolic pathways (cytochrome P-450 enzyme systems) between APs and anticancer or palliative care medications, needs also to be carefully examined when prescribing drugs to psychotic patients with cancer.

J.-H. Kim (✉)
Mental Health Clinic, National Cancer Center, 323 Ilsan-ro, Ilsandong-gu, Goyang, Gyeonggi-do, Republic of Korea
e-mail: psy@ncc.re.kr

C.-K. Fang
Department of Psychiatry, Mackay Memorial Hospital, Taipei, Taiwan, ROC

Hospice and Palliative Care Center (HPCC) & Suicide Prevention Center (SPC), Mackay Memorial Hospital, Taipei, Taiwan, ROC
e-mail: fang0415@yahoo.com.tw

L. Grassi and M. Riba (eds.), *Psychopharmacology in Oncology and Palliative Care*,   229
DOI 10.1007/978-3-642-40134-3_13, © Springer-Verlag Berlin Heidelberg 2014

13.1   Introduction

Psychosis refers to an abnormal mental state with poor insight and impaired reality testing. Psychotic patients typically show perceptual, cognitive, and behavioral symptoms and signs. Key features are positive symptoms (delusion, hallucination, disorganized thinking, or speech) and negative symptoms (apathy, anhedonia, or social withdrawal).

Psychotic disorders may be divided into primary and secondary psychotic disorders. The category of primary psychotic disorders essentially consists of a series of disturbances subsumed under the DSM5 section of schizophrenia spectrum and other psychotic disorders. This section includes schizophrenia, schizoaffective disorder, delusional disorder, and brief psychotic disorder. Secondary psychotic disorders encompass substance/mediation-induced psychotic disorder and psychotic disorder due to another medical condition (DSM-5 2013; Heckers et al. 2013) (Table 13.1).

Schizophrenia, a severe mental illness, is the most common form of primary psychotic disorders. In the oncology and palliative care setting, dealing with patients affected by schizophrenia or primary psychotic disorders is extremely challenging, given the severity of these mental illnesses (Howard et al. 2010; Irwin et al. 2014). The patient's unusual behavior or inappropriate affect and the psychotic symptoms and signs may be unfamiliar and incomprehensible to the medical team. Furthermore, patients with a primary psychotic disorder are often not cooperative with medical team during the process of diagnosis and treatment of cancer (Thomson and Henry 2012), tend to show hostility to caregivers and healthcare workers, and to refuse therapy and/or to be noncompliant care (Hwang et al. 2012). Mechanisms of pathological denial of symptoms may cause delay in diagnosis of cancer, with patients often referred to oncologists or surgeons in a high-stage disease, making treatment difficult and only partial (Farasatpour et al. 2013). Cognitive symptoms (e.g., impaired attention and executive function), quite typical in schizophrenia, may also reduce the patient's capacity to understand the meaning of medical and surgical procedures to treat cancer. Data also show that patients with schizophrenia in an advanced stage of cancer, are less likely to see specialists (other than psychiatrists), less likely to be prescribed analgesics, and less likely to receive palliative care (Chochinov et al. 2012).

Secondary psychotic disorders comprise several different syndromes that are very common in oncology and palliative care setting. Delirium is an example of a disorder with psychotic symptoms secondary to different causes. Distinguishing delirium from the aggravation of underlying psychosis is sometimes difficult. The issues of delirium are dealt with in separate part of this book (see Chap. 12). Cancer patients with brain tumors, extracranial tumors, or paraneoplastic syndrome sometimes manifest psychotic or schizophreniform symptoms. Sometimes psychotic features appear before the diagnosis of cancer (Schönfeldt-Lecuona et al. 2005; Shih et al. 2012; Gesundheit et al. 2008). Antineoplastic agents can cause confusion and acute psychotic symptoms as a side effect (Raison et al. 2005; Kunene and Porfiri 2011; Schellekens et al. 2011). Abrupt onset of psychotic symptoms in

Table 13.1 Diagnoses of psychotic disorders in DSM-5

Key features that define the psychotic disorders
Delusions
Hallucinations
Disorganized thinking (speech)
Grossly disorganized or abnormal motor behavior (including catatonia)
Negative symptoms
Schizophrenia spectrum and other psychotic disorders
Schizotypal personality disorder
Delusional disorder
Brief psychotic disorder
Schizophreniform disorder
Schizophrenia
Schizoaffective disorder
Substance/medication-induced psychotic disorder
Psychotic disorder due to another medical condition
Catatonia associated with another mental disorder (catatonia specifier)
Catatonic disorder due to another medical condition
Unspecified catatonia
Other specified schizophrenia spectrum and other psychotic disorder
Unspecified schizophrenia spectrum and other psychotic disorder

cancer patients without previous history of psychiatric illness requires thorough evaluation of possible causes of secondary psychotic disorder, including cancer, medication, or paraneoplastic syndrome.

In this chapter, the principles of pharmacotherapy for primary psychotic disorders will be discussed. Specific issues including choice of drugs, dosages, side effects, drug–drug interactions, and communication will be dealt with.

13.2 Major Issues

13.2.1 Prescribing Antipsychotics for Psychotic Disorders in General

Pharmacotherapy is the key of management of psychotic disorders, along with psychosocial therapies. Medications that may be used to treat psychotic disorders or symptoms include antipsychotic agents, benzodiazepines, or possibly certain anticonvulsants. First-generation (or typical) antipsychotics are all dopamine receptor blockers, and second-generation (or atypical) drugs have multiple actions on multiple receptors. The former are mostly effective for positive symptoms, whereas the latter may be also effective for negative symptoms. Each antipsychotic drug has its own initial dose and titration schedule. The general characteristics of antipsychotics are discussed elsewhere (see Chap. 2).

13.2.2 Side Effects of Antipsychotics and Their Management

Avoiding adverse effects is the first important issue of prescribing antipsychotic drugs (Yap et al. 2011). Extrapyramidal symptoms (EPS) are the common forms of adverse effects, especially with first-generation antipsychotics (Gerlach 2002). The severest side effect is neuroleptic malignant syndrome (see Chap. 17).

EPS are caused by dopamine antagonism, and encompass acute dystonia, akathisia, parkinsonism-like symptoms, and tardive dyskinesia. EPS are usually controlled with anticholinergic drugs or benzodiazepines. Tardive dyskinesia (TD), a side effect of long-term use, however, has no effective treatment yet. The genotypic variants of dopamine D1 receptors (DRD1) might play a role in the susceptibility of tardive dyskinesia (Lai et al. 2011).

Neuroleptic malignant syndrome is potentially fatal with symptoms of hyperpyrexia, rigidity, confusion, and autonomic instability. If this condition is suspected, antipsychotic drugs must be stopped to prevent mortality (Baba et al. 2013). Cancer patients represent a high risk group for NMS (Kawanishi et al. 2005).

Ziprasidone and sertindole were reported the high risk of prolongation of heart rate-corrected QT interval (Haddad and Sharma 2007), but not reported in cancer care. However, some anticancer agents have the QTc interval-prolonging risk (Brell 2010). The combination of anticancer and antipsychotic therapies should be considered.

13.2.3 Drug–Drug Interaction

Most antipsychotics are metabolized by the cytochrome P-450 enzyme systems in the liver (Nasrallah et al. 2005). In the second-generation antipsychotics, clozapine is metabolized by cytochrome P450 1A2, 2C19, 2D6, and 3A4; risperidone is metabolized by 2D6 and 3A4; olanzapine is metabolized by 1A2, 2D6, and 3A4; quetiapine and ziprasidone are metabolized by 3A4; and aripiprazole is metabolized by 2D6 and 3A4. Only paliperidone and amisulpride are involved in cytochrome P450 system (Urichuk et al. 2008). Patients taking antipsychotics generally do not have to change the dosing of other medications, but the possibility of antipsychotics inhibiting the metabolism of chemotherapeutic agents via cytochrome P450 system can't be excluded.

Some antiemetics including metoclopramide are dopamine agonists. When used in combination with antipsychotics, acute movement disorders may occur. The potentiation of drug-induced prolongation of the QTc interval, elevating the risk of ventricular tachycardia, is other potentially problematic interaction. This can occur when lapatinib is used with antipsychotics that prolong the QTc interval (Howard et al. 2010).

Clozapine is atypical antipsychotic agent which can lead to blood dyscrasias. Although there are little evidences that combined use of antineoplastic agents and clozapine has synergistic effect on agranulocytosis, caution must be required including hematological monitoring (Frieri et al. 2008; Goulet and Grignon 2008).

Table 13.2 Common antipsychotics in the cancer setting

Antipsychotics	Common dosages (mg/day)	Most common side effects					Cytochrome P-450
		EPS	Prolactin	Weight gain	Sedation	Automatic	
Haloperidol	1–20	+++	+++	+	+	+	1A2, 2D6, 3A4
Sulpiride	50–1,000	+	+++	+	+	+	−
Amisulpiride	50–800	+	+++	+	+	+	−
Risperidone	1–9	+	++	+	+	+	2D6, 3A4
Paliperidone	3–12	+	++	+	+	+	−
Quetiapine	25–800	−	−	+	++	+	3A4
Ziprasidone	20–160	++	++	−	+	++	3A4
Aripiprazole	2.5–30	+	+	+	+	+	2D6, 3A4
Zotepine	50–400	+	+	+++	++	+	1A2, 2D6, 3A4
Olanzapine	2.5–20	+	+	+++	++	++	1A2, 2D6, 3A4
Clozapine	25–400	−	−	+++	+++	+++	1A2, 2C19, 2D6, 3A4

+++ severe, ++ moderate, + mild, − none

13.2.4 Use of Antipsychotics for Cancer Patients

Antipsychotics play the most important roles for treatment of psychotic disorders among cancer patients. Cancer patients were significantly more often prescribed antipsychotics along with benzodiazepines and antidepressants (Ng et al. 2013). The use of antipsychotics for advanced cancer patients in the palliative care setting shows a rapid increase recently (Farriols et al. 2012; Sera et al. 2014). It is recommended to maintain antipsychotic medications as simple and minimal as possible, considering the patients' physical conditions and complicated medications (Table 13.2).

Treatment for psychotic disorders should not be stopped for the reason of cancer treatment. Possible relapse of psychosis and increased delirium are major problems of discontinuation of antipsychotic drugs (Howard et al. 2010). Because there are few valid scientific evidences of antipsychotics causing or aggravating cancer, treatment for cancer patients using appropriate antipsychotics can be reassured (Burgess 2012; Fond et al. 2012).

Conclusion

As indicated by Irwin et al. (2014), early psychiatric consultation and communication with the patient's outpatient mental health team are key strategies that are extremely important to optimize the delivery of quality cancer care and to define the several steps in decision-making process, including how to deal with psychopharmacological intervention. Integrated intervention, in multidisciplinary team, is essential to treat patients with severe mental illness and those who developed psychotic disorders as a consequence of cancer. On one side, mental health professionals should be alerted in how to treat psychotic patients in oncology setting because the patients are at risk of aggravating psychotic symptoms in face of major crisis of cancer and/or death. On the other, cancer care professionals should be trained to understand how to communicate and manage patients with psychotic disorders and how to collaborate in integrating anticancer therapy with psychiatric treatment. The use of psychotropic drugs in patients with psychotic disorders or psychotic symptoms and, concurrent cancer, is, for these reasons, extremely important in oncology setting. Side effects and drug–drug interactions should be always taken into consideration before prescribing antipsychotics. For psychotic patients suffering from cancer, the combination with the best anticancer and antipsychotic treatment should be maintained appropriately.

A Clinical Case

Mr. L, 50 years old, was a patient with schizophrenia hospitalized in a psychiatric hospital since 2001. On November 2010 he was brought to a general hospital because of severe constipation. With medical examination, he was diagnosed as colon cancer stage IIIA (T2N1M0).

During his stay in the psychiatric hospital, Mr. L had been taking chlorpromazine 600 mg daily to manage his schizophrenic symptoms. He was withdrawn socially, delusion and hallucination being not prominent. His only daughter discussed with the surgeon on treatment options by proxy, as Mr. L had limited capacity to make a decision. Family history revealed his wife had killed herself 20 years ago while suffering from major depressive disorder. His daughter, Ms. L, was diagnosed with bipolar disorder in 2006 and visits regularly the psychiatric outpatient department at the same general hospital. Being fully informed on the diagnosis and treatment from the surgeon, she accepted the option of colectomy followed by chemotherapy for cure of her father's cancer.

Shortly after he was told that the decision on surgery was made, Mr. L started to hear a woman's voice, saying "I will kill you." and "You are supposed to die tonight." His surgeon consulted with the psychiatrist, who happened to be Ms. L's doctor, for evaluation of the mental condition of Mr. L. After full psychiatric examination, the psychiatrist, taking Mr. L's scheduled chemotherapy into consideration, switched antipsychotic medication from chlorpromazine to amisulpride, as the latter was safer for his liver function. Mr. L was initially prescribed amisulpride 100 mg daily, being slowly increased to the target dosage of 600 mg. Since his psychotic symptoms were relieved and remained in control after 2 weeks of changing medication, the surgical operation was carried out successfully.

(continued)

After Mr. L completed his course of chemotherapy, he was sent to a psychiatric nursing home, taking amisulpride 400 mg daily without any significant side effects. He regularly visits both the psychiatric outpatient and the oncological clinic every 3 months for checkup of his mental and physical states.

▶ **Key Points**

1. Avoiding adverse effects and minimizing drug–drug interactions are important for prescribing antipsychotics for psychotic patients in oncology setting.
2. Based on the misgivings about the metabolism by the cytochrome P-450 189 enzyme systems, the choice of antipsychotics for cancer patients with psychotic disorders should consider their metabolic pathways.
3. To promote the smooth process of cancer treatments, treatment for psychotic disorders should not be stopped for the reason of cancer treatment.

Suggested Further Readings

- Foti ME. Palliative care for patients with serious mental illness. In: Chochinov HM, Breitbart W, editors. Handbook of psychiatry in palliative medicine. New York: Oxford; 2009.
- Ganzini L, Socherman R. Cancer care for patients with schizophrenia. In: Holland JC et al., editors. Psycho-oncology. New York: Oxford; 2010.
- Leigh H. Psychosis. In: Leigh H, Streltzer J, editors. Handbook of consultation-liaison psychiatry. New York: Springer; 2007.

References

American Psychiatric Association: Diagnostic and Statistical Manual forMental Disorders – Fith edition (DSM5). American Psychiatric Publishing, Washington, DC. 2013.

Baba O, Yamagata K, Tomidokoro Y, Tamaoka A, Itoh H, Yanagawa T, Onizawa K, Bukawa H. Neuroleptic malignant syndrome in a patient with tongue cancer: a report of a rare case. Case Rep Dent. 2013;2013:542130.

Brell JM. Prolonged QTc interval in cancer therapeutic drug development: defining arrhythmic risk in malignancy. Prog Cardiovasc Dis. 2010;53(2):164–72.

Burgess DJ. Anticancer drugs: antipsychotic to anticancer agent? Nat Rev Drug Discov. 2012;11 (7):516.

Chochinov HM, Martens PJ, Prior HJ, Kredentser MS. Comparative health care use patterns of people with schizophrenia near the end of life: a population-based study in Manitoba, Canada. Schizophr Res. 2012;141:241–16.

Diagnostic and Statistical Manual of Mental Disorders, 5th ed. DSM-5. American Psychiatric Association; 2013.

Farasatpour M, Janardhan R, Williams CD, Margenthaler JA, Virgo KS, Johnson FE. Breast cancer in patients with schizophrenia. Am J Surg. 2013;206(5):798–804.

Farriols C, Ferrández O, Planas J, Ortiz P, Mojal S, Ruiz AI. Changes in the prescription of psychotropic drugs in the palliative care of advanced cancer patients over a seven-year period. J Pain Symptom Manage. 2012;43(5):945–52.

Fond G, Macgregor A, Attal J, Larue A, Brittner M, Ducasse D, Capdevielle D. Antipsychotic drugs: pro-cancer or anti-cancer? a systematic review. Med Hypotheses. 2012;79(1):38–42.

Frieri T, Barzega G, Badà A, Villari V. Maintaining clozapine treatment during chemotherapy for non-Hodgkin's lymphoma. Prog Neuropsychopharmacol Biol Psychiatry. 2008;32(6):1611–2.

Gerlach J. Improving outcome in schizophrenia: the potential importance of EPS and neuroleptic dysphoria. Ann Clin Psychiatry. 2002;14(1):47–57.

Gesundheit B, Lerer B, Budowski E, Neuman T, Gomori JM, Or R. Sudden psychotic symptoms in a 28-year-old male with thymoma. J Clin Oncol. 2008;26(26):4353–5.

Goulet K, Grignon S. Case report: clozapine given in the context of chemotherapy for lung cancer. Psychooncology. 2008;17(5):512–6.

Haddad PM, Sharma SG. Adverse effects of atypical antipsychotics: differential risk and clinical implications. CNS Drugs. 2007;21(11):911–36.

Heckers S, Barch DM, Bustillo J, Gaebel W, Gur R, Malaspina D, Owen MJ, Schultz S, Tandon R, Tsuang M, Van Os J, Carpenter W. Structure of the psychotic disorders classification in DSM 5. Schizophr Res. 2013;150:11–4. pii: S0920-9964(13)00255-7.

Howard LM, Barley EA, Davies E, Rigg A, Lempp H, Rose D, Taylor D, Thornicroft G. Cancer diagnosis in people with severe mental illness: practical and ethical issues. Lancet Oncol. 2010;11(8):797–804.

Hwang M, Farasatpour M, Williams CD, Margenthaler JA, Virgo KS, Johnson FE. Adjuvant chemotherapy for breast cancer in patients with schizophrenia. Oncol Lett. 2012;3:845–50.

Irwin KE, Henderson DC, Knight HP, Pirl WF. Cancer care for individuals with schizophrenia. Cancer. 2014;120:323–34.

Kawanishi C, Onishi H, Kato D, Yamada T, Onose M, Hirayasu Y. Neuroleptic malignant syndrome in cancer treatment. Palliat Support Care. 2005;3(1):51–3.

Kunene V, Porfiri E. Sunitinib-induced acute psychosis: case report. Clin Genitourin Cancer. 2011;9(1):70–2.

Lai IC, Mo GH, Chen ML, Wang YC, Chen JY, Liao DL, Bai YM, Lin CC, Chen TT, Liou YJ. Analysis of genetic variations in the dopamine D1 receptor (DRD1) gene and antipsychotics-induced tardive dyskinesia in schizophrenia. Eur J Clin Pharmacol. 2011;67 (4):383–8.

Nasrallah H, Dewan N, Keck P. Treating schizophrenia in patients with cancer. The clinical guide to pharmacotherapy for patients with co-occurring medical conditions. Cincinnatti, OH: University of Cincinnati; 2005.

Ng CG, Boks MP, Smeets HM, Zainal NZ, de Wit NJ. Prescription patterns for psychotropic drugs in cancer patients; a large population study in the Netherlands. Psychooncology. 2013;22 (4):762–7.

Raison CL, Demetrashvili M, Capuron L, Miller AH. Neuropsychiatric adverse effects of interferon-alpha: recognition and management. CNS Drugs. 2005;19(2):105–23.

Schellekens AF, Mulder SF, van Eijndhoven PF, Smilde TJ, van Herpen CM. Psychotic symptoms in the course of sunitinib treatment for advanced renal cell cancer. Two cases. Gen Hosp Psychiatry. 2011;33(1):83.e1–3.

Schönfeldt-Lecuona C, Freudenmann RW, Tumani H, Kassubek J, Connemann BJ. Acute psychosis with a mediastinal carcinoma metastasis. Med Sci Monit. 2005;11(1):CS6–8.

Sera L, McPherson ML, Holmes HM. Commonly prescribed medications in a population of hospice patients. Am J Hosp Palliat Care. 2014;31:126–31.

Shih YH, Chen HC, Liao SC, Tseng MC, Lee MB. Psychotic disorder due to phosphaturic mesenchymal tumor with mixed connective tissue variant. Psychosomatics. 2012;53(1):96–7.

Thomson K, Henry B. Oncology clinical challenges: caring for patients with preexisting psychiatric illness. Clin J Oncol Nurs. 2012;16(5):471–80.

Urichuk L, Prior TI, Dursun S, Baker G. Metabolism of atypical antipsychotics: involvement of cytochrome p450 enzymes and relevance for drug-drug interactions. Curr Drug Metab. 2008;9 (5):410–8.

Yap KY, Tay WL, Chui WK, Chan A. Clinically relevant drug interactions between anticancer drugs and psychotropic agents. Eur J Cancer Care. 2011;20(1):6–32.

Treatment of Sleep Disorders

14

Lúcia Monteiro, Andreia Ribeiro, and Salomé Xavier

Abstract

Sleep disturbances have a negative impact over mood, cognition, performance, and well-being. Quality of sleep and sleep physiology can be studied using several methods. There are also many different classifications for sleep disorders (eg: in the DSM-5, the diagnosis of *primary insomnia* has been renamed *insomnia disorder*, in order to avoid the differentiation of primary and secondary insomnia). The impact and nature of sleep problems in the cancer population are presently a hot research topic. The most prevalent sleep problems in the Oncology setting are **Insomnia** (the most common sleep complaint), *Hypersomnolence Disorder (HD)*, and *Restless Legs Syndrome*. Breathing-related sleep Disorder (*Obstructive Sleep Apnea*) is common in head and neck cancer patients. Parasomnias and Narcolepsy are occasionally referred to. In this work, the term **insomnia** will refer to sleep problems (difficulty falling or staying asleep, poor sleep quality, and/or short sleep duration) and insomnia syndrome (the cluster of several and severe sleep), with or without full criteria for insomnia disorder. Despite broad discrepancies in the literature, the most consistent studies have figured a general prevalence of insomnia among cancer patients between 25.9 and 57.9 %.

Insomnia is frequently secondary to multiple and synergistic factors: etiological factors may be directly related to the tumor's biology or symptoms, oncologic treatments, or lifestyle changes. The path between pain and sleep in cancer

L. Monteiro (✉) • A. Ribeiro
Psychiatry Service, Psychosocial Department, Instituto Português de Oncologia Lisboa,
Rua Professor Lima Basto, 1099-023, Lisbon, Portugal
e-mail: lmonteiro@ipolisboa.min-saude.pt; alima@ipolisboa.min-saude.pt

S. Xavier
Psychiatry Service, Hospital Prof. Dr. Fernando Fonseca, IC-19, 2720-276 Amadora, Portugal
e-mail: salome.i.xavier@hff.min-saude.pt

L. Grassi and M. Riba (eds.), *Psychopharmacology in Oncology and Palliative Care*,
DOI 10.1007/978-3-642-40134-3_14, © Springer-Verlag Berlin Heidelberg 2014

patients is bidirectional, as sleep loss also leads to increased pain. Insomnia, depression, and fatigue are often present as a symptom cluster that should be treated overall.

Chemotherapy deregulates immune function, enhances inflammatory response, and interferes with circadian rhythms; when chronic, these effects are predictors of acute and long-term poor quality of sleep either in cancer patients or survivors. Other treatments like synthetic glucocorticoids may disrupt diurnal cortisol rhythms and alter the circadian component of sleep. Considering the medical burden of cancer patients, one should minimize pharmacotherapy only focused on poor sleep and try to scope the health problems altogether. Recent studies highlight the importance of non-pharmacologic approaches like sleep hygiene measures and behavioral interventions. The newer hypnotics are safe, have few side effects, and may help within other cancer symptoms (pain, pruritus, nausea, anorexia, hot flashes, fatigue, and memory decline).

14.1 Introduction to Sleep Disorders

The reason why living beings and specifically humans need to sleep is one of the enduring questions in biology (Allade and Siegel 2008). While the ultimate understanding of the biological function of sleep is still unclear, the consequences of bad sleep are well known. Sleep disturbances have a negative impact over mood, cognition, performance, and well-being. Poor sleep conditions may also affect cardiovascular, endocrine, metabolic, and immunity balances (Lee-Cheong 2008); moreover, it is clearly linked with the higher occurrence of accidents, higher mortality, and reduced quality of life (Moszczynski and Murray 2012).

Sleep may be *good* regarding its quantity and quality. For an average adult, the sleep requirement—the amount of sleep required to remain alert, fully awake, and to function adequately throughout the day—is approximately 7.5–8 h (Chokroverty and Avidan 2012). Quality of sleep assessment is usually based in objective parameters namely *total sleep time, sleep onset latency, total wake time, sleep fragmentation,* and *sleep efficiency* (Table 14.1) (Krystal and Edinger 2008; Page and Johnson 2006).

These parameters can be studied either using sleep questionnaires, like the Pittsburgh Sleep Quality Index (PSQI) (Buysse et al. 1989) or by polysomnography (PSG). The former assesses sleep latency, duration, efficiency, or disturbances, plus the need of sleep medication and daytime dysfunction; the later assesses both sleep quality measurements and architecture. Sleep quality also has a subjective component related to "variations in the experience of sleep itself" (Krystal and Edinger 2008) that may possibly be defined as the *quality of perceived sleep*, the "multidimensional perceptions of length and depth of sleep, feelings of being rested on awakening, and/or the subjective assessment of sufficiency of sleep for daytime functioning" (Page and Johnson 2006).

Table 14.1 Quality of sleep measures

Total sleep time	Number of minutes of sleep while in bed
Sleep onset latency	Number of minutes elapsed from lying in bed and actually falling asleep
Total wake time	Number of minutes awake after sleep onset during the sleep period
Sleep fragmentation	Number of awakenings during the sleep period
Sleep efficiency	Number of minutes of sleep divided by the number of minutes in bed, plus 100

To clearly understand sleep disorders, it is essential to introduce some sleep physiology. Basically, humans have two types of sleep—REM (rapid eye movement) and nREM (non REM sleep)—with different physiology and pathology. For an adult, 80 % of the total sleep time is nREM sleep which is divided in three phases, N1, N2, and N3 (Hypnogram).

N1, 5 % of total sleep, is the transition wake/sleep; N2, 50 % of total sleep, the beginning of sleep or superficial sleep, and N3, 10–20 % of total sleep, the deep sleep, slow wave, or delta sleep (typical delta waves in Electroencephalography EEG), usually occurring during the first third or half of the night. REM sleep's name comes from the typical bursts of eye movements that occur during this period of sleep. It is also associated with the dreaming phenomena. Overnight, nREM and REM sleep alternate between cycles of 90 min, three to five times per night (Reite et al. 2009).

Contemporary authors stress the complexity of sleep/wake cycle regulation. Borbely's two-process model (Borbely 1982) considers that timing, depth, and duration of sleep have a double regulation being either controlled by the day clock (circadian control, process C) and by the duration of prior wakefulness (homeostatic control, process S) (Borbely 1982; Brown et al. 2012).

The pattern of sleep also evolves throughout life. It is relatively stable throughout childhood and adolescence with large amounts of deep, slow-wave sleep per night. With aging, continuity and deepness of sleep tend to deteriorate. Normally, old people have more time of vigil, N1, N2 sleep, and a reduction of N3.

The screening of sleep complaints uses several methods: patient and bed partner interview, sleep chart or diary, sleep self-questionnaires, and rating scales plus objective exams like actigraphy or PSG.

Clinical interviews should be detailed and include questions focused on the sleep problems but also on current sleep/wake schedule, associated symptoms, daytime routines and activities, sleep hygiene and naps; list the current prescribed and non-prescribed drugs and previous treatments to ameliorate sleep; summarize medical and psychiatric history and present stressful circumstances; consider secondary gains and perpetuating factors (Trevorrow 2010).

Talking with the bed partner might be really useful since he/she may disclose symptoms that the patient is unable to detect, e.g., ronchopathy, restless legs, or periods of apnea (Trevorrow 2010).

Sleep diary, a chart where patient writes information about sleep-related behavior—fall asleep/waking schedule, number and time of night awakenings,

Table 14.2 Sleep–Wake Disorders, DSM-IV vs. DSM-5

DSM-IV	DSM-5
Primary sleep disorders	
Dyssomnias	Insomnia disorder
Primary Insomnia	Hypersomnolence disorder
Primary hypersomnia	Narcolepsy
Narcolepsy	Breathing-related sleep disorder
Breathing-related sleep disorder	Circadian rhythm sleep disorder
Circadian rhythm sleep disorder	
Dyssomnia NOS	
Parasomnias	Parasomnias
Nightmare disorder	Non-rapid eye movement sleep
Sleep terror disorder	arousal disorder
Sleepwalking disorder	Nightmare disorder
Parasomnia NOS	Rapid-eye movement sleep behavior
	disorder
Sleep disorders related to another mental disorder	
Insomnia related to . . . [*indicate the Axis I or Axis II Disorder*]	Restless legs syndrome
	Substance/medication-induced sleep
Hypersomnia related to . . . [*indicate the Axis I or Axis II disorder*]	disorders
	Other specified insomnia disorder
	Unspecified insomnia disorder
Other sleep disorders	
Sleep disorder due to . . . [*indicate the general medical condition*]	Other specified hypersomnolence disorder
Substance-induced sleep disorder	Unspecified hypersomnolence disorder
	Other specified sleep–wake disorder
	Unspecified sleep–wake disorder

perceived quality of sleep, day naps, etc.—is a simple and economic method to assess the sleep pattern baseline, its variations and dysfunctions or the outcome under treatment (Trevorrow 2010).

There are many different classifications for sleep disorders. Among the most used in clinical practice are the *International Classification for Sleep Disorders* (ICSD-2, 2005), American Sleep Disorders Association (The International Classification of Sleep Disorders 2005), and the *DSM—Diagnostic and Statistical Manual of Clinical Disorders*, American Psychiatry Association (2013).

The recently edited *DSM-5* includes an entire chapter dedicated to sleep–wake Disorders and introduces many changes on their classification (Table 14.2).

The DSM-5 puts an end to the distinction between primary and secondary (to other mental or medical conditions) sleep disorders to better emphasize that when an individual has a sleep disorder warranting independent clinical attention, in addiction to any medical or mental disorders that might also be present. Consequently, the diagnosis of *primary insomnia* has been renamed *insomnia disorder*, in order to avoid the differentiation of primary and secondary insomnia.

14.2   Sleep Disorders and Cancer

The impact and nature of sleep problems in the cancer population is presently a hot research topic. However, studies are too heterogeneous and rather difficult to compare—whether the diversity of samples (patients with different cancers and/or at different stages), different definitions/classification of the sleep problems, different methods (self-questionnaires vs. objective measures) (Yue and Dimsdale 2010).

The most prevalent sleep problems in the Oncology setting are *Insomnia*, *Hypersomnolence Disorder*, and *Restless Legs Syndrome* (RLS) (Davidson et al. 2002). Breathing-related sleep disorder, in the case *Obstructive Sleep Apnea* (OSA), is common in head and neck cancer patients. Parasomnias and Narcolepsy are occasionally referred to (Yue and Dimsdale 2010).

Insomnia is by far the most common sleep complaint among cancer patients. But reviewing the literature on the subject, there is a broad mismatching in what concerns Insomnia definition and classification, especially when discriminating between *insomnia symptom, problem, and syndrome* (Yue and Dimsdale 2010; Palesh et al. 2012a).

In an effort to try and integrate concepts and designations, we summarized these definitions according to the most consistent authors and systems:

Sleep problems or **insomnia symptoms** (Palesh et al. 2012a): difficulty falling or staying asleep, poor sleep quality, and/or short sleep duration.

Insomnia syndrome: the cluster of several and severe sleep problems (Palesh et al. 2012a).

Based in Morin works, Savard has defined the **Diagnostic Criteria for Insomnia Syndrome** (Table 14.3).

In this work, the term *insomnia* will refer to sleep problems and insomnia syndrome, with or without full criteria for insomnia disorder (Table 14.4).

Despite broad discrepancies in the literature, the most consistent studies have figured a general prevalence of insomnia among cancer patients between 25.9 and 57.9 % (Table 14.5).

Hypersomnolence disorder HD (i.e., excessive daytime sleepiness) often occurs in the cancer population. Davidson et al. found 37 % of HD among patients recently submitted to oncological treatments (CHE, RT, or surgery in less than 6 months) (Davidson et al. 2002). In a prospective study with 93 breast metastatic cancer patients, Palesh et al. found 25 % of the women complaining of HD (Palesh et al. 2007). However, this symptom correlates significantly with stressful life events on baseline evaluation and with depression over the follow-up. Neither prevalence rates nor possible causes for HD among cancer patients are clarified.

Restless legs syndrome RLS consists in strong feelings of restlessness and distressing paresthesia-like sensations in the lower legs, typically at rest, and cause an intense urge to begin moving in order to relieve the discomfort (Sethi and Mehta 2012). It is usually associated with Periodic Limb Movement Disorder

Table 14.3 Diagnostic criteria for insomnia syndrome [Savard (2011), adapted from Morin (1993)]

1. Sleep-onset latency or wake after sleep onset >30 min at least 3 nights per week
2. Sleep efficiency <85 %
3. Duration ≥1 month
4. Insomnia-related impairment daytime functioning or marked distress

Table 14.4 Insomnia disorder

ISCD-2 criteria for general insomnia disorder
1. A complaint of difficulty initiating sleep, maintaining sleep, or waking up too early, turning sleep chronically non restorative or poor in quality
2. The above difficulty occurs despite adequate opportunity and circumstances for sleep
3. At least one of the following forms of daytime impairment related to the night time non restorative sleep is reported by the patient: fatigue or malaise; attention, concentration or memory impairment; social or professional dysfunction or poor school performance; mood disturbance or irritability; daytime sleepiness; reduction of motivation, energy or initiative; proneness to errors or accidents at work or while driving; tension, headaches or gastrointestinal symptoms in response to sleep loss; concerns or worries about sleep
DSM-5 criteria for insomnia disorder
(A) A predominant complaint of dissatisfaction with sleep quantity or quality, associated with one (or more) of the following symptoms:
– Difficulty initiating sleep
– Difficulty maintaining sleep (especially frequent awakenings or problems returning to sleep after them)
– Early-morning awakening with inability to return sleep
(B) The sleep disturbance causes clinically significant distress or impediment in social, occupational, educational, academic, behavioral, or other important areas of functioning
(C) The sleep difficulty occurs at least 3 nights per week
(D) The sleep difficulty is present for at least 3 months
(E) The sleep difficulty occurs despite adequate opportunity for sleep
(F–H) Insomnia is not better explained by nor secondary to other sleep–wake disorder, substance usage, mental or medical condition

(PLMD), where repeated sudden limb movements occur in a periodic fashion within sleep causing its fragmentation and poor quality (Reite et al. 2009).

Davidson et al. (2002) submitted 1,000 cancer patients to a sleep questionnaire and pointed out RLS prevalence of 41 %. Ostacoli et al. (2010) used a structured diagnosis interview (n=257 patients) and found a HD prevalence of 18.3 %. Moreover, these authors found a significant correlation between RLS and female sex, long lasting CHE (more than 3 months) or high levels of anxiety or depression. Saini et al. (2007) also found high prevalence of RLS in a sample of 500 mixed cancer diagnosis: 12 % in male, 22 % in women. The literature often based on case reports highlights the relationship of RLS/PLMD and iron deficiency anemia, especially in GI cancer (Yue and Dimsdale 2010).

Table 14.5 Prevalence of Insomnia in cancer patients

References	Study design: cross-sectional vs. longitudinal	N	Sample's oncological profile	Prevalence	Comments on study methodology
Davidson et al. (2002)	CS	982	Mixed locations; various stages	31 % (insomnia criteria as defined by authors)[a]	"Sleep Survey" questionnaire, developed by authors
Akekushi et al. (2007)	L	209	Mixed locations; palliative care	25.9 % (sleep disturbances); 36.5 % (sub threshold sleep disturbances)	Structured Clinical Interview DSM-III-R insomnia/ hypersomnia item
Palesh et al. (2010)	L	823	Mixed sites; undergoing chemotherapy	36 % insomnia symptoms; 43 % insomnia syndrome (at baseline)	Hamilton Depression Scale, sleep items
Savard et al. (2009a)	L	991	Mixed; peri- and post-surgery	31 % insomnia symptoms; 28.5 % insomnia syndrome (at baseline)	Insomnia diagnostic interview
Colagiuri et al. (2011)	CS	3,343	Breast cancer; 3–4 months after surgery	57,9 % (sleep difficulty defined as PSQI>5)	PSQI
Sharma et al. (2012)	CS	2,862	Mixed sites; various stages	30.2 % (sleep problems)	PHQ-9 (Patient Health Questionnaire-9) sleep item

CS cross-sectional, *L* Longitudinal
[a](a) trouble sleeping in the past 4 weeks; (b) trouble on at least seven of the previous 28 nights; (c) trouble sleeping interfered with daytime functioning

Obstructive sleep apnea OSA is a sleep-related breathing disorder characterized by transitory but recurrent episodes of upper airway obstruction during sleep. OSA is essentially described among head and neck cancer patients whether with primary or metastatic head and neck tumors. The obstruction mechanisms, leading to a lower diameter of upper airways, might be intrinsic (intra-luminal tumor) or extrinsic (external masses compression).

There are very few studies focused on OSA and cancer (Payne et al. 2005; Friedman et al. 2011; Steffen et al. 2009; Stern and Auckley 2007) but these ones convey that OSA may occur in different moments of the disease: whether in the initial phase of diagnosis or after treatments as surgery or RT.

14.3   Etiology of Sleep Disorders in Cancer Patients

Most of the studies analyzing the causes of sleep problems in cancer population focus on *insomnia*, since this is by far the most prevalent problem/dysfunction.

There are multiple factors—some directly related to the tumor's biology and symptoms, its treatments, or secondary to lifestyle changes—that simultaneously or sequentially contribute to damage the quality of sleep in cancer patients; these factors may (inter)play different roles in how they contribute to the insomnia problem: may predispose, precipitate, amplify or perpetuate the insomnia (Spielman et al. 1987; Savard and Morin 2001); several factors may occur along the disease process, isolated or concomitantly; each one's importance or role may vary with time, but ultimately they tend to coexist in a vicious-cycle, synergic association that perpetuates the sleep problem.

14.3.1 Tumor-Related Factors

Pain
Pain is the most unpleasant of cancer symptoms and unfortunately, a common one. In the advanced or metastatic phase of disease, pain has a prevalence rate of 30–60 % (Cleeland et al. 1994; Teunissen et al. 2007).

Chronic pain is a well-known factor for bad sleeping in rheumatic and other chronic patients (McCraken and Iverson 2002); the same is being consistently found in cancer patients where mild or severe, persistent or irruptive, or whatever type of pain eventually is a major cause of insomnia (Bardwell et al. 2008; Grond et al. 1994; Fortner et al. 2002; Rumble et al. 2005; Mercadante et al. 2004). The path between pain and sleep is bidirectional, as sleep loss also leads to increased pain (Stepanski and Burgess 2007).

Normal subjects forced to partial sleep deprivation or interrupted REM sleep show lower pain threshold the following day. Therefore, any clinical condition that may possibly interfere with the amount of total sleep or phase REM periods is expected to increase pain (Roehrs et al. 2006; Kunderman et al. 2004; Moldofsky and Scarisbrick 1976; Onen et al. 2001).

Opioids are common usage in malignant pain palliation and traditionally known for their concomitant sedative effects. Recently though, some studies pointed out the disruptive effect of different opioids on sleep architecture, mainly decreasing REM and slow wave sleep amounts and leading to an increase of nocturnal awakenings (Kay 1975; Kay et al. 1979; Lewis et al. 1970; Dimsdale et al. 2007).

Fatigue
Insomnia has consistently been referred as a cause for Cancer-Related Fatigue (CRF), but the relationship between both symptoms is more complex. Insomnia and fatigue play a mutual synergism whose reciprocal amplification fits better in the notion of cancer cluster symptoms (Miaskowski et al. 2004; Dodd et al. 2001, 2004; Roscoe et al. 2007).

Fatigue may induce insomnia since it promotes napping and therefore, disruption of normal sleep pattern (Theobald 2004). However, Liu et al. (2012) warn that patients may feel more fatigue during chemotherapy treatment, but they actually sleep longer whether day or night time.

Further research is needed to truthfully understand the whole interaction between insomnia and fatigue.

Psychiatric Symptoms and Disorders

Distress

Distress secondary to cancer disclosure is ubiquitous to all recently diagnosed cancer patients. This highly disturbing emotional state usually endures the first medical appointments and discussion of treatment plan. This very first period of coping with a brand new cancer diagnosis is probably the most prevalent, universal, and independent cause of sleep disturbance among cancer patients, occurring whatever the initial cancer site or extension, as much as patient age, personality, social support, or culture.

Fortunately, this state tends to rapidly ameliorate. Activating healthy individual coping skills and encouraged by family and team support, the majority of patients achieve a successful psychological adjustment to the new onset disease. Transitory new onset insomnia related with first knowledge of having a cancer might end in a few days. Nevertheless, between 20 and 30 % of new onset cancer patients evolve into a dysfunctional adjustment syndrome (Alex et al. 2011) where insomnia is usually present besides depression and/or anxiety.

Depression

Chronic insomnia may be a predisposing factor to depression. Opposite, insomnia is a frequent symptom in depressive spectrum disorders. Sometimes "depressive" insomnia seems to have an independent course and endures beyond mood recovery. Actually, depression and insomnia are often associated in a synergic and reverberating cycle, each other worsening the other (Breslau et al. 1996; Gillin 1998; Ford and Kameron 1989). In current psychiatric practice, it is wise to treat both sleep and mood symptoms simultaneously and from the very beginning.

As known in the psycho-oncology setting, 30 % of cancer population suffer from clinical depression whether during the disease process or survivorship (Derogatis et al. 1983; Massie and Holland 1990; Bottomley 1998). Studies designed for Oncology setting detected depression as the most prevalent risk factor for insomnia (Bardwell et al. 2008; Savard et al. 2001). For psycho-oncologists and other clinicians, the notion of symptom cluster is here particularly accurate since patients often present concurrent and synergistic depression, fatigue, and insomnia. The good practice should be to try and treat them altogether in order to rapidly improve patient's quality of life.

Anxiety

Anxiety *symptom* is very common throughout the disease process and peaks in every moment of uncertainty about cancer control or treatment failure. In these situations anxiety is better named as *distress*, and its interference with the quality of sleep may be significant although transient, leading to initial insomnia, EDS, and nightmares. With a satisfactory prospect for diagnosis, prognosis, or other uncertain medical issues, the sleep disturbance ceases spontaneously.

Opposite, Anxiety *disorders* are much less prevalent in the cancer population, around 10 % (Derogatis et al. 1983; Stark et al. 2002), and their correlation with insomnia has not been properly studied.

Delirium

Delirium is a frequent comorbidity in cancer especially in the advanced stages of the disease. Multiple medical problems, hospitalization, pain, and opioid treatment are all often associated with delirium in cancer patients. Sleep–wake cycle disruption is ubiquitous to delirium and is likely to be one of the most distressing symptoms for the patient but also for the family and staff (Bush and Bruera 2009; Fiorentino and Ancoli-Israel 2007).

The CNS global affection is traditionally regarded as the obvious cause of every major sleep problem that might be associated to the delirium condition. However, there might be a reciprocal pathogenic influence. Patients' prolonged sleep deprivation inherent to Intensive Care Units (ICU) or other busy and noisy ward hospitalization may eventually be a major factor in precipitating or worsening their delirium (Weinhouse et al. 2009).

14.3.2 Oncologic Treatment, Iatrogenic Factors

Surgery

There is no consistent data about the real effect of surgery over the quality of sleep in cancer patients (Omne-Ponten et al. 1992; Tsunoda et al. 2007). The sleep disturbance is usually transient and secondary to anticipatory anxiety about the success of the surgery plus the changes of rhythms and behaviors inherent to hospitalization.

Radiotherapy

The studies focused on the effects of RT on the quality of sleep in cancer patients are scarce and poor in design and control of variables. Most of these studies use breast cancer patients in the active phase of RT treatment but do not control concomitant chemo or hormone therapy. Having said that, most of those women referred displayed significant levels of insomnia during the course of RT that got worse in the last period of treatment (Wengstrom et al. 2000; Van Someren et al. 2004).

Even fewer studies are found regarding other large groups of patients whose treatment is usually based on neoadjuvant RT, namely Head and Neck or CNS tumors (Van Someren et al. 2004; Harrison et al. 1997).

Chemotherapy

While chemotherapy is a highly effective cancer treatment, its administration is often associated with negative side effects and a significant impact on patient's quality of life; among some of the most common CHE-related side effects feature fatigue, nausea, pain, anorexia, and insomnia (Palesh et al. 2012a; Hoffman et al. 2004; Cheng and Yeung 2013).

Despite the massive presence of CHE in most oncologic therapeutic protocols and an impressive amount of worldwide research focused on cytostatic side effects and their impact on patients' quality of life, nothing has been effectively studied about their putative sleep damage.

Patients' subjective reports point out CHE as a frequent factor for sleep disruption, either as a precipitating or an amplifying factor of insomnia. Objective studies focused on this issue are scarce, enroll a small number of patients, and their findings are inconsistent (Berger et al. 2003; Payne et al. 2006). There is significant heterogeneity amidst CHE regimens. Each CHE protocol is usually a drug combo which is adjusted to each patient's weight, height, and physical complaints at every administration; each drug may affect sleep differently whether acting alone or in combination with others. When submitted to a CHE regime, patients often take many other medicines to prevent or alleviate its side effects. To be reliable enough studies must compare patients undergoing similar CHE regimen and control concomitant medicines that might interfere with sleep namely HT, immunomodulators, glucocorticoids, opioids, anti-emetics, BZD, and antidepressants.

Having said that and trying to summarize data from actual literature, CHE agents may affect quality of sleep either by *direct* or *indirect effects*. Directly, via inflammatory/immune system/neuroendocrine deregulation; indirectly, secondary to their GI, hormonal and other systemic side effects that *per se* interfere with sleep (Savard and Ivers 2012).

Chemotherapy, inflammation and immune function deregulation Substantial evidence supports a strong bidirectional relationship between immune function and sleep: on one side, sleep deprivation lowers immune responses; acute infection and its subsequent inflammatory cascade reaction impacts on sleep architecture by increasing slow-wave sleep and reducing REM sleep (Majde and Krueger 2005; Kapsimalis et al. 2005; Dantzer et al. 2008; Reyes-Gibby et al. 2008; Seruga et al. 2008; Miller et al. 2008; Mills et al. 2008).

Pro-inflammatory cytokines are possible mediators of CHE-induced systemic symptoms and associated sleep wake disturbances (Dantzer et al. 2008; Reyes-Gibby et al. 2008; Seruga et al. 2008; Miller et al. 2008; Mills et al. 2008).

Inflammation resulting from cancer treatments possibly lead to sleep problems; opposite, deregulation of sleep may lead to altered immune profiles; inasmuch, chronic inflammatory active processes are predictors of acute and long-term poor quality of sleep either in cancer patients or survivors (Wang et al. 2010; Clevenger et al. 2012).

Immune function also interferes with neuroendocrine systems and circadian rhythms; consistently, high levels of circulating pro-inflammatory cytokines such as IL-6, TNF-α, and TGN-α have been shown to be associated with disrupted circadian function in patients with advanced cancer (Miller et al. 2008; Lee et al. 2004; Dantzer and Kelley 2007; Rich et al. 2005). Moreover, an intervention study using cognitive behavioral therapy (CBT) to treat insomnia in cancer patients showed decrease in cytokine-blood levels following successful treatment of insomnia (Stepanski and Burgess 2007; Savard et al. 2005).

Chemotherapy and circadian rhythms Recent literature stresses the evidence that CHE may interfere in circadian rhythms, e.g., cortisol cycle, flattening cortisol slopes which may cause sleep disturbance and more awakenings (Palesh et al. 2008, 2012a; Savard et al. 2009b).

Acute, transient but profound circadian rhythm disruption induced by CHE has been further demonstrated in two studies involving flattened patterns of salivary cortisol, motor activity, and temperature in advanced cancer patients receiving treatment (Ortiz-Tudela et al. 2011, 2012; Innominato et al. 2009). Furthermore, disrupted circadian rhythms blunt biological-clock physiological synchronizers such as light exposure, physical and social activity, and meal schedules, worsening daytime dysfunction due to insufficient night rest (Innominato et al. 2009; Ancoli-Israeli et al. 2012; Liu et al. 2005; Lévi et al. 2010).

Chemotherapy systemic side effects may be potent sleep disruptors *per se*. In women with breast cancer undergoing CHE and consequent iatrogenic ovarian failure, **hot flashes** are likely to be the major factor associated with insomnia (Bardwell et al. 2008; Carpenter et al. 2002; Stein et al. 2000). Hot flushes lead to fragmented sleep because of higher amount of arousals, wake time, and REM latency (Savard et al. 2004).

Glucocorticoids

Synthetic glucocorticoids administered in therapeutic doses or for supportive care (antiemetic and immunosuppressive properties) may disrupt diurnal cortisol rhythms and alter the circadian component of sleep (Innominato et al. 2009, 2010). In fact, in Oncology practice glucocorticoids are ubiquitous drugs and some of the most common agents causing insomnia, frequent awakenings, and overall non-restorative sleep in cancer patients.

Immunotherapy

Agents like α Interferon (IFN α2b) or Interleukin (IL 2) may cause iatrogenic depression which is usually associated with significant levels of insomnia (Capuron et al. 2000).

Nowadays, brand new **Immunossupressores, Immunomodulators,** and **Targeted molecules** are being used on a large scale as neo or co-adjuvant therapies in Oncology protocols. They are often long-term treatments, and their impact on the quality of sleep is unknown.

14.4 Treatment of Sleep Disorders in Cancer Patients

14.4.1 General Procedures

Despite the impact and prevalence of sleep disturbances in cancer, patients tend to underreport them (Engstrom et al. 1999) and physicians tend to ignore, probably because they do not know how to treat them (Laugsand et al. 2011).

Considering the medical burden of cancer patients, one should minimize pharmacotherapy only focused on poor sleep and try to scope the health problems altogether. The efficacy of current sleep medications in specific Oncology setting needs further research. Nevertheless, the newer hypnotics are safe, have few side effects, and may help within other cancer symptoms (pain, pruritus, nausea, anorexia, hot flashes, fatigue, and memory decline) (Caruso et al. 2013). Recent studies highlight the importance of non-pharmacologic approaches like sleep hygiene measures and behavioral interventions.

14.4.2 Psychotropic Drugs (#: These drugs Are Not Available in Portugal)

Antihistamines

Histamine from the tuberomammillary nucleus of the hypothalamus regulates sleep/wake switch, being known as the "on" switch, i.e., the wake promoter. When the pathway is turned on, histamine is released, triggering arousal and inhibiting the sleep promoter (Taylor et al. 2009; Stahl 2008).

Despite having little evidence of efficacy for the treatment of insomnia, sedative antihistamines (AHs) are often used as "over the counter" (OTC) drugs. They can be an option for patients with a history of intolerance to benzodiazepines (BZDs), alcohol or substance abuse, or atopic reactions. Most AHs have significant side effects such as daytime sedation, weight gain, anticholinergic and antimuscarinic actions (additional caution is mandatory in the elderly population), as well as in an addictive profile.

Diphenhydramine (Nytol®, Sominex®, Simply Sleep®, Benadryl®, Drenoflux®): It is a very potent nonselective AH agent, widely used in the United States (US). It has been associated to cognitive impairment in the elderly hospitalized patients. Diphenhydramine has a half-life/duration of action of 6 h at low dose. Suggested doses are 25–100 mg/*q.h.s (quaque hora somni,* i.e., every night at bedtime) po or im (maximum 400 mg/day).

Doxylamine (Unisom®): It has a half-life of 4–12 h and is used in the US at 25–100 mg/*q.h.s.* (Labbate et al. 2010).

Hydroxyzine (Atarax®): Hydroxyzine is related to the antipsychotic phenothiazine (Moszczynski and Murray 2012). The usual hypnotic dosage ranges 50–200 mg/*q.h.s.* po or im (can cause local pain; maximum 600 mg/day) with a half-life of 7–20 h. Paradoxical reactions (excitement) in children and seniors have been reported. Dose reduction is mandatory in renal insufficiency.

Promethazine (Pentazine®, Phenergan®): Promethazine also belongs to the phenothiazine group. Its use as an antipsychotic has been abandoned. Promethazine is also antihistaminic, blocking H1 receptors. It has sedative, hypnotic, and antiemetic effects. It enhances opioid effect when combined with pethidine/meperidine (Mepergan®#) or codeine (syrup presentation, euphoric effects).

Promethazine sedative effect occurs 20 min after oral administration and has a long half-life (4–12 h) with low potential of abuse. It is metabolized by the liver into various metabolites. Additional caution is required in older adults, in epilepsy, high blood pressure or heart disease, respiratory distress, sleep apnea, glaucoma, peptic ulcer, bone marrow depression, pheochromocytoma, enlarged prostate and hypocalcaemia.

The usual adult dose is 25 mg po, iv, or im once; repeat the administration if necessary. In pediatric use (≥2 years) give 0.5–1 mg/kg/dose oral, im, iv, or rectal (do not exceed 25 mg), repeat every 6 h if necessary (in children the dosage should not exceed half of suggested adult dosage).

Benzodiazepine Hypnotics (BDZ-H)

There are several BDZs indicated in the short-term (2–4 weeks) management of insomnia. They have sedative-hypnotic effects, reducing fragmentation and improving latency and duration of sleep (Stahl 2008; Labbate et al. 2010; Bazire 2010).

BDZs act by binding to a specific site on the GABA A (γ-amino butyric acid A) receptor. GABA is the main inhibitory neurotransmitter in the brain, producing inhibition of neuronal firing. The GABA from the ventrolateral preoptic nucleus of the hypothalamus also participates in the sleep/wake switch, acting as the "off" switch, the sleep promoter. Unlike barbiturates, BZDs are relatively safe drugs; their overdose are seldom mortal. Although effective in reducing insomnia, BDZs can cause long-term problems (tolerance, dependence, daytime sedation, memory problems, dizziness, and rebound insomnia when discontinued, or other withdrawal effects). Hence, they should not be used as first-line hypnotic agents and rather be held in reserve when other drugs fail.

When selecting a BDZ, one should consider its pharmacokinetic, dose forms, rate and duration of action, as well as predictable side effects (Table 14.6) (Chesson et al. 1999), (Table 14.7).

In the US there are at least five BDZs approved by FDA for short-term use:

Ultra-long half-lives (24–150 h): **FLurazepam** (Dalmane®, 15–30 mg/night capsule) and **Quazepam** (Doral®,# 7.5–30 mg/night tablet). They can cause drug accumulation with chronic use and have been associated with increased risk of falls, especially in the elderly.

Ultra-short half-life (1–3 h): **Triazolam** (Halcion®, 0.125–0.25 mg/night tablet). May wear off before one needs to awake; may be associated with rebound insomnia.

Moderate half-lives (15–30 h): **Temazepam** (Restoril®, 7.5–30 mg/night capsule) and **Estazolam** (ProSom®, 1–2 mg/night tablet). Can wear off after one has awakened producing sedation and memory problems and useful in treating daytime anxiety.

Table 14.6 Precautions when prescribing BZD

• Initiate with a low dose and keep it at the lowest effective dose
• Avoid every night usage, recommend taking only when really necessary
• Patients should plan a minimum of 8 h of sleep
• Be aware of side-effects like slight functional impairment
• Consider BZD prescription if other psychiatric (anxiety...) and/or medical illnesses (epilepsy, muscle tension and pain...) comorbidities are present
• In early insomnia, prefer drugs with a rapid onset of action
• In intermediate insomnia, it is preferable to use drugs with a slow rate of elimination
• Avoid BZD if: history of alcohol or drug abuse, pregnancy and with possible or known sleep apnea
• Reduce the doses in the elderly
• After 4 weeks, patient should be reevaluated regarding the maintenance of BZD
• A slow discontinuation should be attempted (level of evidence, D)

Nonbenzodiazepine Hypnotics

The "Z" drugs are also GABA A positive allosteric modulators (PAMs) but with a different way of binding. They may not have the long-term effects of BZDs, therefore may be used for chronic treatment in chronic insomnia (level of evidence, A) (Taylor et al. 2009; Stahl 2008; Krystal et al. 2003, 2008). However, according to the UK's NICE (National Institute for Clinical Excellence) guidelines, there are no differences between the two groups, and Z drugs keep the license only for short-term use (Bazire 2010; TA77 2004).

These agents are optimal to induce sleep and have reduced risk of dependence. In RLS with persistent sleep distortion, the augmentation strategy with zolpidem or eszopiclone may be useful.

Z overdoses are not lethal, and they remain safe when prescribed with SSRIs and other nonsedating antidepressants or concomitant to alcohol intake (safer than BZDs-H).

Zolpidem (Stilnox®, Ambien®, Intermezzo®, Zolpimist®: half-life 1–3 h). Usual therapeutic dose: 5–10 mg/*q.h.s.* tablet and oral spray. At higher doses may be associated with next-day anterograde amnesia.

Zolpidem CR, controlled-release formulation (Ambien CR®#: half-life/ duration of action 6 h). Usual therapeutic dose: 6.25–12.5 mg/*q.h.s.* tablet.

Zaleplon (Sonata®#: half-life 1–3 h). Usual therapeutic dose: 5–20 mg/*q.h.s.* capsule. It is a pyrazolopyrimidine hypnotic, a selective full agonist at the δ-1 benzodiazepine receptor. Evidence favors Zolpidem, with longer duration of sleep (Krystal et al. 2003).

Eszopiclone (Lunesta®#: half-life/duration of action 6 h). Usual therapeutic dose: 1–3 mg/*q.h.s.* tablet. Active S enantiomer/isomer of Zopiclone (#) with negative toxicity in preclinical cancer assays, unlike the racemic mixture of R and S isomers (Zopiclone). Studies have demonstrated sleep-improving effects lasting for 6 months with few withdrawal effects.

Table 14.7 Benzodiazepines

Benzodiazepines	Regular bed time doses (mg)	Parental forms	Active metabolite	Onset after oral dose	Distribution half-life	Elimination half-life (h)
Chlordiazepoxide[a] (Librium®)	10–30 (capsule)	No	Many	Slow	–	36–200?
Clonazepam[b](Klonopion®) (off-label)	0.5–2 (tablet) (wafer)	No	Yes	Intermediate	Intermediate	18–40
Lorazepam (Ativan®)	1–3 (tablet)	Yes (20 mg/10 ml; 40 mg/ 10 ml)	No (metabolized only by glucuronidation, less affected by hepatic injury)	Intermediate	Intermediate	10–20
Midazolam (Dormicum®)	7.5–15 (tablet)	Yes (1 mg/ml; 5 mg/ml)	Yes	Intermediate	Rapid	2–3
Oxazepam (Serax®)	10–30 (capsule)	No	No (metabolized only by glucuronidation, less affected by hepatic injury)	Intermediate-slow	Intermediate	8–12

[a]Also used for management of acute alcohol withdrawal syndrome
[b]Also used in the treatment of PLMS and as an augmenter in RLS
Question mark indicates that the values 36–200 are not consensual and are estimated values

Barbiturates

Barbiturates are anticonvulsant drugs and should be reserved as a final option for severe and intractable insomnia in patients already taking them or introduced in other patients for a very short term (2 weeks). They are very high risk drugs for dependence and tolerance and its overdose can be mortal. They are commonly misused drugs, may exacerbate amnesia secondary to alcohol intake, cause hematological effects, and interact with many other drugs. For all these dangerous effects, barbiturates are seldom prescribed in Europe and in the US.

Antidepressants

It is common to prescribe antidepressants for the management of primary or secondary insomnia, essentially if there is a comorbid mood disorder. Antidepressants side effects may also help hindering other cancer-related symptoms.

Trazodone (Azona®, Desyrel®, Devidon®, Oleptro®, Triticum®): It is a serotonin 5-HT2 receptor antagonist with mild inhibition of the serotonin transporter. It is currently used as off-label for insomnia, employing lower doses (50–300 mg po *q.h.s.*) and with an immediate onset of action, but a long half-life. Evidence supports its superiority over placebo. Due to the antagonism of α1-adrenergic receptors, there can be some unpleasant effects like orthostatic hypotension and priapism.

Amitriptyline (Elavil®, ADT®, Adepil®, Amilin®, Amitrip®, Amizol®):, At 10–50 mg po *q.h.s.* doses, it has immediate effects in insomnia or anxiety (level of evidence, A). As a tricyclic antidepressant it can be toxic even in these low doses. It may be a good choice in the presence of neuropathic or chronic pain and is also safe in sleep apnea. One should be aware of its anticholinergic action, cardiac risk, daytime sedation, and long half-life.

Doxepin (Silenor®, Sinequan®, Doxal®, Doxedyn®, Adapin®, Anten®#): Again a sedating tertiary-amine antidepressant unlicensed by UK's British National Formulary (BNF), in spite of showing some efficacy in the management of insomnia. A new Doxepin presentation (1, 3 and 6 mg po) has been reviewed by FDA, especially to treat insomnia.

Mianserin (Athymil®, Lerivon®, Tolvon®): It is an old tetracyclic antidepressant with noradrenergic profile. It has showed efficacy treating depression and comorbid insomnia (30–60 mg po *q.h.s.)* in cancer patients although in poorly controlled studies. Renal and hepatic impairment does not require dose adjustment. It has reported less cardiac and sexual toxicity than with tricyclic drugs.

Mirtazapine (Remeron®): Evidence suggests that mirtazapine (15–45 mg po *q.h.s.*) is effective treating insomnia as well as anxiety and depressive symptoms in cancer patients. However, more systematic research (e.g., placebo-controlled studies) is needed. Being similar to H1 receptors antagonists, it is increases appetite and weight, which might be quite useful in oncologic rehabilitation and palliative care (Cankurtaran et al. 2008).

Paroxetine (Paxil®, Paxil CR®): the SSRI paroxetine seems to be useful to treat sleep disorders both in depressed and nondepressed cancer patients (Palesh et al. 2012b). Its usage can also be extended to comorbid anxiety. Common doses range 20–40 mg po/day. Side effects should be monitored: hyponatremia, altered liver function, autonomic activation, sexual dysfunction, and gastrointestinal symptoms. Be aware of the significant interaction with tamoxifen.

Venlafaxine (Effexor®, Effexor XR®): the SNRI venlafaxine may be especially useful in cancer treatment-induced menopause, decreasing the vasomotor symptoms and nocturnal hot flashes; it is also an adjunctive drug for pain relief (37-5-150 mg po/day) (Joffe et al. 2010).

Melatonergic Agents

Melatonin is the pineal neurotransmitter involved in biological clock regulation and sleep pattern design. Melatonin boosts after dark, peaking at 2–4 h AM and then decreases, encompassing the human light/dark cycle. It has been reported that the elderly with primary insomnia secrete less melatonin and cancer patients have less contrasted melatonin values between day and nighttime. Melatonergic agents seem to be effective in modulating sleep onset and shifting phase circadian rhythms.

Agomelatine (Valdoxan®): It is a melatonin 1 (MT) and 2 receptor antagonist, as well as a serotonin 2C and 2B receptor antagonist, being developed as an antidepressant. Its actions as antidepressant and as hypnotic might be independent. There are low incidence of sexual side effects and discontinuation symptoms. The new EMA (European Medicines Agency) recommendation requires liver function tests before treatment and at 6, 12, and 24 weeks after initiation. The usual dose is 25–50 mg/*q.h.s* (tablet).

Melatonin (Circadin®): It is a synthetic melatonin agonist of the MT1, MT2, and MT3 receptors. In the UK it is licensed for monotherapy of sleep disorders (primary insomnia) only in patients older than 54. It is used in a 21-day course as a prolonged-release formulation, 2 mg po 1–2 h before bedtime and after food intake. Several major trials have conveyed its efficacy whether improving sleep quality, sleep onset, or morning alertness. Melatonin also helps patients with jet lag and with Circadian Rhythm Sleep Disorder (CRSD) (level of evidence, A). It has been shown to be a well-tolerated and safe drug, with no withdrawal symptoms and no impairment in everyday life.

Its use in other age groups is "off-label." There are other melatonin products, immediate-release capsules, tablets, or liquids but are considered unlicensed.

Ramelteon (Rozerem®#): Selectively binds to the MT1 and MT2 receptors in the suprachiasmatic nucleus. It is approved by the FDA for long-term use for insomnia, specifically delayed sleep onset. Ramelteon is metabolized by CYP1A2, showing drug interactions with fluvoxamine, asketoconazole, flucona zole, and rifampin. It is a well-tolerated drug with few side effects except for hyperprolactinemia, which appeared two to three times more often than placebo in clinical trials. It does not have a dependence profile, no abuse potential, or withdrawal syndrome. The usual and maximum dose is 8 mg po 30 min before bedtime and not after a high-fat meal. The clinical trials conducted support its efficacy up to 6 months.

Atypical Antipsychotics

Regarding atypical antipsychotics (AP) frequent adverse effects, there is no indication for use as first-line treatment of insomnia or other sleep disorders (level of evidence, D). However, they can be indicated for adjunctive treatment in refractory patients (off-label), besides in patients with comorbid schizophrenia or bipolar disorder.

Olanzapine (Zyprexa®, Olasek®): It is structurally similar to Clozapine. It has several effects that are helpful in cancer patients, like sedation, weight gain, no hyperprolactinemia, no agranulocytosis, and few extrapyramidal symptoms (EPS). The usual dose in these cases is 2.5–10 mg po *q.h.s.* It could be a first choice drug to treat sleep problems in patients with comorbid *Delirium*.

Quetiapine (Seroquel®): It also has hypnotic properties due to its H1 selective antagonist at normal clinical doses and even at lower doses: 25–200 mg po at night (immediate release formulation). Expected effects are increased weight and improved mood. It is not associated with EPS or prolactin elevations, being a good choice in Parkinson's disease, comorbid *Delirium*, and senior patients.

Dopaminergic Agents

The primary management of PLMS and RLS is the use of dopaminergic agents (DA) agonists. The newer D2 and D3 receptor agonists are better tolerated, but may cause nausea: **Ropinirole** (Requip®) 0.25–2 mg po and **Pramipexole** (Mirapex®) 0.125–0.75 mg po 2–3 h before bedtime (Kushida 2006). Iron replacement is mandatory, and it is still used as **Levodopa/Carbidopa**.

As secondary approaches Gabapentin (300–1,200 mg po *q.h.s.*) or Pregabaline, especially if painful RLS, should be considered. If partial response you should think of low-potency opiods (e.g., acetaminophen with codeine 300 mg/30 mg *q.h.s.*), BZD or GABAA PAMS (see above).

Wake-Promoting Drugs/Psychostimulants

Primary hypersomnia, the rare narcolepsy, and EDS (more frequent in cancer patients, particularly near recent treatment) are treated with:

Dextroamphetamine (Dexedrine®, Dextrostat®#): 10–60 mg po/day.

Modafinil (Modiodal®, Provigil®): 100–400 mg po once a day.

14.4.3 Other Medicines

DORA (dual Orexin 1 and 2 receptor antagonists): under investigation.

Valerian Root/extract *(Valeriana officinalis)*: Valerian is an herbal medicine used for anxiety and sleep difficulties, frequently OTC. Some studies suggest that it is effective but most of them are inconclusive. Long-term valerian treatment may be able to interact with anesthesia and other drugs (chemotherapy, anti-fungal, AHs, BZDs, sedatives, narcotics. . .), although information is still incomplete.

Valerian is a dietary supplement in the US and thus does not obey to the FDA directives. However, the German regulatory agency for herbs approved its usage in sleep problems based on animal studies and some European clinical trials. The usual dosage for sleeping purposes is 300–900 mg tablet, 1–2 h before bedtime, during 4–6 weeks.

Further research is needed to assess valerian's effectiveness and safety (Oxman et al. 2007; Bent et al. 2006; Blumenthal 1998).

Chronomodulated chemotherapy There is a growing interest in the possible linkage between disrupted circadian rhythm and insufficient response to chemotherapy. Studies involving time-adjusted chemotherapy in colorectal cancer patients (chemotherapy delivered at times selected to match greater tumor cell division) demonstrated better response rates and fewer side effects (Levi et al. 1997).

14.4.4 Non-pharmacological

Phototherapy/Light Therapy

For CRSD scheduled light exposure can be used (level of evidence, B/C). Bright white light exposition at adequate time can change endogenous circadian rhythms in order to match the optimal environmental rhythms.

CPAP

Nasal continuous positive airway pressure (CPAP) and bi-level positive airway pressure are the most commonly used nonsurgical approaches for OSA. This condition is common in head and neck cancer patients and less frequently in over weight menopausal breast cancer women. Both systems use a mask that is connected with a machine that generates positive air pressure. CPAP uses continuous pressure throughout inspiration and expiration, and bi-level positive airway pressure uses higher pressure in inspiration than in expiration (Stahl 2008).

Cognitive Behavioral Therapy

CBT-based treatments are effective and should be suggested as a first-line treatment (level of evidence, A) in chronic primary insomnia and in insomnia *not* secondary to medical or psychiatric disorders. Behavioral interventions are recommended to treat primary hypersomnia, narcolepsy, CRSD, parasomnias (use of relaxation and systematic desensitization), as well as in children with disturbed sleep (level of evidence, A). When trying to discontinue long-term hypnotic drug treatment, CBT increases outcome (level of evidence, A). CBT packages include the following (Chesson et al. 1999; Davidson 2012; Langford et al. 2012; Berger et al. 2009) (Table 14.8):

Table 14.8 Sleep hygiene education

1. Sleep hygiene education
• Increase daily exercise (not at evening)
• Reduce/stop daytime napping
• Reduce caffeine (since midday), nicotine or alcohol intake, especially before bedtime
• Use the bed only for sleeping
• Eliminate noise or temperature extremes, and control bright light exposure at night
• Use anxiety management (don't watch the clock. . .) or relaxation techniques
• Develop a regular sleep/wake routine at the same time each day
2. Cognitive therapy: cognitive restructuring, paradoxical intention
3. Relaxation therapy: progressive muscle relaxation, imagery training, yogic breathing techniques
4. Stimulus-control therapy
5. Sleep-restriction therapy

Acupuncture/Acupressure

In one study, acupuncture treatment seemed a feasible alternative for highly motivated breast cancer survivors with sleep problems and hot flashes (Otte et al. 2011). Further confirmation within a larger, randomized, controlled clinical trial is missing.

Clinical Case

- 67-year-old man, no previous psychiatric antecedents.
- Newly diagnosed Multiple Myeloma, multiple bone lesions, and secondary pain.
- After the second CHE treatment (Bortezomib+ Cyclophosphamide+ Dexamethasone 160 mg/treatment), he complained of acute, severe anxiety symptoms and total insomnia, unresponsive to BZD (Diazepam 5 mg po 2×/day + Lorazepam 1 mg po qhs). His mental condition got worse with agitation, helplessness, and suicidal thoughts.
- After first psychiatric evaluation, the glucocorticoid dose was half-reduced and he started Quetiapine 400 mg po/d. He has soon recovered his mood and sleep balance, maintaining those psychotropic dosages throughout the whole chemotherapy (6 months).
- Afterwards, BZD and Quetiapine doses were lowered.
- Early relapse, 3 months after ending the first CHE, demanding a second CHE schedule which included Dexamethasone 160 mg/treatment.
- Immediately after the first treatment, an even more severe psychiatric syndrome appeared, once more with serious insomnia and intense secondary anxiety; he was prescribed higher dose of Quetiapine (600 mg po/d) and proceeded to a different glucocorticoid schedule (8 mg Dexamethasone 2×/week; total 64 mg/treatment).

(continued)

- Favorable outcome with complete remission of both hematological and psychiatric disorders allowed progressive suspension of the psychotropic drugs.

▶ **Key Points**

- Insomnia is the most prevalent sleep problem among cancer patients.
- Insomnia is frequently secondary to multiple and synergistic factors: etiological factors may be directly related to the tumor's biology or symptoms, oncologic treatments, or lifestyle changes.
- Insomnia, depression, and fatigue are often present as a symptom cluster that should be treated overall.
- Chemotherapy deregulates immune function, enhances inflammatory response, and interferes with circadian rhythms; when chronic, these effects are predictors of acute and long-term poor quality of sleep either in cancer patients or survivors.
- Considering the medical burden of cancer patients, one should minimize pharmacotherapy only focused on poor sleep and try to scope the health problems altogether.
- Sleep hygiene measures should be always taught and implemented (Table 14.8).
- Z drugs and BZD are both recommended for short-term use when treating acute insomnia.
- Z drugs are safer than BZD and might be considered in chronic treatment of chronic insomnia (evidence A).
- AD are recommended whether in primary or secondary insomnia treatment, being especially useful when there is a comorbid mood disorder or when hindering other cancer-related symptoms.

References

Akekushi T, et al. Associated and predictive factors of sleep disturbance in advanced cancer patients. Psychooncology. 2007;16:888–94.

Alex J, Chan M, Bhatti H, et al. Prevalence of depression, anxiety, and adjustment disorder in oncological, haematological, and palliative-care settings: a meta-analysis of 94 interview-based studies. Lancet Oncol. 2011;12:160–74.

Allade R, Siegel JM. Unearthing the phylogenetic roots of sleep. Curr Biol. 2008;18(15):670–9.

American Psychiatric Association. Diagnostic and statistical manual of mental disorders. 5th ed. Washington, DC: American Psychiatric Press; 2013.

Ancoli-Israeli S, Rissling M, Neikrug A, et al. Light treatment prevents fatigue in women undergoing chemotherapy for breast cancer. Support Care Cancer. 2012;20(6):1211–9.

Bardwell WA, Profant J, Casden DR, et al. The relative importance of specific risk factors for insomnia in women treated for early-stage breast cancer. Psychooncology. 2008;17(1):9–18.

Bazire S. Psychotropic drug directory 2010. 1st ed. Aberdeen: HealthComm UK Ltd; 2010.

Bent S, Padula A, Moore D, Patterson M, Mehling W. Valerian for sleep: a systematic review and meta-analysis. Am J Med. 2006;119:1005–12.

Berger AM, Von Essen S, Kuhn BR. Adherence, sleep and fatigue outcomes after adjuvant breast cancer chemotherapy: results of a feasibility intervention study. Oncol Nurs Forum. 2003; 30(3):513–22.

Berger AM, Kuhn BR, Farr LA, et al. One-year outcomes of a behavioral therapy intervention trial on sleep quality and cancer-related fatigue. J Clin Oncol. 2009;27(35):6033–40.

Blumenthal M, editor. The complete German Commission E monographs: therapeutic guide to herbal medicines. Austin, TX: American Botanical Council; 1998.

Borbely AA. A two process model of sleep regulation. Hum Neurobiol. 1982;1:195–204.

Bottomley A. Depression in cancer: a literature review. Eur J Cancer Care. 1998;7:181–91.

Breslau N, Roth T, Rosenthal L, Andreski P. Sleep disturbance and psychiatric disorders: a longitudinal epidemiological study of young adults. Biol Psychiatry. 1996;39(6):411–8.

Brown RE, Basheer R, McKenna JT, et al. Control of sleep and wakefulness. Physiol Rev. 2012;92 (3):1087–187.

Bush S, Bruera E. The assessment and management of delirium in cancer patients. Oncologist. 2009;14:1039–49.

Buysse DJ, Reynolds CF, Monk TH, Berman SR, Kupfer DJ. The Pittsburgh Sleep Quality Index (PSQI): a new instrument for psychiatric research and practice. Psychiatry Res. 1989;28: 193–213.

Cankurtaran ES, Ozalp E, Soygur H, et al. Mirtazapine improves sleep and lowers anxiety and depression in cancer patients: superiority over imipramine. Support Care Cancer. 2008;16(11): 1291–8.

Capuron L, Ravaud A, Dantzer R. Early depressive symptoms in cancer patients receiving Interleukin 2 and/or Interferon alfa-2b therapy. J Clin Oncol. 2000;18(10):2143–51.

Carpenter JS, Johnson D, Wagner L, Andrykowski M. Hot flashes and related outcomes in breast cancer survivors and matched comparison women. Oncol Nurs Forum. 2002;29(3):E16–25.

Caruso R, Grassi L, Nanni MG, Riba M. Psychopharmacology in psycho-oncology. Curr Psychiatry Rep. 2013;15(9):393.

Cheng KK, Yeung RM. Impact of mood disturbance, sleep disturbance, fatigue and pain among patients receiving cancer therapy. Eur J Cancer Care (Engl). 2013;22:70–8.

Chesson Jr AL, Anderson WM, Littner M, Davila D, Hartse K, Johnson S, et al. Practice parameters for the nonpharmacologic treatment of chronic insomnia. An American Academy of Sleep Medicine report. Standards of Practice Committee of the American Academy of Sleep Medicine. Sleep. 1999;22(8):1128–33.

Chokroverty S, Avidan AY. Sleep and its disorders. In: Daroff RB, Fenichel GM, Jankovic J, Mazziotta JC, editors. Bradley's neurology in clinical practice. Philadelphia, PA: Elsevier Saunders; 2012. p. 1641.

Cleeland CS, Gonin R, Hatfield AK, et al. Pain and its treatment in outpatients with metastatic cancer. N Engl J Med. 1994;330(9):592–6.

Clevenger L, Schrepf A, Christensen D, et al. Sleep disturbance, cytokines and fatigue in women with ovarian cancer. Brain Behav Immun. 2012;26(7):1037–44.

Colagiuri B, Christensen S, Jensen AB, et al. Prevalence and predictors of sleep difficulty in a national cohort of women with primary breast cancer three to four months postsurgery. J Pain Symptom Manage. 2011;42(5):710–20.

Dantzer R, Kelley KW. Twenty years of research on citokyne-induced sickness behaviour. Brain Behav Immun. 2007;21(2):153–60.

Dantzer R, O'Connor JC, Freund GG, et al. From inflammation to sickness and depression: when the immune system subjugates the brain. Nat Rev Neurosci. 2008;9(1):46–56.

Davidson JR. Sleep disturbance interventions for oncology patients: steps forward and issues arising. Sleep Med Rev. 2012;16:395–6.

Davidson JR, MacLean AW, Brundage MD, et al. Sleep disturbances in cancer patients. Soc Sci Med. 2002;54:1309–21.

Derogatis LR, Morrow GR, Fetting J, et al. The prevalence of psychiatric disorders among cancer patients. JAMA. 1983;249(6):751–7.

Dimsdale JE, Norman D, DeJardin D, Wallace MS. The effect of opioids on sleep architecture. J Clin Sleep Med. 2007;3(1):33–6.

Dodd MJ, Miaskowski C, Paul SM. Symptom clusters and their effect on the functional states of patients with cancer. Oncol Nurs Forum. 2001;28:465–70.

Dodd MJ, Miaskowski C, Lee KA. Occurrence of symptom clusters. J Nat Cancer Inst Monogr. 2004;2004:76–8.

Engstrom CA, Strohl RA, Rose L, Lewandowski L, Stefanek ME. Sleep alterations in cancer patients. Cancer Nurs. 1999;22(2):143–8.

Fiorentino L, Ancoli-Israel S. Sleep dysfunction in patients with cancer. Curr Treat Options Neurol. 2007;9(5):337–46.

Ford DE, Kameron DB. Epidemiologic study of sleep disturbances and psychiatric disorders: an opportunity for prevention. JAMA. 1989;262:1479–84.

Fortner BV, Stepanski EJ, Wang SC, et al. Sleep and quality of life in breast cancer patients. J Pain Symptom Manage. 2002;24:471–80.

Friedman M, et al. The occurrence of sleep-disordered breathing among patients with head and neck cancer. Laryngoscope. 2011;111:1917–9.

Gillin JC. Are sleep disturbances risk factors for anxiety, depressive and addictive disorders? Acta Psychiatr Scand Suppl. 1998;393:39–43.

Grond S, Zech D, Diefenbach C, Bichoff A. Prevalence and pattern of symptoms in patients with cancer pain: a prospective evaluation of 1635cancer patients referred to a pain clinic. J Pain Symptom Manage. 1994;9(6):372–82.

Harrison LB, Zelefsky MJ, Pfister DG, et al. Detailed quality of life assessment in patients treated with primary radiotherapy for squamous cell cancer of the base of the tongue. Head Neck. 1997;19(3):169–75.

Hoffman M, Morrow GR, Roscoe JA, et al. Cancer patients expectations of experiencing treatment related side effects: a university of Rochester Cancer Center-Community Clinical Oncology Program study of 938 patients from community practices. Cancer. 2004;101(4):851–7.

Innominato PF, Focan C, Gorlia T, et al. Circadian Rhythm in rest and activity: a biological correlate of quality of life and a predictor of survival in patients with metastatic colorectal cancer. Cancer Res. 2009;69(11):4700–7.

Innominato PF, Levi FA, Bjarnason GA. Chronotherapy and the molecular clock: clinical implications in oncology. Adv Drug Deliv Rev. 2010;62(9–10):979–1001.

Joffe H, Partridge A, Giobbie-Hurder A, et al. Augmentation of venlafaxine and selective serotonin reuptake inhibitors with zolpidem improves sleep and quality of life in breast cancer patients with hot flashes: a randomized, double-blind, placebo-controlled trial. Menopause. 2010;17(5):908–16.

Kapsimalis F, Richardson G, Opp MR, Kryger M. Cytokines and normal sleep. Curr Opin Pulm Med. 2005;11(6):481–4.

Kay DC. Human sleep during morphine intoxication. Psychopharmacologia. 1975;44(2):117–24.

Kay DC, Pickworth WB, Neidert GL, et al. Opioid effects on computer-derived sleep and EEg parameters in nondependent human addicts. Sleep. 1979;2(2):175–91.

Krystal AD, Edinger JD. Measuring sleep quality. Sleep Med. 2008;9 suppl 1:S10–7.

Krystal AD, et al. Sustained efficacy of eszopiclone over 6 months of nightly treatment: results of a randomized, double-blind, placebo-controlled study in adults with chronic insomnia. Sleep. 2003;26:793–9.

Krystal AD, et al. Long-term efficacy and safety of zolpidem extended-release 12.5mg administered 3 to 7 nights per week for 24 weeks, in patients with chronic primary insomnia:

a 6-month, randomized, double-blind, placebo-controlled, parallel-group, multicenter study. Sleep. 2008;31:79–90.

Kunderman B, Spernal J, Huber MT, et al. Sleep deprivation affects thermal pain threshold but not somatosensory threshold in healthy volunteers. Psychosom Med. 2004;66(6):932–7.

Kushida AC. Ropinirole for the treatment of restless legs syndrome. Neuropsychiatr Dis Treat. 2006;2(4):407–19.

Labbate LA, Fava M, Rosenbaum JF, Arana GW. Handbook of psychiatric drug treatment. 6th ed. Philadelphia, PA: Lippincott Williams & Wilkins; 2010. p. 232–53.

Langford DJ, Lee K, Miaskowski C. Sleep disturbance interventions in oncology patients and family caregivers: a comprehensive review and meta-analysis. Sleep Med Rev. 2012;16: 397–414.

Laugsand EA, Jakobsen G, Kaasa S, Klepstad P. Inadequate symptom control in advanced cancer patients across Europe. Support Care Cancer. 2011;19:2005–14.

Lee BN, Dantzer R, Langley KE, et al. A citokyne-based neuroimmunologic mechanism of cancer-related symptoms. Neuroimmunomodulation. 2004;11(5):279–92.

Lee-Cheong Jr T. Sleep medicine: essentials and review. New York: Oxford University Press; 2008. p. 28–9.

Levi F, Zidani R, Misset JL. Randomized multicenter trial of chronotherapy with oxaliplatin, fluorouracil, and folinic acid in metastatic colorectal cancer. International Organization for Cancer Chronotherapy. Lancet. 1997;350(9079):681–6.

Lévi F, Okyar A, Dulong S, et al. Circadian timing in cancer treatments. Annu Rev Pharmacol Toxicol. 2010;50:377–421.

Lewis SA, Oswald I, Evans JI, Akindale MO. Heroin and human sleep. Electroencephalogr Clin Neurophysiol. 1970;28(4):429.

Liu L, Marler MR, Parker BA, et al. The relationship between fatigue and light exposure during chemotherapy. Support Cancer Care. 2005;13(12):1010–7.

Liu L, Rissling M, Natarajan L, et al. The longitudinal relationship between fatigue and sleep in breast cancer patients undergoing chemotherapy. Sleep. 2012;35(2):237–45.

Majde JA, Krueger JM. Links between the innate immune system and sleep. J Allergy Clin Immunol. 2005;116(6):1188–98.

Massie MJ, Holland JC. Depression and the cancer patient. J Clin Psychiatry. 1990;51:12–7. discussion 18–19.

McCraken LM, Iverson GL. Disrupted sleep patterns and daily functioning in patients with chronic pain. Pain Res Manag. 2002;7(2):75–9.

Mercadante S, Girelli D, Casuccio A. Sleep disorders in advanced cancer patients: prevalence and factors associated. Support Care Cancer. 2004;12:355–9.

Miaskowski C, Dodd MJ, Lee KA. Symptom clusters: the new frontier in symptom management research. J Natl Cancer Inst Monogr. 2004;2004:17–21.

Miller AH, Ancoli-Israle S, Bower JE, et al. Neuroendocrine-immune mechanisms of behavioural comorbidities in patients with cancer. J Clin Oncol. 2008;26(6):971–82.

Mills PJ, Ancoli-Israel S, Parker B, et al. Predictors of inflammation in response to anthracycline-based chemotherapy for breast cancer. Brain Behav Immun. 2008;22(1):98–104.

Moldofsky H, Scarisbrick P. Induction of neurasthenic musculoskeletal pain syndrome by selective sleep stage deprivation. Psychosom Med. 1976;38(1):35–44.

Morin CM. Insomnia: psychological assessment and management. New York, NY: The Guilford Press; 1993.

Moszczynski A, Murray BJ. Neurobiological aspects of sleep physiology. Neurol Clin. 2012;30: 963–85.

Omne-Ponten M, Holmberg L, Burns T, et al. Determinants of psychosocial outcome after operation for breast cancer. Results of prospective comparative interview study following mastectomy and breast conservation. Eur J Cancer. 1992;28A(6–7):1062–7.

Onen SH, Alloui A, Gross A, et al. The effects of total sleep deprivation, selective sleep interruption and sleep recovery on pain tolerance threshold in healthy subjects. J Sleep Res. 2001;10(1):35–42.

Ortiz-Tudela EIP, Iurisci I, Karaboué A et al. Chemotherapy-induced circadian disruption in cancer patients. XII congress of European Biological Rhythms Society; 20–26 Aug 2011; Oxford, UK.

Ortiz-Tudela EIP, Rol MA, Madrid JA, Levi F. Circadian patterns in integrated wrist temperature, rest activity and position (TAP) as a biomarker for personalized cancer chronotherapeutics. SRBR meeting. 19–23 May 2012; Florida, USA.

Ostacoli L, Saini A, Ferini-Strambi L, et al. Restless legs syndrome and its relationship with anxiety, depression, and quality of life in cancer patients undergoing chemotherapy. Qual Life Res. 2010;19(4):531–7.

Otte JL, Carpenter JS, Zhong X, Johnstone PA. Feasibility study of acupuncture for reducing sleep disturbances and hot flashes in postmenopausal breast cancer survivors. Clin Nurse Spec. 2011;25(5):228–36.

Oxman AD, Flottorp S, Håvelsrud K, et al. A televised, web-based randomized trial of an herbal remedy (valerian) for insomnia. PLoS One. 2007;2:e1040.

Page MS, Johnson LB. Putting evidence into practice: evidence-based interventions for sleep-wake disturbances. Clin J Oncol Nurs. 2006;10(6):753–67.

Palesh OG, Collie K, Batiuchok D, et al. A longitudinal study of depression, pain, and stress as predictors of sleep disturbance among women with metastatic cancer. Biol Psychol. 2007; 75(1):37–44.

Palesh O, Zeitzer JM, Conrad A, et al. Vagal regulation, cortisol and sleep disruption in women with metastatic breast cancer. J Clin Sleep Med. 2008;4(5):441–9.

Palesh OG, Roscoe JA, Mustian KM, et al. Prevalence, demographics, and psychological associations of sleep disruption in cancer patients: University of Rochester Cancer Center Community Clinical Oncology Program. J Clin Oncol. 2010;28:292–8.

Palesh OG, Peppone L, Innominato PF, et al. Prevalence, putative mechanisms, and current management of sleep problems during chemotherapy for cancer. Nat Sci Sleep. 2012a;4: 151–62.

Palesh OG, Mustian KM, Peppone LJ, et al. Impact of paroxetine on sleep problems in 426 cancer patients receiving chemotherapy: a trial from the University of Rochester Cancer Center Community Clinical Oncology Program. Sleep Med. 2012b;13(9):1184–90.

Payne RJ, et al. High prevalence of obstructive sleep apnea among patients with head and neck cancer. J Otolaryngol. 2005;34:304–11.

Payne J, Piper B, Rabinowitz I, Zimmerman B. Biomarkers, fatigue, sleep and depressive symptoms in women with breast cancer; a pilot study. Oncol Nurs Forum. 2006;33(4):775–83.

Reite M, Weissberg M, Ruddy J. Clinical manual for evaluation and treatment of sleep disorders. 1st ed. Arlington, VA: American Psychiatric Publishing; 2009. p. 17–26.

Reyes-Gibby CC, Wu X, Spitz M, et al. Molecular epidemiology, cancer related symptoms and cytokines pathway. Lancet Oncol. 2008;9(8):777–85.

Rich T, Innominato PF, Boerner J, et al. Elevated serum cytokines correlated with altered behaviour, serum cortisol rhythm and dampened 24-hour rest-activity patterns in patients with metastatic colorectal cancer. Clin Cancer Res. 2005;11(5):1757–64.

Roehrs T, Hyde M, Blaisdell B, et al. Sleep loss and REM sleep loss are hyperalgesic. Sleep. 2006;29:145–51.

Roscoe JA, Kaufman ME, Matteson-Rusby SE, et al. Cancer-related fatigue and sleep disorders. Oncologist. 2007;12 suppl 1:35–42.

Rumble ME, Keefe FJ, Edinger JD, et al. A pilot study investigating the utility of the cognitive-behavioral model of insomnia in early stage lung cancer patients. J Pain Symptom Manage. 2005;30:160–9.

Saini A, Ostacoli E, Sguazzotti S, et al. High prevalence of restless legs syndrome in cancer patients undergoing chemotherapy: relationship with anxiety, depression and quality of life perception. JCO ASCO Annual meeting proceedings Part I. 2007; 25 (18S).

Savard J. Insomnia. In: Davis MP, Feyer PC, Ortner P, Zimmermann C, editors. Supportive oncology. Philadelphia, PA: Elsevier Saunders; 2011. p. 187–99.

Savard J, Ivers H. The initiation of chemotherapy but not radiation therapy coincides with increased insomnia. Psychooncology. 2012;21:37–8.

Savard J, Morin CM. Insomnia in the context of cancer: a review of a neglected problem. J Clin Oncol. 2001;19(3):895–908.

Savard J, Simard S, Blanchet J, et al. Prevalence, clinical characteristics and risk factors for insomnia in the context of breast cancer. Sleep. 2001;24(5):583–90.

Savard J, Davidson JR, Ivers H, et al. The association between nocturnal hot flashes and sleep in breast cancer survivors. J Pain Symptom Manage. 2004;27(6):513–22.

Savard J, Simard S, Ivers H, et al. Randomized study on the efficacy of cognitive-behavioral therapy for insomnia secondary to breast cancer, part II: immunologic effects. J Clin Oncol. 2005;23:6097–106.

Savard J, Villa J, Ivers H, et al. Prevalence, natural course and risk factors of insomnia comorbid with cancer over a 2-month period. J Clin Oncol. 2009a;27:5233–9.

Savard J, Liu L, Natarajan L, et al. Breast cancer patients have progressively impaired sleep-wake activity rhythms during chemotherapy. Sleep. 2009b;32(9):1155–60.

Seruga B, Bernstein LJ, Tannock IF. Cytokines and their relationship to the symptoms and outcome of cancer. Nat Rev Cancer. 2008;8(11):887–99.

Sethi KD, Mehta SH. A clinical primer on restless legs syndrome: what we know and what we don't know. Am J Manag Care. 2012;18(5 Suppl):S83–8.

Sharma N, Hansen CH, O'Connor M, et al. Sleep problems in cancer patients: prevalence and association with distress and pain. Psychooncology. 2012;21(9):1003–9.

Spielman AJ, Caruso LS, Glovinsky PB. A behavioural perspective on insomnia treatment. Psychiatr Clin North Am. 1987;10(4):541–53.

Stahl SM. Stahl's essential psychopharmacology—neuroscientific basis and practical applications. 3rd ed. New York: Cambridge University Press; 2008.

Stark D, Kiely M, Smith A, et al. Anxiety disorders in cancer patients: their nature, associations, and relation to quality of life. J Clin Oncol. 2002;20(14):3137–48.

Steffen A, Graefe H, Gehrking E, König IR, Wollenberg B. Sleep apnoea in patients after treatment of head neck cancer. Acta Otolaryngol. 2009;129(11):1300–5.

Stein KD, Jacobsen PB, Hann DM, et al. Impact of hot flashes on quality of life among postmenopausal women being treated for breast cancer. J Pain Symptom Manage. 2000; 19(6):436–45.

Stepanski EJ, Burgess HJ. Sleep and cancer. Sleep Med Clin. 2007;2:67–75.

Stern TM, Auckley D. Obstructive sleep apnea following treatment for head and neck cancer. ENT J. 2007;86(2):101–3.

TA77: Guidance on the use of zaleplon, zolpidem and zopiclone for the short-term management of insomnia. National Institute for Health and Care Excellence (NICE), April 2004.

Taylor D, Paton C, Kapur S. The Maudsley—prescribing guidelines. 10th ed. London: Informa Healthcare; 2009.

Teunissen SC, Wesker W, Kruitwagen C, et al. Symptom prevalence in patients with incurable cancer: a systematic review. J Pain Symptom Manage. 2007;34(1):94–104.

The International Classification of Sleep Disorders. Diagnostic and coding manual. Westchester, IL: American Academy of Sleep Medicine; 2005.

Theobald DE. Cancer pain, fatigue, distress, and insomnia in cancer patients. Clin Cornerstone. 2004;6(suppl 1D):S15–21.

Trevorrow T. Assessing sleep problems of older adults. In: Lichtenberg PA, editor. Handbook of assessment in clinical gerontology. Philadelphia, PA: Elsevier Saunders; 2010. p. 410–4.

Tsunoda A, Nakao K, Hiratsuka K, Kusano M. Prospective analysis of quality of life in the first year after colorectal surgery. Acta Oncol. 2007;46(1):77–82.

Van Someren EJ, Swart-Heikens J, Endert E, et al. Long term effects of cranial irradiation for childhood malignancy on sleep in adulthood. Eur J Endocrinol. 2004;150(4):503–10.

Wang XS, Shi Q, Williams LA, et al. Inflammatory cytokines are associated with the development of symptom burden in patients with NSCLC undergoing concurrent chemoradiation therapy. Brain Behav Immun. 2010;24(6):968–74.

Weinhouse G, Schwab R, Watson P, et al. Bench-to-bedside review: Delirium in ICU patients—importance of sleep deprivation. Crit Care. 2009;13:234. doi:10.1186/cc8131.

Wengstrom Y, Haggmark C, Strander H, Forsberg C. Perceived symptoms and quality of life in women with breast cancer receiving radiation therapy. Eur J Oncol Nurs. 2000;4(2):78–88. discussion 89–90.

Yue HJ, Dimsdale JE. Psycho-oncology. 2nd ed. New York, NY: Oxford University Press; 2010.

Substance Abuse in Oncology

15

Steven D. Passik, Nicholas Miller, Matthew Ruehle, and Kenneth L. Kirsh

Abstract

Historically, problems related to the prevalence and impact of substance use disorders of all kinds have been underestimated in psycho-oncology. This is ironic, because if one practices outside the confines of the tertiary care academic medical center, the rate of SUDs that the psycho-oncologist will encounter is shockingly high. And the impact of unchecked substance and alcohol abuse on adherence with potentially lifesaving and life extending cancer treatments can be among the most profound of any psychiatric morbidity psycho-oncologists are likely to confront. The growing problem of prescription drug abuse has shined a light on the need for the application of addiction medicine techniques and interventions when opioids are used in people with pain in general, and now that the differences between the treatment of cancer and non-cancer pain are narrowing, psycho-oncologists need to learn to employ strategies learned from colleagues working in the field of chronic pain. And pain and symptom management are hardly the only areas of oncology affected by SUD. Yet, psycho-oncologists of virtually every discipline lack specific training in the addictions and so there is an enormous gap between the prevalence of these problems and the expertise available to assist these patients. It is hoped this chapter will help to begin to fill this gap.

15.1 Introduction

Until very recently, discussing the management of substance use in the person with cancer might have been seen as having only minor clinical relevance. Certainly, the relief of anxiety, pain and other distressing symptoms has been identified as a top

S.D. Passik (✉) • N. Miller • M. Ruehle • K.L. Kirsh
Millennium Laboratories, 16981 Via Tazon, San Diego, CA 92127
e-mail: Steven.Passik@millenniumlabs.com; Nicholas.Miller@millenniumlabs.com; Matthew.Ruehle@millenniumlabs.com; Kenneth.Kirsh@millenniumlabs.com

L. Grassi and M. Riba (eds.), *Psychopharmacology in Oncology and Palliative Care*, DOI 10.1007/978-3-642-40134-3_15, © Springer-Verlag Berlin Heidelberg 2014

priority for clinicians, and the use of medications, even those with abuse potential, has been deemed essential. Much of the literature on this subject suggests that problems of substance abuse are only infrequently encountered in oncology. Perhaps this underestimation of the problem stems from the fact that much of this academic work has come from tertiary care settings—where those with histories of addiction are less frequently encountered because of economic and insurance barriers to care. Or perhaps it has been that cancer typically remains a disease of later life, whereas addiction overwhelmingly manifests earlier, making it unlikely to emerge de novo in a person first exposed to substances with abuse potential when they are older and ill (Cicero et al. 2012; Minozzi et al. 2013). Or perhaps it has been because cancer used to follow an almost uniformly fast and fatal trajectory, and so any exposure to controlled substances was likely to be brief and occur during a period of time that the person was becoming increasingly disabled. Thus, even if the exposure to such drugs might trigger a relapse in a person who suffered with the disease of addiction before they became ill with cancer, the dysfunctional behaviors that might have been set in motion would be mediated and limited by the relentless impact of the cancer itself. Or perhaps it was simply the trivialization of addiction that characterized the early rhetoric accompanying the increase in opioid prescribing which led to this being such a neglected topic (Passik 2001).

During recent years, in response to the public health crisis that is chronic pain in our aging society, the prescribing of opioids and other controlled substances has increased dramatically. Unfortunately, a parallel set of public health crises has arisen, the problems of prescription drug abuse, diversion, overdose, and death. Now that people with cancer are routinely living longer at all stages of disease, including those with painful but stable disease and those who go onto remission but are left with chronic pain issues from chemotherapy and other factors, exposures to controlled substances are considerably longer than they once were and thus there is greater opportunity for those who come to the disease with a history of SUD to lose control, overuse, or even have the problem of addiction fully rekindled (Lowery et al. 2013; Modesto-Lowe et al. 2012). Finally, of additional concern for those prescribing controlled substances and treating pain, anxiety, and other symptoms in people with cancer including older patients, their medications are increasingly sought after by younger drug abusers in their family or environment (including grandchildren and caregivers).

There is a certain irony in the fact that the use of opioids in non-cancer pain grew out of recognition that people with cancer pain (at least those seeking treatment at tertiary care facilities) appeared to be able to take these medications with generally positive results. That is, their pain was controlled, side effects manageable, functional status improved or stabilized, and problems of misuse or addiction minimal. Opioid prescribing then increased dramatically in North America, to the much more diverse population of those with chronic pain—more diverse in terms of age, psychiatric and addiction histories and comorbidities, and duration of exposure (Kirsh et al. 2012). Not surprisingly, the results of this effort were decidedly more mixed. Rather than the self-titration model based on the assumption that risk of misuse and addiction is uniformly minimal across patients (generally a cancer pain model), a risk stratification model emerged for the delivery of opioid therapy. Younger age, personal or family history of addiction, history of sexual trauma, and active psychiatric comorbidity were seen as risks for a poor outcome in opioid therapy, unless the delivery of this therapy was tailored to the needs of the individual (with the employment of safeguards such as urine drug testing, prescription monitoring programs, and the like as well as consultations with psychiatric and addictions professionals to assure safety). This type of risk stratification is somewhat foreign to oncology pain management, but it seems that the time is right to close the loop and for the therapy that initially influenced non-cancer pain practice to adopt strategies developed therein, especially now that many of the differences between cancer and non-cancer pain patients have narrowed (Kircher et al. 2011).

Pain and anxiety management are hardly the only aspects of cancer care affected by the presence of a substance use disorder. Indeed, because unchecked drug or alcohol abuse can cause spotty or complete non-adherence to potentially lifesaving cancer treatments, virtually every step along the disease trajectory, from diagnosis to palliative care, can be threatened. And if the psycho-oncologist is working outside of a tertiary care academic center, the frequency with which they will be confronted with substance use disorders is shockingly high, due to the high base rate of these disorders in this population which is so much more reflective of the population as a whole. If one considers that substance use can be a risk factor for cancer, one would expect substance abusers to be over, not under, represented in the oncology population. So many psycho-oncologists from nearly all of the disciplines represented in this group of practitioners from psychiatry to psychology to nursing to social work are lacking in their knowledge of addictions. There is an enormous gap between the prevalence of these problems and the expertise in caring for cancer patients who are struggling with them. It is hoped that this chapter helps to bridge this gap.

15.2   Major Issues

15.2.1 Prevalence

Substance use disorders are a consistent phenomenon in the United States over time, with estimated base rates of 6–15 % (Muirhead 2000; Gfroerer and Brodsky 1992; Colliver and Kopstein 1991; Regier et al. 1984; SAMHSA 2011a, b, c). This prevalence of drug abuse certainly touches medically ill patients and can negatively influence how patients are treated. Although few studies have been conducted to evaluate the epidemiology of substance abuse in patients with advanced illness, substance use disorders appear to be relatively rare within the tertiary care population with cancer and other advanced diseases (Kirsh and Passik 2013; Passik and Kirsh 2013; Passik and Portenoy 1998b). However, the prevalence of alcoholism in major cancer centers is most likely underestimated. A study by Bruera and colleagues (1995) of 100 terminally ill alcoholic cancer patients found that despite multiple hospital admissions and screenings, only one-third had documentation of alcoholism in their medical records.

The belief that aging drug habits would diminish and vanish with age is no longer held with the certainty of past belief. An early study supporting this belief showed 50 % of individuals addicted to narcotics were no longer active drug users by age 32, and over 99 % were no longer users by age 67 (Winick 1962). However, as the "baby boom" cohort ages, the extent of alcohol and medication misuse is predicted to significantly increase because of the combined effect of the growing population of older adults and cohort-related differences in lifestyles and attitudes (Patterson and Jeste 1999). One study suggested that the number of illicit drug users aged 50 years or older will approximately double from the year 2000 to the year 2020 because of an anticipated 52 % increase in this segment of the population and the attendant shift in attitudes and historical experiences with substance use in this cohort (Colliver et al. 2006).

15.2.2 Prescription Drug Abuse

The use of illicit drugs and the nonmedical use of prescription opioids have increased significantly in the general population over the last decade, with the highest prevalence among younger adult men (Manchikanti and Singh 2008; SAMHSA 2012). Such estimates, however, belie alarming trends emerging among older adults. Among adults aged 50 or older, nearly five million, roughly 5 % of that age group, report using illicit drugs in the past year (SAMHSA 2011b). Marijuana is the most abused drug in the US, but among adults aged 60 or older, the abuse of prescription drugs is equally common. A changing pattern of cannabis use among older adults suggests that as an individual ages the social incentive to smoke marijuana decreases while the attempt to use it medicinally increases (Taylor and Grossberg 2012). In the oncology setting this might include an attempt to self-medicate nausea, anorexia, pain, anxiety, or combinations of these common symptoms (Borgelt et al. 2013). More alarming than rates of cannabis use, emergency room visits related to pharmaceutical abuse more than doubled from 2004 to 2008 among adults aged 50 or older, and a fifth of these were among adults aged 70 or older (SAMHSA 2010a). Prescription opioids were the most common culprit, followed by benzodiazepines. Although ER visits in 2008 related to illicit drug use among adults 50 and older were a little less than half that of pharmaceuticals (118,495 vs. 256,097 visits), they were not uncommon (SAMHSA 2010a, b). The majority of those visits were related to cocaine, followed by heroin. Consistent with this, one study demonstrated marijuana, cocaine, and opioid use in 2.4 %, 1.9 %, and 11.6 % of elderly men, respectively (Rockett et al. 2006). Substance use treatment admissions among adults aged 50 and older have nearly doubled in recent years, from 6.6 % of all admissions in 1992 to 12.7 % in 2009 (SAMHSA 2011a). During this same time period, alcohol as the only substance of abuse being treated decreased from 87.6 to 58.0 %, while the addition of other drugs to alcohol increased from 12.4 to 42.0 %. Also around this time, treatment admissions involving heroin more than doubled, from 7.2 to 16.0 %, and those reporting multiple drugs of abuse nearly tripled (SAMHSA 2010c).

Even as the baby boomer population continues to age, and more frequently experiencing pain, there is a paucity of information on older patients and the risk of comorbid pain and SUDs. A survey in Denmark revealed that 22.5 % of men and 27.8 % of women aged 65 and older reported chronic pain (Sjorgren et al. 2009). Out of these men and women, 35 % of them were not satisfied with the pain treatment that was offered. This can lead to alternative methods for relieving pain such as taking non-prescribed medications. In one study of 100 patients with chronic pain (average age near 50), 23 tested positive for illicit drugs and 12 tested positive for opioids even though they had no prescription and denied taking opioids (Manchikanti et al. 2004). In another study of primary care patients in a Veterans Affairs facility who were receiving opioids for the treatment of chronic pain (average age 59), 78 % reported at least one indicator of medication misuse during the prior year, with significantly more of those who misused pain medications reporting comorbid substance use disorder (Morasco and Dobscha 2008). This is consistent with a more recent examination of a subset of data from the Researched Abuse, Diversion and Addiction-Related Surveillance system (RADARS) that found that though severe chronic pain is common in adults entering treatment for prescription opioid abuse, it is exponentially more prevalent in adults older than 45 years (70 %) relative to adults aged 18–24 (45 %) (Cicero et al. 2012). Clearly, to the extent that chronic pain and SUDs are comorbid or mutually exacerbating problems, older adults would appear to represent a particularly vulnerable population. This might be especially true in the oncology culture, wherein performing a risk assessment has been historically uncommon and decreasing patients' wariness about using opioids aggressively when needed has been the biggest concern.

Thus, the emerging pattern, consistent with the aging of the "baby boom" generation and their greater likelihood of exposure to various types of drugs, is that illicit and prescription drug misuse and abuse, along with the need for treatment, is expected to have doubled by 2020 (relative to 1990s prevalence estimates) among older adults (Colliver et al. 2006; Gfroerer et al. 2003), with the greatest changes reflecting the increasing rates of emergency room visits and treatment admissions related to prescription opioids, benzodiazepines, heroin, and cocaine. Knowledge of these trends should assist oncology providers in identifying and managing problems in a more age-appropriate manner.

15.2.3 Alcohol

There have been relatively few studies that have examined the prevalence of alcoholism in an oncology population. The prevalence likely varies widely from one cancer to another with the highest rate found in the head and neck cancer population. One study found that greater than 25 % of patients admitted to a palliative care unit were found to have problems with alcohol abuse (Bruera et al. 1995). Socioeconomic barriers such as low income or unemployment, lack of health insurance, and possibly even attempts to self-medicate early signs of malignancies may preclude patients from seeking care at tertiary care centers. Alcohol abuse obviously complicates cancer care. For example, postsurgical withdrawal and delirium tremens (DTs) can be life threatening. Unfortunately, many patients are unrecognized prior to undergoing surgery. Integrating screening for alcoholism and offering detoxification ahead of surgery is an unanswered and ongoing problem.

15.2.4 Defining Abuse and Addiction in the Medically Ill

It is difficult to define substance abuse and addiction in patients with cancer, as the definitions of both terms have been adopted from addicted populations without medical illness. Furthermore, the pharmacological phenomena of tolerance and physical dependence continue to be commonly confused with abuse and addiction. The use of these terms is so strongly influenced by sociocultural considerations that it may lead to confusion in the clinical setting. Therefore, the clarification of this terminology is necessary to improve the diagnosis and management of substance abuse when treating patients with advanced disease (Hamrick et al. 2013; Passik and Portenoy 1998a).

Substance abuse Psychosocial, physical, and vocational harm that occurs from drug taking.
• Identifying harmful drug-taking behaviors is more difficult when patients are receiving potentially abusable drugs for legitimate purposes.

Substance dependence A normal phenomenon for many patients taking medication for chronic conditions.
• "Tolerance" occurs when a higher dosage of a drug is required to achieve the same effect.
• "Physical Dependence" occurs when a patient begins to require a drug in order to function normally and can lead to withdrawal symptoms when medication administration ceases.

Because substance abuse is increasingly widespread in the population at large, patients with cancer who have used illicit drugs are more frequently encountered in medical settings. Illicit drug use, actual or suspected misuse of prescribed medication, or actual substance use disorders create the most serious difficulties in the clinical setting, complicating the treatment of pain management. However, the management of substance abuse is fundamental to adherence to medical therapy and safety during treatment. Also, adverse interactions between illicit drugs and medications prescribed as part of the patient's treatment can be dangerous. Continuous substance abuse may alienate or weaken an already tenuous social support network that is crucial for alleviating the chronic stressors associated with advanced disease and its treatment. Therefore, a history of substance abuse can impede treatment and pain management and increase the risk of hastening morbidity and mortality among advanced patients, which can only be alleviated by a therapeutic approach that addresses drug-taking behavior while expediting the treatment of the malignancy and distressing symptoms, as well as addiction (Kirsh and Passik 2013; Passik and Kirsh 2013).

Important factors when assessing drug-taking behavior in cancer patients.
- Undertreatment of associated issues, particularly pain disorders
- Sociocultural differences in defining "aberrant" drug taking

15.2.5 Pseudoaddiction

Various studies have provided compelling evidence that pain is poorly treated in many oncology patients (Ramer et al. 1999; Glajchen et al. 1995; Ward et al. 1993). Clinical experience indicates that the inadequate management of symptoms and related pain may be the motivation for aberrant drug-taking behaviors.

Pseudoaddiction Distress and aberrant drug seeking behaviors that produce a similar pattern as addicts; however, these behaviors actually stem from the patient seeking relief from untreated pain (Passik et al. 2011).
- Patients are often attempting to "self-medicate" and behaviors can be considered pseudoaddictive if sufficient pain relieve eliminate these behaviors.
- Physical dependence can often lead to pseudoaddictive behaviors, as clinicians do not compensate for growing tolerance to medications and therefore underdose patients.

More recent scientific advances have also provided new insight into behaviors that may be considered pseudoaddiction. Pharmacogenetic variances in the enzymes that metabolize pain medications help to explain individual differences in medication response and side effects experienced. If a patient is an ultrarapid metabolizer, they may complain that the medication is effective for a shorter period of time than is common for that medication. If a patient is a poor metabolizer, they may complain that the medication is not working or possibly continue to ask for increased amount of medication. Pharmacogenetic variations should be considered and pharmacogenetic testing implemented when a patient has an unusual response to a medication, more than expected side effect profile, and/or inefficacy at usual dosages (Argoff 2010).

The potential for pseudoaddiction creates a challenge for the assessment of a known substance abuser with an advanced illness. Clinical evidence indicates that aberrant behaviors impelled by unrelieved pain can become so dramatic in this population that some patients appear to return to illicit drug use as a means of self-medication. Others use more covert patterns of behavior, which may also cause concerns regarding the possibility of true addiction. Although it may not be obvious that drug-related behaviors are aberrant, the meaning of these behaviors may be difficult to discern in the context of unrelieved symptoms (Kirsh and Passik 2013; Passik and Kirsh 2013; Passik and Portenoy 1998b).

15.2.6 Aberrant Drug Taking Behaviors

When a drug is prescribed for a medically diagnosed purpose, less assuredness exists as to the behaviors that could be deemed aberrant, thereby increasing the potential for a diagnosis of drug abuse or addiction. The ability to categorize these questionable behaviors as apart from social or cultural norms is also based on the assumption that certain parameters of normative behavior exist. Although it is useful to consider the degree of aberrancy of a given behavior, it is important to recognize that these behaviors exist along a continuum, with certain behaviors being less aberrant (such as aggressively requesting medication) and other behaviors more aberrant (such as injection of oral formulations) (See Table 15.1). If a large portion of patients were found to engage in a certain behavior, it may be normative, and judgments regarding aberrancy should be influenced accordingly (Kirsh and Passik 2013; Passik and Kirsh 2013; Passik and Portenoy 1998b).

We know more scientifically about aberrant behaviors, their prevalence, and meaning today than we did in the mid-1990s. We know that many patients will have at least a few aberrant behaviors in a 6-month period (Passik et al. 2005). We also know that once a patient has demonstrated four behaviors in their lifetime, they have an 85 % likelihood of meeting diagnostic criteria for substance use disorder (Fleming et al. 2007). But there is still much to be learned, confirmed, replicated, and studied.

15.2.7 Disease-Related Variables

Changes caused by progressive diseases, such as cancer, also challenge the principal concepts used to define addiction. Alterations in physical and psychosocial functioning caused by advanced illness and its treatment may be difficult to distinguish from the morbidity associated with drug abuse. In particular, alterations in functioning may complicate the ability to evaluate a concept that is vital to the diagnosis of addiction: "use despite harm." For example, discerning the questionable behaviors can be difficult in a patient who develops social withdrawal or cognitive changes after brain irradiation for metastases. Even if diminished cognition is clearly related to pain medication used in treatment; this effect might only reflect a narrow therapeutic window rather than the patient's use of analgesic to acquire these psychic effects (Hamrick et al. 2013; Passik et al. 1998a; Passik and Portenoy 1998a). To accurately assess drug-related behaviors in patients with advanced disease, explicit information is usually required regarding the role of the drug in the patient's life. Therefore, the presence of mild mental clouding or the time spent out of bed may have less meaning than other outcomes, such as noncompliance with primary therapy related to drug use or behaviors that threaten relationships with physicians, other healthcare professionals, and family members (Hamrick et al. 2013; Passik et al. 1998a; Passik and Portenoy 1998a).

Table 15.1 Examples of Aberrant drug-taking behaviors and severity

Examples of clearly aberrant behaviors	Examples of potentially aberrant behaviors
Illicit drug use	Requests for early medication refills
Intravenous injection of oral formulations	Requesting specific medications
Recurrent prescription "losses"	Patient taking extra doses of medication

15.2.8 Definitions of Abuse and Addiction for Advanced Illness

Abuse Use of an illicit drug or prescription medication with medical indication.

Addiction The compulsive use of a substance resulting in physical, psychological, or social harm to the user and continued "use despite the harm." (Rinaldi et al. 1988)
- This definition of addiction emphasizes the psychological and behavioral nature of this syndrome (Hamrick et al. 2013; Passik et al. 1998a; Passik and Portenoy 1998a).

A differential diagnosis should also be considered if questionable behaviors occur during treatment. A true addiction (substance dependence) is only one of many possible interpretations. A diagnosis of pseudoaddiction should also be taken into account if the patient is reporting distress associated with unrelieved symptoms. Impulsive drug use may also be indicative of another psychiatric disorder, the diagnosis of which may have therapeutic implications. On occasion, aberrant drug-related behaviors appear to be causally remotely related to a mild encephalopathy, with perplexity concerning the appropriate therapeutic regimen. On rare occasions, questionable behaviors imply criminal intent. These diagnoses are not mutually exclusive (Hamrick et al. 2013; Passik et al. 1998a; Passik and Portenoy 1998a).

Varied and repeated observations over a period of time may be necessary to categorize questionable behaviors properly (See Table 15.2). Perceptive psychiatric assessment is crucial and may require evaluation by consultants who can elucidate the complex interactions among personality factors and psychiatric illness.

Patients with borderline personality disorders, for example, may impulsively use prescription medications that regulate inner tension or improve chronic emptiness or boredom and express anger at physicians, friends, or family. Psychiatric assessment is vitally important for both the population without a prior history of substance abuse and the population of known substance abusers who have a high incidence of psychiatric comorbidity (Khantzian and Treece 1985).

Risks in Patients with Current or Remote Histories of Drug Abuse
There is a lack of information regarding the risk of abuse or addiction during or subsequent to the therapeutic administration of potentially abusable drugs to medically ill patients with a current or remote history of abuse or addiction (Hamrick et al. 2013; Passik and Portenoy 1998a). The possibility of successful long-term opioid therapy in patients with cancer or chronic nonmalignant pain has been

Table 15.2 Differential diagnoses to consider when interpreting aberrant drug-taking behaviors

Possible alternate diagnoses for aberrant drug-taking behaviors
Anxiety
Depression
Insomnia
Problems of adjustment (such as boredom caused by decreased ability to engage in usual activities)
Borderline personality disorder

indicated by anecdotal reports, particularly if the abuse or addiction is remote (Dunbar and Katz 1996; Gonzales and Coyle 1992; Macaluso et al. 1988).

Because it is commonly accepted that the likelihood of aberrant drug-related behavior occurring during treatment for medical illness will be greater for those with a remote or current history of substance abuse, it is reasonable to consider the possibility of abuse behaviors occurring when using different therapies. For example, although no clinical evidence exists to support that the use of short-acting drugs or the parenteral route is more likely to cause questionable drug-related behaviors than other therapeutic strategies, it may be prudent to avoid such therapies in patients with histories of drug abuse (Hamrick et al. 2013; Passik and Portenoy 1998a).

15.3 Clinical Management of Substance Use Disorders in Oncology

The most challenging issues in caring for patients with advanced disease typically arise from patients who are actively abusing alcohol or other drugs. This is because patients who are actively abusing drugs experience more difficulty in managing pain (Kemp 1996). Patients may become caught in a cycle where pain functions as a barrier to seeking treatment for addiction with another addiction, possibly complicating treatment for chronic pain (Savage 1993). Also, because pain is undertreated, the risk of binging with prescription medications and/or other substances increases for drug-abusing patients (Kemp 1996).

15.3.1 General Guidelines

The following guidelines can be beneficial, whether the patient is actively abusing drugs or has a history of substance abuse. The principles outlined assist clinicians in establishing structure, control, and monitoring of addiction-related behaviors, which may be helpful and necessary at times in all pain treatment (Kirsh and Passik 2013).

Recommendations for the long-term administration of potentially abusable drugs, such as opioids, to patients with a history of substance abuse are based exclusively on clinical experience. Research is needed to ascertain the most effective strategies and to empirically identify patient subgroups which may be most responsive to different approaches. The following guidelines broadly reflect the types of interventions that might be considered in this clinical context (Hamrick et al. 2013; Passik et al. 1998a, b).

15.3.2 Multidisciplinary Approach

Pain and symptom management is often complicated by various medical, psychosocial, and administrative issues in the population of advanced patients with a substance use disorder. The most effective team may include a physician with expertise in pain/palliative care, nurses, social workers, and, when possible, a mental healthcare provider with expertise in the area of addiction medicine (Kirsh and Passik 2013; Passik and Kirsh 2013).

15.3.3 Assessment of Substance Use History

In an effort to not offend, threaten, or anger patients, many times clinicians avoid asking patients about drug abuse. There is also often the expectation that patients will not answer truthfully. However, obtaining a detailed history of duration, frequency, and desired effect of drug use is vital. Adopting a nonjudgmental position and communicating in an empathetic and truthful manner is the best strategy when taking patients' substance abuse histories (Kirsh and Passik 2013; Passik and Kirsh 2013; Passik and Portenoy 1998b).

In anticipating defensiveness on the part of the patient, it can be helpful for clinicians to mention that patients often misrepresent their drug use for logical reasons, such as stigmatization, mistrust of the interviewer, or concerns regarding fears of undertreatment. It is also wise for clinicians to explain that in an effort to keep the patient as comfortable as possible, by preventing withdrawal states and prescribing sufficient medication for pain and symptom control, an accurate account of drug use is necessary (Kirsh and Passik 2013; Passik and Kirsh 2013; Passik and Portenoy 1998b).

Taking an accurate, detailed history from the patient is essential for the proper assessment and treatment of alcohol and drug abuse as well as any comorbid psychiatric disorders. It is also important to ask information regarding duration, frequency, and desired effect of the drug or alcohol consumption. In the wake of current pressures to treat the majority of patients in the ambulatory setting, and to admit patients on the morning of major surgery, the quick identification of alcoholism and initiation of plans for social, medical, and physiological needs of the patient must begin upon initial contact.

The use of a careful, graduated-style interview can be beneficial in slowly introducing the assessment of drug abuse. This approach begins with broad and general inquiries regarding the role of drugs in the patient's life, such as caffeine and nicotine and gradually proceeds to more specific questions regarding illicit drugs. This interview style can also assist in discerning any coexisting psychiatric disorders, which can significantly contribute to aberrant drug-taking behavior. Once identified, treatment of comorbid psychiatric disorders can greatly enhance management strategies and decrease the risk of relapse (Kirsh and Passik 2013; Passik and Kirsh 2013; Passik and Portenoy 1998b).

15.3.4 Use of Risk Assessment Tools

As stated above, potential opioid use must be accompanied by risk stratification and management. Given time constraints, a full psychiatric interview may not be feasible and thus time sensitive measures are clearly needed to help in this endeavor. Many screening tools contain items on personal and family history of addiction as well as other history-related risk factors, such as pre-adolescent sexual abuse, age, and psychological disease. These are tools for clinical decision-making and should not be viewed as necessarily diagnostically accurate (Passik et al. 2008; Smith and Kirsh 2009). Whatever tool the clinician chooses, it is advised that the screening process be presented to the patient with the assurance that no answers will negatively influence effective treatment.

15.3.5 Setting Realistic Goals for Therapy

The rate of recurrence for drug abuse and addiction is high in general. The stress associated with cancer and the easy availability of centrally acting drugs increases this risk. Therefore, total prevention of relapse may be impossible in this type of setting. Gaining an understanding that compliance and abstinence are not realistic goals may decrease conflicts with staff members in terms of management goals. Instead, the goals might be perceived as the creation of a structure for therapy that includes ample social/emotional support and limit-setting to control the harm done by relapse (Kirsh and Passik 2013; Passik and Kirsh 2013; Passik and Portenoy 1998b).

There may be some subgroups of patients who are unable to comply with the requirements of therapy because of severe substance use disorders and comorbid psychiatric diagnoses. In these instances, clinicians must modify limits on various occasions and endeavor to develop a greater variety and intensity of supports. This may necessitate frequent team meetings and consultations with other clinicians. However, pertinent expectations must be clarified, and therapy that is not successful should be modified (Kirsh and Passik 2013; Passik and Kirsh 2013; Passik and Portenoy 1998b).

15.3.6 Evaluation and Treatment of Comorbid Psychiatric Disorders

Extremely high comorbidity of personality disorders, depression, and anxiety disorders exist in alcoholics and other patients with substance abuse histories (Khantzian and Treece 1985). Individuals who are with a history of alcohol abuse have been found to be at higher risk for other psychiatric disorders. The most common comorbid mental disorders associated with alcoholism are anxiety disorders (19.4 %), antisocial personality disorder (14.3 %), affective disorder (13.4 %), and schizophrenia (3.8 %) (Regier et al. 1990). The occurrence of comorbid mental disorders in alcoholics may contribute to poor treatment compliance and success due to cognitive limitations and premorbid (in relation to the diagnosis of cancer) pain and neurological deficits. The same is true of opioid abuse where 85 % of addicts have a comorbid, nondrug abuse-related psychological disorder (Khantzian and Treece 1985). Thus, the psycho-oncologist assessing the cancer patient with addiction or alcoholism must identify and treat any comorbid disorders present. The treatment of depression and anxiety can increase patient comfort and decrease the risk of relapse or aberrant drug taking (Kirsh and Passik 2013; Passik and Kirsh 2013; Passik and Portenoy 1998b).

15.4 Alcohol Withdrawal Syndrome

Alcohol withdrawal is dangerous and can seriously complicate cancer treatment. In some instances, it is fatal. The first symptoms of withdrawal typically appear in the first few hours following the cessation of alcohol consumption and may consist of tremors, agitation, and insomnia. In cases of mild to moderate withdrawal, these symptoms tend to dissipate within 1–2 days without recurrence. However, in cases of severe withdrawal, autonomic hyperactivity, hallucinations, and disorientation may follow. The onset of delirium tremens marks the individual's progression from the withdrawal state to a state of delirium that represents a serious medical emergency.

Delirium tremens Characterized by agitation, hallucination, delusions, incoherence, and disorientation, typically within the first 72–96 h of withdrawal.
- Occurs in approximately 5–15 % of patients with alcohol withdrawal (Maxmen and Ward 1995).
- Is self-limiting and often ends with the patient entering a deep sleep with amnesia for most of the episode.
- DT can increase the risk of further complications in medically ill patients.

Wernicke–Korsakoff's syndrome Indicative of thiamine deficiency that causes permanent cognitive impairment.
- Frequently under-diagnosed
- Symptoms

- Fixed upward gaze
- Alcoholic neuropathy
- "Stocking-glove" paresthesia
- Autonomic instability
- Delirium encephalopathy

15.4.1 Medical Treatment of Withdrawal

While a full discussion of the pharmacological approach to alcohol withdrawal is beyond the scope of this chapter, a basic approach to the treatment of this syndrome is given. The use of hydration, benzodiazepines, and, in some cases, neuroleptics are appropriate for the management of alcohol withdrawal syndrome (see Table 15.3). The administration of a vitamin–mineral solution is indicated to counteract the effects of malnutrition that results from the alcohol itself and poor eating habits. Thiamine 100 mg administered intra-muscularly or intravenously for 3 days before switching to oral administration for the duration of treatment to prevent the development of Korsakoff's syndrome and alcoholic dementia. A daily oral dose of folate 1 mg. should also be given throughout the course of treatment. In cases of mild withdrawal, hydration alone may be sufficient. Benzodiazepines (lorazepam, midazolam, diazepam, and chlordiazepoxide) are the drugs of choice for the management of alcohol withdrawal because of their sedative effects (see Table 15.4) (Erstad and Cotugno 1995; Newman et al. 1995). Careful consideration must be given to route, absorption, potency, and dose of benzodiazepine prescribed. Dose should be based upon estimated alcohol consumption and the type of setting of detoxification (see below). Insufficient administration of benzodiazepines (too low dose; or too rapid taper) may allow the progression of withdrawal to a state of delirium tremens. The development of seizures is life threatening, and they may repeatedly recur in the patient while unconscious. The non-benzodiazepine anticonvulsants are not prescribed prophylactically. In cases of severe withdrawal and confusion, neuroleptics (i.e., haloperidol 0.5–5.0 mg IV every 8 h) are added to the treatment regimen. Commonly, alcoholic patients report to the hospital either intoxicated or in the early stages of withdrawal. From a surgical perspective, serious complications can arise from the presence of alcohol withdrawal, and its acute management is the primary treatment goal. Unfortunately, clinicians are frequently provided insufficient lead time to properly detoxify the patient prior to surgery (typically less than 24 h); the patient stands at an increased risk for the postoperative development of organic mental disorders, seizure, and delirium tremens. Since alcoholic cancer patients are already at high risk for delirium postoperatively due to poor nutrition, prior head trauma, and brain injury from excessive alcohol consumption, the development of seizures and delirium tremens adds to the risk of fatality. It is important to note that since it is desirable for the patient to be alert postoperatively for ambulation and use of pulmonary toilet, the amount of sedation required for detoxification is much lower than the desired level of sedation in a nonsurgical alcoholic patient.

Table 15.3 Guidelines for the treatment of alcohol withdrawal

Continual close monitoring of withdrawal status
Utilization of benzodiazepines
Taper dose slowly (generally not by more than 25 % per 24 h period)
Administration of thiamine 100 mg Im or IV qid
Administration of folate 1 mg po qid
Monitor for signs of the potential onset of delirium tremens
Consideration should be given to a loading dose of phenytoin for patients with a history of withdrawal seizures or for patients in whom seizures are likely (i.e., patients with brain metastases)

Table 15.4 Types and characteristics of benzodiazepines for treatment of alcohol withdrawal

Drug	Dose	Duration of action	Half-life (h)
Chlordiazepoxide	25–100 mg every 3 h IV	Short	5–30
Diazepam	10–20 mg every 1–4 h IV	Short	20–100
Lorazepam	1–2 mg every 1–4 h IV	Intermediate	10–20
Midazolam	1–5 mg every 1–2 h IV	Very short	1–4

15.4.2 Preventing and Minimizing Withdrawal Symptoms

Because many patients with drug abuse histories use multiple drugs, it is necessary to conduct a complete drug-use history to prepare for the possibility of withdrawal. Delayed abstinence syndromes, such as those that may occur after abuse of some benzodiazepine drugs, may be particularly diagnostically challenging (Kirsh and Passik 2013; Passik and Kirsh 2013; Passik and Portenoy 1998b).

15.4.3 Considering the Therapeutic Impact of Tolerance

Patients who are active substance abusers may be tolerant to drugs administered for therapy, which will make pain management more difficult. The magnitude of this tolerance is never known. Therefore, it is best to begin with a conservative dose of therapeutic drug and then rapidly titrate the dose, with frequent reassessments until the patient is comfortable (Hamrick et al. 2013; Passik and Portenoy 1998a; Macaluso et al. 1988). Also, it must be remembered that opioids, pharmacologically speaking, still have no ceiling (Coluzzi et al. 2005). Cancer patients and those with progressive disease can still be treated with gradually increasing doses, and opioids can still be titrated to effect or toxicity with no arbitrary number of milligrams constituting a limit. Tolerance to a variety of opioid effects can be reliably observed in animal models (Ling et al. 1989), and tolerance to non-analgesic effects, such as respiratory depression and cognitive impairment (Bruera et al. 1989), occurs regularly in the clinical setting. However, analgesic tolerance does not appear to routinely interfere with the clinical efficacy of opioid drugs.

15.5 Psychopharmacology Approaches

Disulfiram (Antabuse) is a pharmacological agent that has been approved by the Food and Drug Administration (FDA) since 1951 for the treatment of alcoholism. Antabuse serves as a deterrent by inducing an unpleasant physical state characterized by nausea or vomiting when alcohol is consumed, thus ideally leading to alcohol cessation (Suh et al. 2006). The practicality and effectiveness of Antabuse are questionable, however, since its use has been limited by difficulties with patient adherence for continued use of the drug (Weinrieb and O'Brien 1997).

There have been a number of studies that have shed light on subgroups of patients who have been shown to benefit the most from treatment with Antabuse. The findings have shown that patients with the following characteristics generally experience the most long-term benefits from Antabuse: (1) older than 40 years of age; (2) longer drinking histories; (3) socially stable; (4) highly motivated; (5) prior attendance of Alcoholics Anonymous; (6) cognitively intact; and (7) able to maintain and tolerate dependent or treatment relationships (Fuller and Gordis 2004; Banys 1988; Hughes and Cook 1997). Further research is needed to ascertain what factors and patient characteristics will increase the likelihood of successful treatment. A greater understanding has the potential to significantly enhance clinicians' ability to select those patients who will experience optimal effectiveness.

15.5.1 Methadone Maintenance

Methadone maintenance therapy (MMT) is superior to illegal heroin use, in part, because the extreme highs and lows felt by heroin users (related to the waxing and waning of serum heroin levels) are avoided by the long-acting properties of methadone. The term "agonist blockade" was coined to describe the phenomenon of significantly limited or blunted effects after administration of "usual" doses of mu opioid agonists to subjects on high-dose methadone (e.g., 80–120 mg/day).

In humans, all opiates suppress the hypothalamic–pituitary–adrenal (HPA) axis when given acutely, and this effect persists during chronic, intermittent exposure to short-acting opioids during chronic cycles of heroin addiction (Kreek et al. 1978).

The endogenous mu opioid receptor-mediated opioid system in humans appears to constitutively provide tonic inhibition of the HPA axis (Kreek et al. 1978; Schluger et al. 1998). Thus, administration of mu opioid receptor antagonists to healthy human volunteers leads to activation of the HPA axis (Culpepper-Morgan et al. 1992; Rosen et al. 1996; Schluger et al. 1998; King 2002; Culpepper-Morgan and Kreek 1997). Similarly, the HPA axis is activated in opioid withdrawal, or with administration of mu opioid receptor antagonists to opioid-dependent individuals, or during acute cocaine or alcohol consumption (Schluger et al. 1998; King 2002).

Kreek and colleagues (Kreek and Vocci 2002; Schluger et al. 2001) proposed that the suppression of the HPA axis through administration of intermittent or binge-type short-acting opioids (e.g., heroin) and then with repeated alternating short cycling of suppression (e.g., with heroin administration), followed by activation (e.g., with heroin withdrawal [i.e., just before next dose]) may lead to and/or exacerbate atypical responsivity to stress/stressors as well as addictive-type behavior (with resultant self-administration/relapse). Adequate methadone maintenance treatment permits normalization of the HPA axis—including response to a chemically induced stress of metyrapone challenge (Kreek 1973a, b). In an optimal situation, stabilized methadone-maintained former heroin addicts treated in high quality methadone maintenance treatment programs (e.g., associated with psychosocial interventions) with effective methadone doses experience the following: markedly reduced drug craving, reduced or eliminated heroin use, improved or normalized stress-responsive hypothalamic–pituitary–adrenal axis, as well as reproductive, gastrointestinal, and immunologic functions with relatively normal responses to acute pain (Kling et al. 2000; Kreek 2000).

15.5.2 Buprenorphine and Naltrexone

Two other therapies used in the medication-assisted treatment (MAT) of those with opioid addiction and alcoholism are not without their complexities if they are to be used in people with cancer.

Buprenorphine is a partial opioid agonist that has significantly advanced MAT for opioid addiction on an international level. Available as a pill, sublingual film (with and without naltrexone), and as an implant for addiction treatment, its use in people with cancer can complicate the treatment of pain in the setting of disease progression and require dose escalation that could "bump up against" the drug's ceiling effect or in the treatment of acute pain requiring the use of a pure mu agonist. However, there are also reports of the successful use of buprenorphine in its oral and transdermal form for chronic and breakthrough cancer pain in nonaddicts (Atkinson et al. 2013). If a person with cancer also has a history of opioid addiction and is to be managed with continuation of their buprenorphine treatment, a consultation should be sought from an addiction medicine expert (who also has the appropriate certification to prescribe it where necessary).

The opioid antagonist naltrexone is used orally to treat alcohol cravings and opioid addiction and is also available as a monthly depot injection for addiction treatment. While ultralow dose naltrexone has been used to augment opioids for cancer-related pain and for the treatment of side effects such as constipation, little has been written about the use of this therapy for addiction treatment in people with cancer. While one can imagine antagonist therapy having a role in, for example, people surviving cancer who struggle with addiction (and in whom pain severe enough to require opioids is not part of the clinical picture), in those with pain and with active disease its role is limited. There has been a paucity of data and direct clinical experience on which specific recommendations might be made.

15.6   Selecting Appropriate Drugs and Route of Administration for the Symptom and Setting

The use of long-acting analgesics in sufficient amounts may help to minimize the number of rescue doses needed, lessen cravings, and decrease the risk of abuse of prescribed medications, given the possible difficulty of using short-acting formulations in patients with substance abuse histories. Rather than being overly concerned regarding the choice of drug or route of administration, the prescription of opioids and other potentially abusable drugs should be carried out with limits and guidelines (Kirsh and Passik 2013; Passik and Kirsh 2013; Passik and Portenoy 1998b).

Many clinicians now respond to particularly high doses with rotation to another opioid. This practice is based on capitalizing on incomplete cross-tolerance, or the unique pharmacology of methadone in particular, to bring doses down while maintaining or improving efficacy and changing the balance of efficacy to toxicity (Wirz et al. 2006; Zimmermann et al. 2005). Some clinicians set arbitrary dose limits for the various opioids. Others stopped using certain opioids they perceived as of higher risk or street value. Still others became so disillusioned as to stop using opioids altogether.

15.6.1 Recognizing Specific Drug Abuse Behaviors

In an effort to monitor the development of aberrant drug-taking behaviors, all patients who are prescribed potentially abusable drugs must be evaluated over time. This is particularly true for those patients with a remote or current history of drug abuse, including alcohol abuse. Should a high level of concern exist regarding such behaviors, frequent visits and regular assessments of significant others who can contribute information regarding the patient's drug use may be required. To promote early recognition of aberrant drug-related behaviors, it may also be necessary to have patients who have been actively abusing drugs in the recent past submit urine specimens for regular screening of illicit, or licit but non-prescribed, drugs. When informing the patient of this approach, explain that it is a method of monitoring that can reassure the clinician and provide a foundation for aggressive symptom-oriented treatment, thus enhancing the therapeutic alliance with the patient (Kirsh and Passik 2013; Passik and Kirsh 2013; Passik and Portenoy 1998b).

15.6.2 Using Nondrug Approaches as Appropriate

The most effective psychotherapeutic treatment approach with medically ill people appears to be one that focuses on the development of effective coping skills, relapse prevention, and most importantly, treatment compliance. Alcohol or the specific substance being abused is representing one of the dependent patient's primary, albeit, maladaptive coping tools. As a result, the improvement of coping skills in these individuals is critical. When compounded with the stress associated with having cancer, the cessation can be overwhelming and contributes to noncompliance and discontinuation of treatment. Teaching specific, illness-related coping methods with an emphasis upon containing episodes of consumption is essential. Further, the recognition and treatment of anxiety and depression may decrease the patients need and desire for alcohol or substances. As an alternative to the abstinence approach, a harm reduction with crisis intervention as a central component should be utilized. The fundamental aims being enhancement of social support, maximization of treatment compliance, and to contain harm associated with episodic relapses. Further, minimizing the frequency and intensity of the patients use and consumption are the broad goals of treatment. Thereby, further damage to the patient will be reduced as well as the facilitation of treatment compliance.

Another psychotherapeutic approach that is beneficial for this population of patients are support groups and 12 step programs. The problem lies in that traditional 12-step groups are based on an abstinence only policy. This poses a problem for the patients who are being treated with opioids for pain-related syndromes. More recently, support groups have been tailored for this specific population.

Many nondrug approaches can be used to assist patients in coping with chronic pain in advanced illness. Such educational interventions may include relaxation techniques, ways of thinking of and describing the experience of pain, and methods of communicating physical and emotional distress to staff members. Although nondrug interventions may be helpful adjuvants to management, they should not be perceived as substitutes for drugs targeted at treating pain or other physical or psychological symptoms (Kirsh and Passik 2013; Passik and Kirsh 2013; Passik and Portenoy 1998b).

15.6.3 Inpatient Management Plan

In designing the inpatient management of an actively abusing patient with advanced illness, it is helpful to use structured treatment guidelines. Although the applicability of these guidelines may vary from setting to setting, they provide a set of strategies that can ensure the safety of the patient and staff, control possible manipulative behaviors, allow for supervision of illicit drug use, enhance appropriate use of medications for pain and symptom control, and communicate an understanding of pain and substance abuse management (Kirsh and Passik 2013; Passik and Kirsh 2013; Passik and Portenoy 1998b).

Under certain circumstances, such as actively abusing patients who are scheduled for surgery, patients should be admitted several days in advance, when possible, to allow for the stabilization of the drug regimen. This time can also be used to avoid withdrawal and to provide an opportunity to assess whether modifications to the established plan are necessary (Kirsh and Passik 2013; Passik and Kirsh 2013).

Once established, the structured treatment plan for the management of active abuse must proceed conscientiously. In an effort to assess and manage symptoms, frequent visits are usually necessary. It is also important to avoid drug withdrawal, and to the extent possible, prescribed drugs for symptom control should be administered on a regularly scheduled basis. This helps to eliminate repetitive encounters with staff that center on the desire to obtain drugs (Kirsh and Passik 2013; Passik and Kirsh 2013; Passik and Portenoy 1998b).

Treatment management plans must be designed to represent the clinician's assessment of the severity of drug abuse. Open and honest communication between clinician and patient to stress that the guidelines were established in the best interest of the patient is often helpful. However, in cases where patients are unable to follow these guidelines despite repeated interventions from the staff, discharge should be considered. Clinicians should discuss this decision for patient discharge with the staff and administration, while considering the ethical and legal ramifications of this action (Kirsh and Passik 2013; Passik and Kirsh 2013; Passik and Portenoy 1998b).

15.6.4 Outpatient Management Plan

Alternative guidelines may be used in the management of the actively abusing patient with advanced illness who is being treated on an outpatient basis. In some instances, the treatment plan can be coordinated with referral to a drug rehabilitation program. However, patients who are facing end-of-life issues may have difficulty participating in such programs. Using the following approaches may be helpful for managing the complex and more difficult-to-control aspects of care.

Case Study

A 36-year-old White male with stage IV lung cancer (pancoast tumor) that was locally advanced and widely metastatic. His sister had died of the same disease at age 35 and he had a history of significant substance abuse and drug dealing. He was presented late after a 35 lb weight loss. The patient complained of out of control pain and lack of willingness of any local providers to prescribe pain medication. The patient was inflexible about acceptance of any other treatments (i.e., nerve block, epidural) other than OxyContin™. The patient's pain was 10/10 from brachial plexopathy with mixed neuropathic/somatic/visceral components.

Patient was titrated to effect over time. The maximum dose reached 800 mg BID at the time of death with 100 mg liquid MSO4 q1h rescues. Although the patient was dying, structured management was required because of his history. The structured management plan was as follows: Hospice nurses delivered 1 day supply, unscheduled visits for pill counts,

(continued)

urine screens, and a reliable family member was identified to lock up pain medication supply.

The patient settled down and with renewed trust was willing to add nortriptyline which helped with neuropathic pain, steroids for nausea, cachexia, and fatigue.

15.7   Guidelines for Prescribing

Patients who are actively abusing must be seen weekly to build a good rapport with staff and afford evaluation of symptom control and addiction-related concerns. Frequent visits allow the opportunity to prescribe small quantities of drugs, which may decrease the temptation to divert and provide a motive for not missing appointments (Kirsh and Passik 2013; Passik and Kirsh 2013; Passik and Portenoy 1998b).

Procedures for prescription loss or replacement should be explicitly explained to the patient, with the stipulation that no renewals will be given if appointments are missed. The patient should also be informed that any dose changes require prior communication with the clinician. Additionally, clinicians who are covering for the primary care provider must be advised of the guidelines that have been established for each patient with a substance abuse history to avoid conflict and disruption of the treatment plan (Kirsh and Passik 2013; Passik and Kirsh 2013; Passik and Portenoy 1998b).

15.7.1 Using 12-Step Programs

Depending on the patient's stage of advanced illness and functional capabilities, the clinician may want to consider referring the patient to a 12-step program with the stipulation that attendance be documented for ongoing prescription purposes. If the patient has a sponsor, the clinician may wish to contact the patient's sponsor, depending on the stage of illness and individual capabilities, in an effort to disclose the patient's illness and that medication is required in the treatment of the illness. This contact will also help to decrease the risk of stigmatizing the patient as being noncompliant with the ideals of the 12-step program (Kirsh and Passik 2013; Passik and Kirsh 2013; Passik and Portenoy 1998b). If the patient is unable to participate in a 12-step Program, other psychosocial and/or spiritual team members can provide care that supports sobriety.

15.7.2 Urine Medication Monitoring

One of the most commonly utilized tools in risk management in chronic non-cancer pain management and adherence monitoring/sobriety in addiction treatment is urine drug testing (UDT). Depending upon the method employed, UDT can be used to gauge whether the patient is adherent to their prescribed medication; whether or not they are also taking non-prescribed licit medications; and/or whether they are using illicit drugs and alcohol (Passik and Kirsh 2011). Indeed, one study in which primary care doctors were taught to employ a "menu" of risk management techniques including UDT and then studied over time to exam their use of them found that UDT was the most commonly retained practice element on 6 month follow up (Brown et al. 2011).

It is safe to say UDT is underutilized in the treatment of people with cancer and addiction as well as those being treated with opioids for cancer-related pain. Perhaps oncologists (and even psycho-oncologists), due to their unfamiliarity with the evolution in methods and mindset that had occurred in the laboratory and clinic in the last decade, think of UDT in only its forensic incarnation. In that view, it is a means to find out if "bad people" are "doing bad things," as seen in a prior chart review study (Passik et al. 2000). Thus, they are fearful that introducing it to their patients and integrating it into patient management will be offensive. And they fear they also lack a vocabulary for discussing results with their patients. The forensic method, from which more modern clinical testing sprung, tends to rely on immunoassay (IA) testing which offers fast but only class level (not drug specific) results with high cutoffs. It is meant to detect recent use of classes of drugs that would impair, for example, a truck driver from driving. Cutoffs are high because of the legal and other consequences that could follow and to avoid falsely accusing people. In recent years gas chromatography and liquid chromatography with mass spectrometry have become capable of giving highly accurate drug-specific results and return them in a timely fashion (1–2 days as opposed to 10 days—2 weeks). Such results can be used to gauge whether a patient is misusing a range of drugs or alcohol and gauge their adherence with specific medications and controlled substances that are being prescribed for them. There is a paucity of data on how such techniques might influence the management of cancer patients and more data is needed in this arena, but the use of UDT for those with pain and/or substance use disorder is well documented (Chou et al. 2009; Christo et al. 2011; FSMB 2004; Pesce et al. 2012; Trescot et al. 2006).

15.7.3 Family Sessions and Meetings

The clinician, in an effort to increase support and function, should involve family members and friends in the treatment plan. These meetings will allow the clinician and other team members to become familiar with the family and additionally assist the team to identify family members who are using illicit drugs. Offering referral of these identified family members to drug treatment can be portrayed as a method of gathering support for the patient. The patient should also be prepared to cope with family members or friends who may attempt to buy or sell the patient's medications. These meetings will also assist the team in identifying dependable individuals who can serve as a source of strength and support for the patient during treatment (Kirsh and Passik 2013; Passik and Kirsh 2013; Passik and Portenoy 1998b). These published guidelines generally advocate an approach to UDT based on risk stratification (i.e., frequency of testing and choice of methods is aimed at matching the approach to the level of risk of abuse, addiction, and diversion in an individualized way to each patient). Such an approach seeks to maximize the benefit of testing while also managing cost. As psycho-oncologists and other oncology professionals learn to integrate UDT into treatment of the person with cancer and addiction or the management of chronic opioid therapy, there is no reason to think that the adaptation of a similar approach might not be a reasonable way to proceed.

Conclusion

Treating oncology patients who are experiencing chronic pain and a substance use disorder is both complicated and challenging, since each can significantly complicate the other. Whether they respond to cancer treatments or go on to have life limiting disease, we are no longer able to justify high dose opioid therapy in a vacuum without trying to assess and manage addiction and abuse behaviors. Using a treatment plan that involves a team approach that recognizes and responds to these complex needs is the optimum strategy to facilitate treatment. While pain management may continue to be challenging even when all treatment plan procedures are implemented, the healthcare team's goal should be providing the highest level of pain management for all patients with substance use disorders.

References

Argoff CE. Clinical implications of opioid pharmacogenetics. Clin J Pain. 2010;26(1 Suppl): S16–20.

Atkinson TJ, Fudin J, Pandula A, Mirza M. Medication pain management in the elderly: unique and underutilized analgesic treatment options. Clin Ther. 2013;35(11):1669–89.

Banys P. The clinical use of disulfiram (Antabuse): a review. J Psychoactive Drugs. 1988;20(3): 243–61.

Borgelt LM, Franson KL, Nussbaum AM, Wang GS. The pharmacologic and clinical effects of medical cannabis. Pharmacotherapy. 2013;33(2):195–209.

Brown J, Setnik B, Lee K, Wase L, Roland CL, Cleveland JM, Siegel S, Katz N. Assessment, stratification, and monitoring of the risk for prescription opioid misuse and abuse in the primary care setting. J Opioid Manag. 2011;7(6):467–83.

Bruera E, Macmillan K, Hanson JA, et al. The cognitive effects of the administration of narcotic analgesics in patients with cancer pain. Pain. 1989;39:13.

Bruera E, Moyano J, Seifert L, Fainsinger RL, Hanson J, Suarez-Almazor M. The frequency of alcoholism among patients with pain due to terminal cancer. J Pain Symptom Manage. 1995;10(8):599–603.

Chou R, Fanciullo GJ, Fine PG, Miaskowski C, Passik SD. Opioids for chronic noncancer pain: prediction and identification of aberrant drug-related behaviors: a review of the evidence for an American Pain Society and American Academy of Pain Medicine clinical practice guideline. J Pain. 2009;10:131–46.

Christo P, Manchikanti L, Ruan X, Bottros M, Hansen H, Solanki D, Jordan A, Colson J. Urine drug testing in chronic pain: comprehensive review. Pain Physician. 2011;14:123–43.

Cicero TJ, Surratt HL, Kurtz S, Ellis MS, Inciardi JA. Patterns of prescription opioid abuse and comorbidity in an aging treatment population. J Subst Abuse Treat. 2012;42(1):87–94.

Colliver JD, Compton WM, Gfroerer J, Condon T. Projecting drug use among aging baby boomers in 2020. Ann Epidemiol. 2006;16:257–65.

Colliver JD, Kopstein AN. Trends in cocaine abuse reflected in emergency room episodes reported to DAWN. Public Health Rep. 1991;106:59–68.

Coluzzi F, Pappagallo M, National Initiative on Pain Control. Opioid therapy for chronic noncancer pain: practice guidelines for initiation and maintenance of therapy. Minerva Anestesiol. 2005;71(7–8):425–33.

Culpepper-Morgan JA, Inturrisi CE, Portenoy RK, Foley K, Houde RW, Marsh F, Kreek MJ. Treatment of opioid-induced constipation with oral naloxone: a pilot study. Clin Pharmacol Ther. 1992;52(1):90–5.

Culpepper-Morgan JA, Kreek MJ. Hypothalamic-pituitary-adrenal axis hypersensitivity to naloxone in opioid dependence: a case of naloxone-induced withdrawal. Metabolism. 1997;46(2):130–4.

Dunbar SA, Katz NP. Chronic opioid therapy for nonmalignant pain in patients with a history of substance abuse: report of 20 cases. J Pain Symptom Manage. 1996;11:163–71.

Erstad BL, Cotugno CL. Management of alcohol withdrawal. Am J Health Syst Pharm. 1995; 52(7):697–709.

Federation of State Medical Boards of the United States, Inc. Model policy for the use of controlled substances for the treatment of pain. J Pain Palliat Care Pharmacother. 2004;19: 73–8.

Fleming MF, Balousek SL, Klessig CL, Mundt MP, Brown DD. Substance use disorders in a primary care sample receiving daily opioid therapy. J Pain. 2007;8(7):573–82.

Fuller RK, Gordis E. Does disulfiram have a role in alcoholism treatment today? Addiction. 2004;99(1):21–4.

Glajchen M, Fitzmartin RD, Blum D, Swanton R. Psychosocial barriers to cancer pain relief. Cancer Pract. 1995;3(2):76–82.

Gfroerer J, Brodsky M. The incidence of illicit drug use in the United States 1962–1989. Br J Addict. 1992;87:1345–51.

Gfroerer J, Penne M, Pemberton M, Folsom R. Substance abuse treatment need among older adults in 2020: the impact of the aging baby-boom cohort. Drug Alcohol Depend. 2003;69(2):127–35.

Gonzales GR, Coyle N. Treatment of cancer pain in a former opioid abuser: fears of the patient and staff and their influences on care. J Pain Symptom Manage. 1992;7:246–9.

Hamrick JR, Passik SD, Kirsh KL. Substance abuse issues in palliative care. In: Berger AM, Shuster JL, Roenn V, editors. Principles and practice of palliative care and supportive oncology. 4th ed. Philadelphia, PA: Lippincott Williams & Wilkins; 2013. p. 575–89.

Hughes JC, Cook CC. The efficacy of disulfiram: a review of outcome studies. Addiction. 1997;92: 381–95.

Kemp C. Managing chronic pain in patients with advanced disease and substance related disorders. Home Healthc Nurse. 1996;14(4):255–61.

Khantzian EJ, Treece C. DSM-III psychiatric diagnosis of narcotic addicts. Arch Gen Psychiatry. 1985;42:1067–71.

King AC. Role of naltrexone in initial smoking cessation: preliminary findings. Alcohol Clin Exp Res. 2002;26(12):1942–4.

Kircher S, Zacny J, Apfelbaum SM, Passik SD, Kirsh KL, Burbage M, Lofwall M. Understanding and treating opioid addiction in a patient with cancer pain. J Pain. 2011;12(10):1025–31. doi:10.1016/j.pain.2011.07.006.

Kirsh KL, Passik SD. Chapter 13: Patients with a history of substance abuse. In: Smith HS, editor. Opioid therapy in the 21st century. 2nd ed. New York: Oxford University Press; 2013. p. 255–62.

Kirsh KL, Peppin JF, Coleman J. Characterization of prescription opioid abuse in the United States: focus on route of administration. J Pain Palliat Care Pharmacother. 2012;26(4):348–61. doi:10.3109/15360288.2012.734905.

Kling M, Carson R, Borg L, et al. Opioid receptor imaging with positive emission tomography and [18f]cyclofoxy in long-term, methadone-treated former heroin addicts. J Pharmacol Exp Ther. 2000;295:1070–6.

Kreek MJ. Medical safety and side effects of methadone in tolerant individuals. J Am Med Assoc. 1973a;223:665–8.

Kreek MJ. Plasma and urine levels of methadone. Comparison following four medication forms used in chronic maintenance treatment. N Y State J Med. 1973b;73:2773–7.

Kreek MJ, Oratz M, Rothschild MA. Hepatic extraction of long- and short- acting narcotics in the isolated perfused rabbit liver. Gastroenterology. 1978;75:88–94.

Kreek MJ. Methadone-related opioid agonist pharmacotherapy for heroin addiction: history, recent molecular and neurochemical research and future in mainstream medicine. Ann N Y Acad Sci. 2000;909:186–216.

Kreek MJ, Vocci FJ. History and current status of opioid maintenance treatments: blending conference session. J Subst Abuse Treat. 2002;23:93–105.

Ling GSF, Paul D, Simantov R, et al. Differential development of acute tolerance to analgesia, respiratory depression, gastrointestinal transit and hormone release in a morphine infusion model. Life Sci. 1989;45:1627.

Lowery AE, Starr T, Dhingra LK, Rogak L, Hamrick-Price JR, Farberov M, Kirsh KL, Saltz LB, Breitbart WS, Passik SD. Frequency, characteristics and correlates of pain in a pilot study of colorectal cancer survivors 1-10 years post-treatment. Pain Med. 2013;14:1673–80. doi:10. 1111/pme.12223.

Macaluso C, Weinberg D, Foley KM. Opioid abuse and misuse in a cancer pain population [abstract]. J Pain Symptom Manage. 1988;3:S24–31.

Manchikanti L, Damron KS, McManus CD, Barnhill RC. Patterns of illicit drug use and opioid abuse in patients with chronic pain at initial evaluation: a prospective, observational study. Pain Phys. 2004;7:431–7.

Manchikanti L, Singh A. Therapeutic opioids: a ten-year perspective on the complexities and complications of the escalating use, abuse, and nonmedical use of opioids. Pain Phys. 2008;11: S63–8.

Maxmen JS, Ward NG. Substance-related disorders. In: Maxmen JS, Ward NG, editors. Essential psychopathology and its treatment. New York: WW. Norton and Company; 1995. p. 132–72.

Minozzi S, Amato L, Davoli M. Development of dependence following treatment with opioid analgesics for pain relief: a systematic review. Addiction. 2013;108(4):688–98.

Modesto-Lowe V, Girard L, Chaplin M. Cancer pain in the opioid-addicted patient: can we treat it right? J Opioid Manag. 2012;8(3):167–75.

Morasco B, Dobscha S. Prescription medication misuse in substance use disorder in VA primary care patients with chronic pain. Gen Hosp Psychiatry. 2008;30:93–9.

Muirhead G. Cultural issues in substance abuse treatment. Patient Care. 2000;5:151–9.

Newman JP, Terris DJ, Moore M. Trends in the management of alcohol withdrawal syndrome. Laryngoscope. 1995;105(1):1–7.

Passik SD. Responding rationally to recent report of abuse/diversion of Oxycontin. J Pain Symptom Manage. 2001;21(5):359.

Passik SD, Kirsh KL. What approaches should be used to minimize opioid diversion and abuse in palliative care? In: Goldstein N, Morrison S, editors. Evidence-based practice of palliative medicine. Philadelphia, PA: Elsevier; 2013. p. 87–92.

Passik SD, Kirsh KL. Ethical considerations in urine drug testing. J Pain Palliat Care Pharmacother. 2011;25(3):265–6.

Passik SD, Kirsh KL, Casper D. Addiction-related assessment tools and pain management: instruments for screening, treatment planning, and monitoring compliance. Pain Med. 2008; 9(S2):S145–66.

Passik SD, Portenoy RK. Substance abuse issues in palliative care. In: Berger A, Portenoy R, Weissman D, editors. Principles and practice of supportive oncology. Philadelphia, PA: Lippincott-Raven; 1998a. p. 513–24.

Passik SD, Portenoy RK. Substance abuse disorders. In: Holland JC, editor. Psycho-oncology. New York, NY: Oxford University Press; 1998b. p. 576–86.

Passik SD, Portenoy RK, Ricketts PL. Substance abuse issues in cancer patients part 1: prevalence and diagnosis. Oncology. 1998a;12(4):517–21.

Passik SD, Portenoy RK, Ricketts PL. Substance abuse issues in cancer patients part 2: evaluation and treatment. Oncology. 1998b;12(5):729–34.

Passik SD, Schreiber J, Kirsh KL, Portenoy RK. A chart review of the ordering and documentation of urine toxicology screens in a cancer center: do they influence patient management? J Pain Symptom Manag. 2000;19(1):40–4.

Passik SD, Webster L, Kirsh KL. Pseudoaddiction revisited: a commentary on clinical and historical considerations. Pain Manage. 2011;1(3):239–48.

Passik SD, Kirsh KL, Whitcomb LA, Schein JR, Kaplan M, Dodd S, Kleinman L, Katz NP, Portenoy RK. Monitoring outcomes during long-term opioid therapy for non-cancer pain: results with the pain assessment and documentation tool. J Opioid Manag. 2005;1(5):257–66.

Patterson TL, Jeste DV. The potential impact of the baby-boom generation on substance abuse among elderly persons. Psychiatr Serv. 1999;50(9):1184–8.

Pesce A, Gonzales E, Almazan P, Mikel C, Latyshev S, West C, Strickland J. Medication and illicit substance use analyzed using liquid chromatography tandem mass spectrometry (LC-MS/MS) in a pain population. J Anal Bioanal Tech. 2012;3:3.

Ramer L, Richardson JL, Cohen MZ, Bedney C, Danley KL, Judge EA. Multimeasure pain assessment in an ethnically diverse group of patients with cancer. J Transcult Nurs. 1999; 10(2):94–101.

Regier DA, Myers JK, Kramer M, Robins LN, Blazer DG, Hough RL, Eaton WW, Locke BZ. The NIMH epidemiology catchment area program. Arch Gen Psychiatry. 1984;41:934–41.

Regier DA, Farmer ME, Rae DS. Comorbidity of mental disorders with alcohol and other drug abuse. JAMA. 1990;264:2511.

Rinaldi RC, Steindler EM, Wilford BB. Clarification and standardization of substance abuse terminology. JAMA. 1988;259:555–7.

Rockett IR, Putnam SL, Jia H, Smith GS. Declared and undeclared substance use among emergency department patients: a population-based study. Addiction. 2006;101(5):706–12.

Rosen MI, McMahon TJ, Woods SW, Pearsall HR, Kosten TR. A pilot study of dextromethorphan in naloxone-precipitated opiate withdrawal. Eur J Pharmacol. 1996;307(3):251–7.

SAMHSA. Emergency department visits involving illicit drug use by older adults: 2008. Rockville, MD: Drug Abuse Warning Network (DAWN); 2010a.

SAMHSA. The DAWN report: drug-related emergency department visits involving pharmaceutical misuse and abuse by older adults. Rockville, MD: Substance Abuse and Mental Health Services Administration, Center for Behavioral Health Statistics and Quality; 2010b.

SAMHSA. Treatment episode data set (TEDS). Changing substance abuse patterns among older admissions: 1992 and 2008. Rockville, MD: Substance Abuse and Mental Health Services Administration (SAMHSA); 2010c.

SAMHSA. Managing chronic pain in adults with or in recovery from substance use disorders. Treatment Improvement Protocol (TIP) Series 54. HHS Publication No. (SMA) 12-4671. Rockville, MD: Substance Abuse and Mental Health Services Administration; 2011a.

SAMHSA. Treatment episode data set (TEDS): Older adult admissions reporting alcohol as a substance of abuse: 1992 and 2009. Rockville, MD: Substance Abuse and Mental Health Services Administration; 2011b.

SAMHSA. National survey on drug use and health: Illicit drug use among older adults. Rockville, MD: Substance Abuse and Mental Health Services Administration; 2011c.

SAMHSA. Results from the 2012 national survey on drug use and health: Summary of national findings. Rockville, MD: Substance Abuse and Mental Health Services Administration; 2012.

Savage SR. Addiction in the treatment of pain: significance, recognition, and management. J Pain Symptom Manage. 1993;8(5):265–77.

Schluger JH, Ho A, Borg L, Porter M, Maniar S, Gunduz M, Perret G, King A, Kreek MJ. Nalmefene causes greater hypothalamic-pituitary-adrenal axis activation than naloxone in normal volunteers: implications for the treatment of alcoholism. Alcohol Clin Exp Res. 1998;22(7):1430–6.

Schluger JH, Borg L, Ho A, Kreek MJ. Altered HPA axis responsivity to metyrapone testing in methadone maintained former heroin addicts with ongoing cocaine addiction. Neuropsychopharmacology. 2001;24(5):568–75.

Sjorgren P, Okholm O, Peuckmann V, Gronbaek M. Epidemiology of chronic pain in Denmark: an update. Eur J Pain. 2009;13:287–92.

Smith HS, Kirsh KL. Identifying and managing the risk of opioid misuse. Therapy. 2009;6 (5):685–93.

Suh JJ, Pettinati HM, Kampman KM, O'Brien CP. The status of disulfiram: a half of a century later. J Clin Psychopharmacol. 2006;26(3):290–302.

Taylor MH, Grossberg GT. The growing problem of illicit substance abuse in the elderly: a review. Prim Care Companion CNS Disord. 2012;14(4):1–16.

Todd KH, Deaton C, D'Adamo AP, Goe L. Ethnicity and analgesic practice. Ann Emerg Med. 2000;35(1):11–6.

Trescot AM, Boswell MV, Atluri SL, Hansen HC, Deer TR. Opioid guidelines in the management of chronic non-cancer pain. Pain Physician. 2006;9:1–39.

Ward SE, Goldberg N, Miller-McCauley V, Mueller C, Nolan A, Pawlik-Plank D, Robbins A, Stormoen D, Weissman DE. Patient-related barriers to management of cancer pain. Pain. 1993; 52:319–24.

Weinrieb RM, O'Brien CP. Current research in the treatment of alcoholism in liver transplant recipients. Liver Transpl Surg. 1997;3(3):328–36.

Winick C. Maturing out of narcotic addiction. Bull Narc. 1962;14:1–7.

Wirz S, Wartenberg HC, Elsen C, Wittmann M, Diederichs M, Nadstawek J. Managing cancer pain and symptoms of outpatients by rotation to sustained-release hydromorphone: a prospective clinical trial. Clin J Pain. 2006;22(9):770–5.

Zimmermann C, Seccareccia D, Booth CM, Cottrell W. Rotation to methadone after opioid dose escalation: how should individualization of dosing occur? J Pain Palliat Care Pharmacother. 2005;19(2):25–31.

Treatment of Sexual Disorders Following Cancer Treatments

16

Catherine Benedict and Christian J. Nelson

Abstract

Sexual dysfunction following cancer treatment is highly prevalent, though often overlooked by healthcare providers. Cancer-related changes in sexual function are associated with worsened mental health for men and women including increased distress, depression, and anxiety. The research in male sexual medicine is more advanced than female sexual medicine. The treatments for men focus primarily on erectile function and include a number of approved pharmacological treatments, whereas treatments for women are primarily behavioral in nature and generally target dyspareunia or vaginismus. Interventions for both genders work best when they include both medical and psychological modalities to address the myriad of factors that may affect sexuality and intimacy in cancer survivors. Educational and psychosocial interventions and support resources may be used in conjunction with medical strategies to facilitate sexual recovery and promote satisfying sexual experiences for patients. It is strongly encouraged that interventions address sexual dysfunction from an individual and relational standpoint when a partner is involved or with consideration to patients' perspectives on future partners.

16.1 Introduction

With the development of more effective cancer treatments over the past 20–30 years, the management of treatment side effects has become increasingly more important. Unfortunately, the impact these treatments have on sexual functioning for both men and women has generally been overlooked. Indeed, a recent report released by the Institute of Medicine in the USA titled, "Cancer Care for the Whole

C. Benedict (✉) • C.J. Nelson
Department of Psychiatry and Behavioral Sciences, Memorial Sloan-Kettering Cancer Center,
614 Lexington Avenue, 7th Floor, New York, NY 10022, USA
e-mail: benedicc@MSKCC.ORG; nelsonc@MSKCC.ORG

L. Grassi and M. Riba (eds.), *Psychopharmacology in Oncology and Palliative Care*,
DOI 10.1007/978-3-642-40134-3_16, © Springer-Verlag Berlin Heidelberg 2014

Patient: Meeting the Psychosocial Health Needs" discussed the standard of care to improve quality of life for cancer patients and failed to mention sexual functioning (Sanchez-Varela et al. 2011). This is disappointing since many cancer survivors will report sexual problems following cancer treatments. At least 50 % of survivors of breast and gynecological cancers report alterations of their sexual functioning following treatment, as well as up to 90 % of men treated for prostate cancer will report problems with the ability to obtain and maintain an erection (Schover 2005; Schover et al. 2002). For colorectal cancer patients, 30–70 % of patients have impaired sex lives, depending on the surgical procedure, gender, and age (Schover 2005). Although sexual dysfunction rates for other cancer sites are lower than those stated above, typically up to 20 % of men and women with these other cancers that do not involve the pelvic area or breasts report that their cancer treatments lead to some type of sexual problem (Schover 2005). As a result of the widespread impact cancer treatments can have on sexual function, most cancer professionals will see many patients who have had deterioration in their sexual function. For this reason, it is important for cancer professionals to understand the current treatments for sexual dysfunction and to be able to discuss these possible treatments with their patients. It is best if the management and treatment of sexual dysfunction is coordinated by professionals specifically trained in sexual medicine and sexual health. Still, patients often need additional support and encouragement to pursue these treatments, and the mental health professional can play a pivotal role in facilitating these treatments.

Although the treatments for sexual dysfunction are not psychopharmacological treatments, helping patients pursue and use these treatments may also assist in lowering the distress, depression, and anxiety that may be associated with sexual dysfunction. It is now well established that erectile dysfunction (ED) and male sexual dysfunction are associated with depressive symptoms (Shabsigh et al. 1998; Araujo et al. 1998; Shiri et al. 2007; Nelson et al. 2010). The rate of depression in men with ED has been reported to be as high as 56 %, and the relationship between ED and depression has been demonstrated in three large, well-designed, population-based studies of aging men in the USA, Finland, Brazil, Japan, and Malaysia. Often times it is assumed that as men grow older they will be less concerned with sexual functioning; however, these studies have been conducted in men ranging in age from 40 to 70 years (similar to the age range of men with prostate cancer) and all controlled for age in their analyses. When focusing on prostate cancer, some have argued that ED distress is mitigated to some extent as patients focus more on the lifesaving nature of treatment (Penson et al. 2003). However, data confirms significant depression and ED bother after prostate cancer treatments (Nelson et al. 2010, 2011). In women, negative body image, damage to a core sense of femininity, and a reduction in relationship closeness tend to be the most highly reported symptoms (Fobair et al. 2006; Figueiredo et al. 2004). Women with breast cancer have reported an association between sexual dysfunction and negative body image, and up to 67 % percent of women who have surgery for breast cancer report significant concerns related to body image. These issues are also present in women treated for colorectal and gynecologic cancers (Sanchez-Varela et al. 2011; Jayne et al. 2007). It should come as no surprise that these feelings are accompanied by feelings of distress and unattractiveness (Ganz 2005; Bloom et al. 2004; Arora et al. 2001). When considering the negative emotional impact sexual dysfunction can have on cancer patients, the need to help these patients understand the appropriate treatments and assist them in pursuing these treatments becomes apparent.

The treatments for men focus primarily on erectile function and include a number of pharmacological treatments. The research in male sexual medicine is more advanced than female sexual health, and there are a number of approved medical treatments for men. The treatments for women generally target dyspareunia (vaginal pain during intercourse) or vaginismus (the inability to engage in any vaginal penetration). The primary treatments are more behavioral in nature, and as a whole there are not as many approved medical treatments for female sexual health. Regardless of the gender, interventions work best when they include both medical and psychological modalities (Mercadante et al. 2010). This allows the treatment team to appropriately address the myriad of factors that may affect sexuality and intimacy in cancer survivors. Other research has highlighted the need to involve partners in order to effect long-lasting improvements (Mercadante et al. 2010).

16.2 Treating Sexual Dysfunction in Women

Women may experience a number of changes in sexual function and feelings about sex as a result of cancer and its treatment. Sexual dysfunction may be the direct result of treatments (e.g., menopausal symptoms that cause vaginal dryness) or related to psychological factors (e.g., body image problems, anxiety, or depression) (McKee and Schover 2001; Wilmoth and Botchway 1999; Roth et al. 2010). Women may also worry about how their partners will react to their lowered sexual function or experience anticipatory anxiety with the thought of a potential new partner. Most interventions have targeted breast cancer patients. Interventions for women who experience sexual dysfunction associated with treatment for gynecologic cancers have primarily focused on providing education and managing symptoms (Katz 2009).

Standard treatments for sexual health problems include different strategies to improve vaginal and physiologic function and provide information about the sexual response cycle and anatomy, effects of cancer treatment on sexual function, and availability of treatment options. Education and counseling on optimal use of vaginal lubricants and/or moisturizers may be a sufficient first step in resolving many of the sexual problems women experience (Carter et al. 2011). Providers should also normalize the experience of sexual problems, encourage patients and couples to explore alternative ways to maintain intimacy such as nonsexual touch, and address any barriers patients may have to treatments (e.g., embarrassment) (Sanchez-Varela et al. 2011). For example, discussions may involve the generation of problem-solving strategies to negotiate discomfort with novel sexual practices or cognitive restructuring techniques to address maladaptive beliefs associated with sexual dysfunction or expectations of recovery. Sexual health should be viewed within the context of the individual patient as well as her relationship with her sexual partner or expectations related to a potential future partner.

During the course of guiding patients through sex interventions, providers should assess patients' comfort level and openness to treatments. Women may feel nervous using devices or introducing new sexual practices into their relationship. Embarrassment and fear have been shown to decrease compliance with sexual rehabilitation therapies (Roth et al. 2010). Simple strategies, such as methods to create a relaxing environment, may help women feel more comfortable with treatment recommendations. More extensive problem-solving and cognitive restructuring techniques may be required if patients express multiple or rigid barriers to engaging in recommended sexual health strategies. Couples may benefit from addressing communication difficulties or partners' maladaptive beliefs regarding patients' sexuality or treatments.

16.2.1 Vaginal Health Solutions

Vaginal moisturizers and lubricants Vaginal moisturizers and lubricants are a safe, accessible, and easily administered first-line treatment for vaginal dryness. There are important differences between moisturizers and lubricants and many women need both to prevent vaginal discomfort and pain during sexual activity (Carter et al. 2011). Vaginal moisturizers are used to hydrate the vaginal mucosa and improve overall vaginal health, and can be beneficial regardless of whether a women is sexually active. Women may use moisturizers several times a week and should apply it at night before bed to optimize absorption. Vaginal lubricants are intended to minimize friction and irritation during intercourse and prevent mucosal tears that may be painful and increase the chance of vaginal and urinary tract infections (Carter et al. 2011). The lubricant can be applied to both the patient and her partner's genital area prior to vaginal penetration, and can be reapplied during sexual activity as needed. Anesthetic gels may also be used to reduce pain or discomfort (Brotto et al. 2008). There are a number of moisturizers and lubricants on the market and patients should be encouraged to try several types to find the one they most prefer. Products with perfumes or flavors should be avoided, as they are more likely to irritate the tissue or the genital area. Lubricants that contain glycerin and those that are petroleum based are also not recommended as they may increase the risk of vaginal infection. Examples of over-the-counter lubricant products include Astroglide, KY, and Eros for women. Moisturizers may be hormonal or nonhormonal. Examples of nonhormonal moisturizers include Vitamin E capsules, Replens, and Liquibeads, whereas examples of hormonal replacement includes Vagiform (requires prescription; may be medically contraindicated).

Pelvic floor and Kegel exercises Pain with intercourse may be lessened if women learn to relax their pelvic floor muscles surrounding the vaginal entrance, anus, and urethra (Brotto et al. 2008). Kegel exercises may help women develop greater awareness of when muscles are tense versus relaxed and gain better control of their pelvic floor muscles. As women gain better awareness and control over these muscles, they are better equipped to stay relaxed during sexual activity. Kegel exercises typically have women tighten their muscles for a count of three and then relax, which is repeated at least ten times, several times a day (Brotto et al. 2008). Women may also be instructed to tense and relax without the count of 3. The Kegel squeeze should be limited to vaginal muscles and should not include the thighs or whole stomach and patients should be made aware that they should not hold their breath while doing the exercises. Women who have difficulty learning these techniques or are unable to gain better control of pelvic floor muscles may benefit from seeing a physical therapist that uses pelvic biofeedback to promote awareness and control of pelvic floor muscles (Carter et al. 2011).

Vaginal dilator therapy Women often experience discomfort or pain with intercourse as a result of vaginal atrophy due to premature menopause, particularly related to radiation treatment. In extreme cases, women may develop complete vaginismus. Vaginal dilators may be used to mechanically stretch the vagina to prevent narrowing or shortening, keep the vagina more elastic, and facilitate vaginal intercourse (Krychman and Millheiser 2013; Schover 2005). Similar to pelvic floor and Kegel exercises, dilators may help women become more aware of being in a tense versus relaxed state and gain better control of pelvic floor muscles. Women often tense these muscles reflexively when they experience pain, which increases friction, pain, and tissue inflammation, and may exacerbate vaginal atrophy (Carter et al. 2011). The use of dilator therapy has been shown to prevent the development of vaginal stenosis (Denton and Maher 2003). Although many physicians are familiar with dilator therapy and may encourage their patients to try it, women often discontinue use due to lack of success and frustration (Schover 2005; Jeffries et al. 2006). Patients often need education and instruction in the proper use of dilators and to manage expectations regarding their effects. Dilator therapy is a gradual process in which patients start with a very small (narrow diameter) dilator and progress to increasingly larger diameters over time. It has been suggested that dilator therapy may be most effective when combined with pelvic floor exercises (Roth et al. 2010; Carter et al. 2011). Providers need to remind patients that insertion should be slow and gradual and should not be painful. Patients who have difficulty or require additional support may benefit from referrals to a sexual health specialist, psychologist trained in treating vaginismus, or pelvic floor physical therapist (Jeffries et al. 2006).

Vaginal estrogen therapy Another approach to address vaginal atrophy is through the use of estrogen therapy. Examples of products that deliver a localized (vaginal delivery) estrogen dose include Estrace Vaginal Cream (an estradiol cream), Premarin Vaginal Cream (a conjugated estrogens vaginal cream), Estring (a sustained release Silastic ring that releases estradiol), and Vagifem (a micronized estradiol hemihydrate vaginal pill) (Sanchez-Varela et al. 2011). Some evidence supports the efficacy of low dose, local estrogen therapy in treating vaginal atrophy among postmenopausal women with limited systemic absorption (Sanchez-Varela et al. 2011). Systemic absorption of estrogen from low dose vaginal estrogen therapy products appears to be minimal (Schover 2005). However, it is unknown how even low levels of absorption may affect women with hormone-dependent cancers, and their use is debated (Labrie et al. 2009; Rossouw et al. 2002; Anderson et al. 2004; Jick et al. 2009). For example, even minimal elevation in systemic serum estrogen levels may interfere with aromatase inhibitor treatment in some women (Simon et al. 2008). Results of a Cochrane review indicated that conjugated estrogen creams resulted in higher levels of estradiol (though levels were within the normal postmenopausal range) compared with the estradiol tablet, which had higher levels compared with the estradiol ring (Farquhar et al. 2005). Further research is needed to clarify situations in which estrogen therapy may be contraindicated. Providers may decide to discuss the risks and benefits with patients on an individual basis, depending on the severity of vaginal atrophy and degree to which sexual dysfunction interferes with psychosocial well-being and quality of life. Women often refuse to use estrogen therapy due to the risks, particularly breast cancer survivors (Ganz et al. 1999; Biglia et al. 2003). Nonhormonal vaginal lubricants and/or moisturizers may be used as an initial treatment strategy, followed by pelvic floor and Kegel exercises, and estrogen therapy only if symptoms persist.

Testosterone therapy Low sexual desire (libido) is a common sexual problem for women after cancer treatment, particularly among women who undergo treatments that affect functioning of the ovaries or experience premature menopause. Fifty percent of circulating testosterone is produced in the ovaries. Treatments that directly impact ovarian function or cause menopausal symptoms may therefore result in low sexual desire or hypoactive sexual desire disorder (HSDD). Testosterone therapy has been shown to be an effective treatment for low sexual desire and may be used with or without concomitant estrogen (Sanchez-Varela et al. 2011; Buster et al. 2005). Randomized, controlled trials have shown that use of a testosterone patch (300 µg) with concomitant estrogen treatment in premenopausal women may improve sexual function in surgically induced and naturally menopausal women with HSDD (Schover 1991). Notably, the use of testosterone to treat desire problems has also been debated. A review of the literature concluded that testosterone therapy should not be used in women due to the risk of long-term adverse effects, primarily breast cancer risk (Schover 1991). Testosterone therapy among breast cancer patients is highly controversial, particularly if the cancer is hormone positive or if women are on an Aromatase Inhibitor or Tamoxifen. Providers should be aware of and communicate potential risks to their patients and be prudent in recommendations for select patient populations (e.g., breast cancer survivors). Low sexual desire is often multifactorial, however, and providers should assess whether psychological or relational difficulties appear to be causing or exacerbating desire problems. For example, mood disorders and their psychopharmacological treatments may both affect sexual function, particularly sexual desire. Depression is often associated with low sex drive. Likewise, antidepressants such as serotonin-specific reuptake inhibitors (SSRIs) and serotonin-norepinephrine reuptake inhibitors (SNRIs) are known to negatively affect libido (Roth et al. 2010). When appropriate, providers may consider targeting these factors if testosterone therapy is not a suitable choice.

Clitoral therapy device A relatively new treatment for female sexual dysfunction is a FDA-approved, non-pharmaceutical clitoral therapy device (EROS Therapy, Urometrics, St. Paul, MN) (Josefson 2000). The CTD is placed over the clitoris and creates a gentle suction thereby increasing blood flow and sensation. The patient activates the device via a battery-powered pump, which creates a vacuum to draw blood into the clitoris and induces successive vasocongestion of the larger genitalia region. The device causes vascular engorgement first in the clitoris and then the vagina and leads to increased vaginal lubrication and stimulation of sensory nerve endings. Anatomically, women are thus more likely to reach orgasm. The CTD has been shown to be particularly effective in women who are postmenopausal, have had a hysterectomy, or have surgically induced menopause (Josefson 2000). Billups et al. reported increased genital/clitoral sensation, vaginal lubrication, ability to have an orgasm, and sexual satisfaction, among women with and without a sexual disorder after 3 months of use (Billups et al. 2001). Similar results were shown in a pilot study of women with a history of irradiated cervical cancer with significant improvements observed in all sexual domains (desire, arousal, lubrication, orgasm, sexual satisfaction, and reduced pain) as well as objective measures of vaginal elasticity, mucosal color and moisture, and decreased bleeding and ulcerations (observed via gynecologic exams) (Schroder et al. 2005). Patients improved from being at the 10th percentile of normal sexual function at baseline to the normalcy cutoff at 3-month follow-up (Schroder et al. 2005). Although findings need to be confirmed with larger, randomized, controlled trials, providers may consider the use of CTD for patients who are interested.

16.3 Treating Sexual Dysfunction in Men

Although there are a number of sexual side effects that may impact men following cancer treatment, the primary concern is erectile functioning. Since prostate cancer is the most common cancer in men, most research related to the rates of sexual dysfunction have been reported in this group. The rates of ED following radical prostatectomy range from 14 to 90 % (Schover et al. 2002; Burnett et al. 2007). This variation is due to multiple methodological limitations in the literature (Burnett et al. 2007). Despite the wide variation, the general conclusion is that RP has a severe impact on erectile functioning and the majority of rates are on the higher end of this range. For example, Schover et al. reported that out of 1,236 men (4.3 years post-early-stage treatment), 85 % stated they had problems with erections (Schover et al. 2002). This percentage is confirmed in a recent longitudinal study which reported that only 16 % of men after radical prostatectomy will be able to achieve erections similar to their erections presurgery without the use of some erectile aid. When focusing on men over 60 years of age, this percentage drops to 4 % (Nelson et al. 2013a). Because of the significant impact cancer treatments can have on erections, the primary focus in treatment of sexual dysfunction in men is on treating erectile dysfunction.

16.3.1 Treatments for Erectile Dysfunction

PDE5 inhibitors The first line of treatment for ED are the oral PDE5 inhibitors (PDE5i) (Hatzichristou 1998). Oral medications are less invasive and easier to use than other available treatments. The most common types of PDE5i are sildenafil, tadalafil, and vardenafil. The mechanism of action for these medications involves nitric oxide (NO). A primary mechanism for erections is the NO secreted from the cavernous nerves that run bilaterally along the prostate. NO promotes smooth muscle relaxation in the penis producing an erection. PDE5 is a chemical that breaks down NO, and as their names imply, oral medications inhibit PDE5, leaving more NO available to produce an erection (Walsh and Donker 1982). A man should take a PDE5i on an empty stomach and wait approximately 2 h before sexual activity. Many men take these medications incorrectly, and as a result, the medications are ineffective. A PDE5i will not increase a man's sexual desire, and sexual stimulation is needed to produce an erection.

Penile injections Penile injection therapy is considered a second-line treatment option for ED. This treatment delivers intracavernosal vasodilators (prostaglandin, phentolamine, and papaverine) at the base of the penis with a 29 gauge needle. It generally takes 10 min for the medication to work and produces an erection that lasts for 20–30 min. Penile injections produce excellent results and are effective for 94 % of injection users (Linet and Neff 1994). Since the medication is injected into the shaft of the penis and works locally, those men who do not respond to a PDE5i have a good chance to responding to penile injections. The common notion is that these injections will be painful. However, since a 29 gauge needle is used and the injection site is in the shaft of the penis, these injections generally produce minimal pain. In fact, on a 0–10 point pain rating scale where 0 represents no pain and 10 represents pain as bad as you can image, 59 % of men rate the pain of the penile injection as ≤ 2 (Nelson et al. 2013b). If a man is interested in penile injections, he should see an urologist who can train him to use the injections. Whenever possible, it is best for these men to see an urologist who specializes in sexual medicine.

Vacuum devices Vacuum devices are placed over a man's penis, and create a vacuum inside the cylinder of the device which pulls blood into the penis creating an erection. Once the penis is erect, the man removes the device, and places a rubber ring around the base of his penis to hold the blood in the penis, which will sustain the erection (Brison et al. 2013). In general, the ring should only be left in place for about 30 min. The blood pulled into the penis by the vacuum device is oxygen-depleted blood, and as a result, the erection can feel cool to the touch and the skin may look darker as compared to a normal erection (Brison et al. 2013). It is important to note that it is difficult for the vacuum device to fill blood in the base of the penis, and this may cause some instability in the erection (often called a hinge effect). The man should be aware of this and potentially adjust the way he thrusts during intercourse.

Intraurethral suppositories Intraurethral suppositories contain the medication prostaglandin, one of the medications used with penile injections (Lewis 2000). These suppositories are small tablets that are inserted in the urethra with a plastic applicator. These should be inserted after urination, as the moisture will help the applicator slide down the urethra. The applicator is inserted about one inch into the urethra and a button on top of the applicator releases the suppository tablet. The man should then massage his penis for 2–3 min. Since the drug is a vasodilator, this will help pull blood into the penis creating an erection. In general, it takes about 30–60 min for the medication to produce a firm erection (Lewis 2000). Penile injections tend to produce more consistent and reliable erections, and as a result, penile injections are usually suggested as a treatment prior to suppositories (Lewis 2000). However, suppositories may be an option if a man is unable to use penile injections.

Inflatable penile prostheses (IPPs) An IPP is a system that is surgically implanted into the penis (Lewis 2000). The surgeon places two cylinders in the shaft of the penis, and a round reservoir in the scrotum. When a man wants an erection he pumps the reservoir transferring fluid (generally saline) from the reservoir into the two cylinders in the shaft of the penis. This creates a firm, erect penis. When the man has completed sexual activity, he then manually releases a valve that lets the saline travel from the cylinders back into the reservoir. This allows a man to have a flaccid penis. The IPP should be the last option when seeking solutions for erectile dysfunction. Men who do not respond to the previously mentioned treatments or men who are not satisfied with the other treatments are candidates for implant surgery. For men who do get to the point of needing a penile implant, most are very satisfied with the procedure. In fact, the satisfaction with penile implant surgery tends to be very high with more that 85 % of men reporting that they are satisfied with the IPP (Falcone et al. 2013).

16.3.2 Penile Rehabilitation Following Radical Prostatectomy: The State of the Art

For men who have had a radical prostatectomy (RP) for prostate cancer as well as men who have had a cystectomy for bladder cancer, the concept of "penile rehabilitation" is currently the best practice for the treatment of erectile dysfunction. These surgeries generally use nerve sparing surgical techniques, which save the cavernous nerves that help produce an erection and run bilaterally along the prostate. Although these nerves are spared, they are also injured interoperatively and can take 18–24 months to heal following surgery (Mulhall et al. 2005). Since these nerves are responsible for erections, natural erections via sexual stimulation and nocturnal erections may also be absent in the 18 to 24 months following surgery. In a normal state, erections serve the purpose of pulling oxygen-rich blood into the penile tissue, keeping this tissue healthy. Men who fail to have natural erections post-RP also fail to oxygenate their penile tissue which can cause atrophy and permanent structural alterations. This may lead to venous leak which, once present, is irreversible and will cause ED (Mulhall et al. 2005).

The first-line treatments for erections are oral PDE5i. Unfortunately, only about 12–17 % of men will respond to these oral medications in the first 6 months following RP (Mulhall et al. 2005). The reason these oral medications are generally ineffective is because their mechanism of action uses the NO secreted from the cavernous nerves (Rabbani et al. 2000). As these nerves are healing, there is reduced NO secretion, which removes the mechanism for these oral medications.

This has led to the use of penile injections prophylactically to sustain penile tissue health in the recovery period post-RP. In 1997, Montorsi completed the first study looking at prophylactic ED treatment administered immediately post-RP. In a randomized, controlled study, penile injection therapy was used by 15 men three times per week compared to 15 men who underwent no postoperative ED therapy (Montorsi et al. 1997). Six months after surgery, 67 % of those who used the injection therapy returned to spontaneous erectile function versus 20 % in men who had no treatment (RR = 3.35). Our group, Mulhall et al. (2005), reported similar results in a study with 58 men who used penile injections three times per week for ED post-RP compared to 74 men who used no ED treatment (Mulhall et al. 2005). At 18 months post-RP, 52 % of the men who used penile injections returned to spontaneous erections compared to 12 % who used no ED treatment (RR = 4.33). Additional data suggests that immediate initiation of ED treatment post-RP is critical for successful maintenance of healthy penile tissue (Fraiman et al. 1999);

low dose PDE5 inhibitors, although not successful in producing an erection, help in the healing of the cavernous nerves (McCullough et al. 2008).

These findings have led to the concept of "penile rehabilitation" post-RP where men who achieve consistent erections after surgery have an increased chance of retaining natural erectile functioning 24 months post-surgery. Penile rehabilitation programs instruct men to achieve medication-assisted erections two to three times per week following RP in the 18–24 month recovery period. It is important to note that these erections do not need to be used for sexual activity. Penile rehabilitation is now the best practice treatment for men following surgery as 89 % of sexual medicine professionals are utilizing some type of penile rehabilitation (Tal et al. 2011). Since oral medications will most likely not be effective during this period, penile injections have become a cornerstone of rehabilitation programs. Some programs prefer to use vacuum devices; however, the current research on penile rehabilitation supports the use of penile injections versus vacuum devices. Penile injections pull oxygen-rich blood into the penile tissue as opposed to oxygen-depleted blood pulled by vacuum devices. In fact, vacuum devices have been found to be generally ineffective in a penile rehabilitation setting (Kohler et al. 2007).

16.4 Educational and Psychosocial Intervention Techniques for Individuals and Couples

Although the strategies described above are often effective in improving sexual health, both men and women may experience a number of psychological or emotional difficulties that impact their sexuality. For example, patients may have anticipatory anxiety regarding resumption of sexual activity in the aftermath of cancer treatment. They may wonder how they will perform or worry how their partner will react to changes in their appearance or function. Excessive worrying may further exacerbate sexual difficulties. Likewise, having a negative experience may discourage patients from further engaging in sexual activity and lead to a pattern of avoidance. If there is unclear communication between partners, this may lead to avoidance of other acts of intimacy. Research suggests that patients want to discuss changes in sexuality with their providers (Hordern and Street 2007a) but are often disappointed by the lack of information, support, and practical strategies they receive (Hordern and Street 2007b). Providers should be knowledgeable about sexual rehabilitation strategies as well as psychosocial factors that may play a role in sexuality and intimacy for the individual patient as well as his/her partner. Couples should be educated regarding rehabilitation strategies that will improve sexual function and also encouraged to explore ways of achieving intimacy and satisfaction when intercourse is not possible. Sexual satisfaction may be achieved through expanding the repertoire of their typical sexual practices as well as through increased communication about sexual difficulties to promote feelings of love and support. It may be helpful for couples to begin slowly in their initiation of sexual activity (e.g., hugging, kissing, massage, nongenital touching), until they feel comfortable progressing to genital touch and intercourse. Alternatively, patients may feel more comfortable with self-stimulation practices to rediscover their post-cancer bodies without the added pressure of a partner present. Educational and psychosocial intervention strategies and support resources may be used in conjunction with treatment strategies discussed above to facilitate sexual recovery and promote satisfying sexual experiences. It is strongly encouraged that interventions address sexual dysfunction from an individual and relational standpoint.

Cancer survivors are often unaware of treatment options such as those described above and benefit from the provision of this information as well as the opportunity to discuss negative feelings associated with sexual dysfunction and barriers to using rehabilitation techniques (e.g., embarrassment, discomfort). A number of interventions that aim to provide information, normalize sexual difficulties and negative experiences, and address maladaptive cognitive and/or behavioral factors related to sexuality and intimacy have shown promising results across a range of cancer populations (Brotto et al. 2010). Brief psycho-educational interventions have been shown to increase compliance with sexual rehabilitation therapies and decrease fear related to sexual activity (Jeffries et al. 2006; Robinson et al. 1999). Couple-based interventions have also been shown to be effective (Baucom et al. 2009; Christensen 1983; Kalaitzi et al. 2007; Scott et al. 2004; Scott and Kayser 2009).

Providers should impart to their patients that sexual health problems are manageable and encourage self-efficacy in their sexual recovery. Provision of education materials regarding sexual and pelvic anatomy and sexual response is a critical first step in sexual rehabilitation (Krychman and Millheiser 2013). Information regarding normal variability in anatomy and arousal response may normalize patients' experiences and improve sexual self-esteem (Krychman and Millheiser 2013). Educational materials concerning sexual anatomy and function may be provided to patients to facilitate their learning (e.g., pelvic models, educational booklets, videos, or DVDs). Materials may be useful for partners as well to increase their knowledge, reduce the onus on patients to communicate information to partners, and facilitate joint coping for couples going through the sexual rehabilitation process (Canada et al. 2005). Partners often want to be helpful and supportive of patients' sexual recovery but may be unsure of patients' wishes or how to best be involved. Providers may offer guidance to couples to help them access educational and support resources. Patients and partners should be encouraged to ask questions of the clinician and also to communicate their fears and concerns with one another. It is important for providers to have an understanding of the couples' pre-cancer sexual relationship, expectations for post-cancer sexuality, and how they have communicated and coped with sexual changes thus far. Assessment of these factors will help identify barriers to sexual rehabilitation and guide further intervention strategies. Patients who are not partnered may likewise benefit from feeling open to pose questions, discuss their concerns, and practice communication strategies with potential future partners. They may be unsure as to how and when to disclose their cancer experiences in the context of dating and lack confidence initiating new sexual relationships. Having the opportunity to discuss their fears and practice, difficult conversations with potential new partners may be beneficial in reducing anticipatory anxiety and promoting optimal sexual experiences in the future (Roth et al. 2010). Most of the strategies reviewed may be adapted for individuals or couples depending on patients' relationship status and comfort level.

16.4.1 Body Awareness and Relaxation Techniques

Intervention strategies that encourage patients to become more aware of body feelings and sensations include Kegel exercises (as described above for women) as well as other exercises to focus on pleasurable sensations without intercourse. Sensate focus exercises may include sensuous massages and nongenital touching. The focus is on giving and receiving pleasure that enhances sensuous feelings but is not connected to an end result such as reaching orgasm (Roth et al. 2010; Hughes 2008). Similarly, outer-course exercises allow patients to enjoy stimulation and sexual contact without intercourse. Patients and their partners may enjoy sexual experiences and feelings of intimacy without the pressure and anxiety that can occur with the anticipation of intercourse (e.g., self-consciousness, self-evaluation) or feeling like orgasm *should* be achieved. The objective is to learn to enjoy pleasurable touch without feeling distressed about the goal of sexual performance. For women who experience pain or who are not ready to have intercourse, these strategies may offer ways to maintain sexual pleasure and intimacy both for patients and their partners. Likewise, men with lowered erectile function may benefit from activities that are not focused on intercourse, thereby reducing cause for performance anxiety related to erectile function. Exercises may also encourage communication between partners regarding painful, problematic, or emotionally sensitive areas of the body. Patients and couples learn to take the emphasis off of goal-oriented sex and discover new ways to expand their sexual repertoire to still have satisfying sexual experiences.

16.4.2 Self-Stimulation

For patients who are anxious about how their partners may react to sexual changes in the relationship or for patients without a partner, self-stimulation offers several advantages. Self-stimulation allows patients to become comfortable with their post-cancer bodies and to explore ways of feeling sexually satisfied despite cancer-related changes in sexual functioning (Krychman and Millheiser 2013). Patients may learn to enjoy sexual contact without the added pressure of having a partner present and worrying about his/her pleasure or reactions. For example, women may feel self-conscious about scars or other changes in appearance, which may interfere with getting aroused with a partner. Women may buy over-the-counter vibrators and other self-stimulators in drug stores or through online vendors if additional stimulation of the vagina or clitoris is needed. Some vibrators have suction cup devices to increase vasocongestion in the clitoral tissue and may be particularly helpful for cervical, rectal, and vaginal cancer patients (Krychman and Millheiser 2013). Providers should assess whether patients hold any maladaptive cognitions regarding masturbation (e.g., cultural or religious taboos) and encourage them to view self-pleasuring activities as a part of the sexual rehabilitation process.

16.4.3 Problem-Solving Techniques

There are a number of difficulties that can emerge as patients engage in sexual rehabilitation and become acquainted with the changes and limitations of their post-cancer sexual functioning. Some of these difficulties may simply require problem-solving strategies to address barriers with sexual rehabilitation once they have been identified. For example, patients should be encouraged to explore different sexual positions to find out which is most comfortable and pleasurable. Positions that avoid placing pressure on scars or ostomy bags should be considered. For women, positions that allow them to have control over the depth and speed of penetration may be most comfortable and optimize the likelihood of sexual satisfaction with intercourse. There are several considerations that patients with colostomies or ileostomies should be aware of to reduce discomfort and promote sexual enjoyment. Providers should educate patients on limiting food intake prior to sexual activity and types of foods that should be avoided if sexual activity is anticipated, emptying the ostomy appliance before sexual activity to reduce the chance of leakage, and having a plan in case the appliance does leak (American Cancer Society 2011; United Ostomy Associations of America 2013). Patients may be embarrassed about their ostomy bag or worry that it will interfere with sexual activity, become dislodged, or damage the stoma. Other considerations may include decorative covers and special lingerie or undergarments (such as those with a support barrier to eliminate leakage), pouches with filters to control odors or use of deodorant tablets or liquids, and pouches that are smaller or hang sideways to facilitate movement (United Ostomy Associations of America 2013). Providers should provide information regarding these simple strategies, as they are relatively easy to implement but may significantly improve sexual experiences. All patients may benefit from other strategies aimed to create a comfortable and relaxing environment to practice interventions such as taking a shower or bath, listening to music, or using candles for a soft atmosphere. Although these measures may seem commonplace or self-evident, patients may have difficulty generating problem-solving strategies on their own. Providers should encourage patients to identify barriers to sexual rehabilitation and discuss problem-solving strategies together to generate solutions or alternatives. These discussions may involve the partner, which not only allows him/her to gain knowledge of the patient's sexual experiences and needs but also may foster intimacy within the couple.

16.4.4 Cognitive Restructuring Techniques

Barriers to sexual rehabilitation may include patients (or their partners) holding inaccurate or maladaptive beliefs regarding their sexual health and recovery. For example, patients may have unrealistic expectations regarding the timeline of recovery or place undue pressure on themselves that can lead to significant distress. Cancer-related body changes that impact patients' sense of self and identity may affect how they perceive themselves sexually and negatively impact intimate relationships and emotional well-being (Carpenter et al. 2009; Campbell et al. 2012). Providers should assess whether patients exhibit signs of low confidence or self-esteem and determine whether emotional distress is related to unrealistic or irrational cognitions. Cognitive restructuring techniques may be used to identify problematic cognitions (automatic thoughts) or cognitive distortions, promote awareness of how cognitions lead to emotional distress or negative behaviors, and teach patients how to replace irrational beliefs with more realistic, positive ways of thinking. Cognitive behavioral interventions have been shown to be effective in improving sexual function (McCabe 2001; McCabe et al. 2008; Molton et al. 2008; Penedo et al. 2007). Acceptance-based techniques may also be used in conjunction to facilitate adjustment to long-term or permanent changes in sexuality (e.g., body image difficulties, feeling less like a man). Providers may wish to refer patients to a mental health specialist or psychologist if cognitions appear firmly entrenched or are causing marked distress.

16.5   Referral to Sexual Health Specialist or Support Group

- American Association of Sex Educators Counselors and Therapists (AASECT)
  - http://www.aasect.org
- American Sexual Health Association (ASHA)
  - http://www.ashastd.org
- International Society for Sexual Medicine
  - http://www.issm.info
- International Society for the Study of Women's Sexual Health
  - http://www.isswsh.org
- North American Menopause Society
  - http://www.menopause.org
- American College of Obstetricians and Gynecologists
  - http://www.acog.org
- American Cancer Society
  - http://www.cancer.org
- National Cancer Institute
  - http://www.cancer.net
- International Psycho-Oncology Society
  - http://www.ipos-society.org
- Psychoeducation or support resources (U.S.)

- Cancer care
- Gilda's Club
- Wellness Community

References

American Cancer Society. Colostomy: a guide. In: Society AC, editor. 2011. American Cancer Society. http://www.cancer.org/

Anderson GL, et al. Effects of conjugated equine estrogen in postmenopausal women with hysterectomy: the Women's Health Initiative randomized controlled trial. JAMA. 2004;291 (14):1701–12.

Araujo AB, et al. The relationship between depressive symptoms and male erectile dysfunction: cross-sectional results from the Massachusetts Male Aging Study. Psychosom Med. 1998;60 (4):458–65.

Arora NK, et al. Impact of surgery and chemotherapy on the quality of life of younger women with breast carcinoma: a prospective study. Cancer. 2001;92(5):1288–98.

Baucom DH, et al. A couple-based intervention for female breast cancer. Psychooncology. 2009;18(3):276–83.

Biglia N, et al. Menopause after breast cancer: a survey on breast cancer survivors. Maturitas. 2003;45(1):29–38.

Billups KL, et al. A new non-pharmacological vacuum therapy for female sexual dysfunction. J Sex Marital Ther. 2001;27(5):435–41.

Bloom JR, et al. Then and now: quality of life of young breast cancer survivors. Psychooncology. 2004;13(3):147–60.

Brison D, Seftel A, Sadeghi-Nejad H. The resurgence of the vacuum erection device (VED) for treatment of erectile dysfunction. J Sex Med. 2013;10(4):1124–35.

Brotto LA, et al. A psychoeducational intervention for sexual dysfunction in women with gynecologic cancer. Arch Sex Behav. 2008;37(2):317–29.

Brotto L, Yule M, Breckon E. Psychological interventions for the sexual sequelae of cancer: a review of the literature. J Cancer Surviv. 2010;4(4):346–60.

Burnett AL, et al. Erectile function outcome reporting after clinically localized prostate cancer treatment. J Urol. 2007;178(2):597–601.

Buster JE, et al. Testosterone patch for low sexual desire in surgically menopausal women: a randomized trial. Obstet Gynecol. 2005;105(5 Pt 1):944–52.

Campbell LC, et al. Masculinity beliefs predict psychosocial functioning in African American prostate cancer survivors. Am J Mens Health. 2012;6(5):400–8.

Canada AL, et al. Pilot intervention to enhance sexual rehabilitation for couples after treatment for localized prostate carcinoma. Cancer. 2005;104(12):2689–700.

Carpenter K, et al. Sexual self schema as a moderator of sexual and psychological outcomes for gynecologic cancer survivors. Arch Sex Behav. 2009;38(5):828–41.

Carter J, Goldfrank D, Schover LR. Simple strategies for vaginal health promotion in cancer survivors. J Sex Med. 2011;8(2):549–59.

Christensen DN. Postmastectomy couple counseling: an outcome study of a structured treatment protocol. J Sex Marital Ther. 1983;9(4):266–75.

Denton AS, Maher EJ. Interventions for the physical aspects of sexual dysfunction in women following pelvic radiotherapy. Cochrane Database Syst Rev. 2003; (1): Cd003750.

Falcone M, et al. Prospective analysis of the surgical outcomes and patients' satisfaction rate after the AMS Spectra penile prosthesis implantation. Urology. 2013;82(2):373–6.

Farquhar CM, et al. Long term hormone therapy for perimenopausal and postmenopausal women. Cochrane Database Syst Rev. 2005;3, CD004143.

Figueiredo MI, et al. Breast cancer treatment in older women: does getting what you want improve your long-term body image and mental health? J Clin Oncol. 2004;22(19):4002–9.

Fobair P, et al. Body image and sexual problems in young women with breast cancer. Psychooncology. 2006;15(7):579–94.

Fraiman MC, Lepor H, McCullough AR. Changes in penile morphometrics in men with erectile dysfunction after nerve-sparing radical retropubic prostatectomy. Mol Urol. 1999;3(2):109–15.

Ganz PA. Breast cancer, menopause, and long-term survivorship: critical issues for the 21st century. Am J Med. 2005;118(Suppl 12B):136–41.

Ganz PA, et al. Are older breast carcinoma survivors willing to take hormone replacement therapy? Cancer. 1999;86(5):814–20.

Hatzichristou DG. Current treatment and future perspectives for erectile dysfunction. Int J Impot Res. 1998;10 Suppl 1:S3–13.

Hordern AJ, Street AF. Communicating about patient sexuality and intimacy after cancer: mismatched expectations and unmet needs. Med J Aust. 2007a;186(5):224–7.

Hordern A, Street A. Issues of intimacy and sexuality in the face of cancer: the patient perspective. Cancer Nurs. 2007b;30(6):E11–8.

Hughes MK. Alterations of sexual function in women with cancer. Semin Oncol Nurs. 2008;24 (2):91–101.

Jayne DG, et al. Randomized trial of laparoscopic-assisted resection of colorectal carcinoma: 3-year results of the UK MRC CLASICC Trial Group. J Clin Oncol. 2007;25(21):3061–8.

Jeffries SA, et al. An effective group psychoeducational intervention for improving compliance with vaginal dilation: a randomized controlled trial. Int J Radiat Oncol Biol Phys. 2006;65 (2):404–11.

Jick SS, et al. Postmenopausal estrogen-containing hormone therapy and the risk of breast cancer. Obstet Gynecol. 2009;113(1):74–80.

Josefson D. FDA approves device for female sexual dysfunction. BMJ. 2000;320(7247):1427.

Kalaitzi C, et al. Combined brief psychosexual intervention after mastectomy: effects on sexuality, body image, and psychological well-being. J Surg Oncol. 2007;96(3):235–40.

Katz A. Interventions for sexuality after pelvic radiation therapy and gynecological cancer. Cancer J. 2009;15(1):45–7.

Kohler TS, et al. A pilot study on the early use of the vacuum erection device after radical retropubic prostatectomy. BJU Int. 2007;100(4):858–62.

Krychman M, Millheiser LS. Sexual health issues in women with cancer. J Sex Med. 2013;10 Suppl 1:5–15.

Labrie F, et al. Effect of one-week treatment with vaginal estrogen preparations on serum estrogen levels in postmenopausal women. Menopause. 2009;16(1):30–6.

Lewis R. Review of intraurethral suppositories and iontophoresis therapy for erectile dysfunction. Int J Impot Res. 2000;12 Suppl 4:S86–90.

Linet OI, Neff LL. Intracavernous prostaglandin E1 in erectile dysfunction. Clin Investig. 1994;72 (2):139–49.

McCabe MP. Evaluation of a cognitive behavior therapy program for people with sexual dysfunction. J Sex Marital Ther. 2001;27(3):259–71.

McCabe MP, et al. Evaluation of an internet-based psychological intervention for the treatment of erectile dysfunction. Int J Impot Res. 2008;20(3):324–30.

McCullough AR, Levine LA, Padma-Nathan H. Return of nocturnal erections and erectile function after bilateral nerve-sparing radical prostatectomy in men treated nightly with sildenafil citrate: subanalysis of a longitudinal randomized double-blind placebo-controlled trial. J Sex Med. 2008;5(2):476–84.

McKee Jr AL, Schover LR. Sexuality rehabilitation. Cancer. 2001;92(4 Suppl):1008–12.

Mercadante S, Vitrano V, Catania V. Sexual issues in early and late stage cancer: a review. Support Care Cancer. 2010;18(6):659–65.

Molton IR, et al. Promoting recovery of sexual functioning after radical prostatectomy with group-based stress management: the role of interpersonal sensitivity. J Psychosom Res. 2008;64 (5):527–36.

Montorsi F, et al. Recovery of spontaneous erectile function after nerve-sparing radical retropubic prostatectomy with and without early intracavernous injections of alprostadil: results of a prospective, randomized trial [see comment]. J Urol. 1997;158(4):1408–10.

Mulhall JP, et al. The use of an erectogenic pharmacothoerapy regimen following radical prostatectomy improves recovery of spontanious erectile function. J Sex Med. 2005;2:532–40.

Nelson CJ, et al. Sexual bother following radical prostatectomyjsm. J Sex Med. 2010;7(1 Pt 1):129–35.

Nelson CJ, Mulhall JP, Roth AJ. The association between erectile dysfunction and depressive symptoms in men treated for prostate cancer. J Sex Med. 2011;8(2):560–6.

Nelson CJ, et al. Back to baseline: erectile function recovery after radical prostatectomy from the patients' perspective. J Sex Med. 2013a;10(6):1636–43.

Nelson CJ, et al. Injection anxiety and pain in men using intracavernosal injection therapy after radical pelvic surgery. J Sex Med. 2013b;10(10):2559–65.

Penedo FJ, et al. Cognitive behavioral stress management intervention improves quality of life in Spanish monolingual hispanic men treated for localized prostate cancer: results of a randomized controlled trial. Int J Behav Med. 2007;14(3):164–72.

Penson DF, et al. Is quality of life different for men with erectile dysfunction and prostate cancer compared to men with erectile dysfunction due to other causes? Results from the ExCEED data base. J Urol. 2003;169(4):1458–61.

Rabbani F, et al. Factors predicting recovery of erections after radical prostatectomy [see comment]. J Urol. 2000;164(6):1929–34.

Robinson JW, Faris PD, Scott CB. Psychoeducational group increases vaginal dilation for younger women and reduces sexual fears for women of all ages with gynecological carcinoma treated with radiotherapy. Int J Radiat Oncol Biol Phys. 1999;44(3):497–506.

Rossouw JE, et al. Risks and benefits of estrogen plus progestin in healthy postmenopausal women: principal results from the Women's Health Initiative randomized controlled trial. JAMA. 2002;288(3):321–33.

Roth AJ, Carter J, Nelson CJ. Sexuality after cancer. In: Holland JC, Breitbart WS, Jacobsen PB, Lederberg MS, Loscalzo MJ, McCorkle R, editors. Psycho-oncology. New York: Oxford University Press; 2010.

Sanchez-Varela V, Nelson CJ, Bober SL. Sexual problems in cancer patients. In: DeVita VT, Hellman S, Rosenberg SA, editors. Cancer: principles and practice of oncology. Philadelphia, PA: Lippincott; 2011.

Schover LR. The impact of breast cancer on sexuality, body image, and intimate relationships. CA Cancer J Clin. 1991;41(2):112–20.

Schover LR. Reproductive complications and sexual dysfunction in the cancer patient. In: Chang AG, Ganz PA, Hayes DF, Kinsella T, Pass HI, Schiller JH, Stone R, Strecher V, editors. Oncology: an evidence-based approach. New York: Springer; 2005. p. 1580–600.

Schover LR. Sexuality and fertility after cancer. Hematology Am Soc Hematol Educ Program. 2005: 523–7. http://asheducationbook.hematologylibrary.org/content/2005/1/523.long.

Schover LR, et al. Defining sexual outcomes after treatment for localized prostate carcinoma [see comment]. Cancer. 2002;95(8):1773–85.

Schroder M, et al. Clitoral therapy device for treatment of sexual dysfunction in irradiated cervical cancer patients. Int J Radiat Oncol Biol Phys. 2005;61(4):1078–86.

Scott JL, Kayser K. A review of couple-based interventions for enhancing women's sexual adjustment and body image after cancer. Cancer J. 2009;15(1):48–56.

Scott JL, Halford WK, Ward BG. United we stand? The effects of a couple-coping intervention on adjustment to early stage breast or gynecological cancer. J Consult Clin Psychol. 2004;72 (6):1122–35.

Shabsigh R, et al. Increased incidence of depressive symptoms in men with erectile dysfunction. Urology. 1998;52(5):848–52.

Shiri RR, et al. Bidirectional relationship between depression and erectile dysfunction. J Urol. 2007;177(2):669–73.

Simon J, et al. Effective treatment of vaginal atrophy with an ultra-low-dose estradiol vaginal tablet. Obstet Gynecol. 2008;112(5):1053–60.

Tal R, Teloken P, Mulhall JP. Erectile function rehabilitation after radical prostatectomy: practice patterns among AUA members. J Sex Med. 2011;8:2370-6.

United Ostomy Associations of America, I. 2013 [cited 2 Dec 2013]. http://www.ostomy.org/

Walsh PC, Donker PJ. Impotence following radical prostatectomy: insight into etiology and prevention. J Urol. 1982;128(3):492–7.

Wilmoth MC, Botchway P. Psychosexual implications of breast and gynecologic cancer. Cancer Invest. 1999;17(8):631–6.

Part III

Special Issues

Psychiatric Emergencies

17

Rachel Y. Lynn and Alan D. Valentine

Abstract

The complexity of oncology and supportive care is such that psychotropic drugs are themselves potential causes of urgent or emergent clinical problems. Polypharmacy and medication interactions increase the risk of drug-related emergencies. Serotonin syndrome is characterized by mental status changes, autonomic hyperactivity, and neuromuscular abnormalities varying from mild to life-threatening. Use of standardized diagnostic criteria can be helpful. Neuroleptic malignant syndrome presents with muscle rigidity, mental status changes, autonomic instability, and hyperpyrexia. Treatment of both syndromes is focused on removal of the precipitating agents and supportive interventions. Psychotropic drugs that are well tolerated in healthy persons are potentially dangerous in high acuity and end stage disease settings. Overdose and intoxication with psychotropic drugs are usually accidental or idiosyncratic in oncology and supportive care though the medications might be used in suicide attempts. Benzodiazepine intoxication risks hypotension, decreased respiratory drive, and exacerbation of delirium. Antipsychotic drugs may cause or exacerbate anticholinergic delirium. Typical and second generation antipsychotics may cause or exacerbate dangerous cardiac conduction delays including torsades de pointes. Antidepressants, frequently involved in suicides, are variably toxic or lethal between classes. Tricyclic antidepressants and monoamine oxidase inhibitors are particularly dangerous. In all cases of psychotropic drug intoxication or overdose treatment involve withdrawal of offending agents and support of affected organ systems. Emergencies related to psychotropic drugs are

R.Y. Lynn (✉) • A.D. Valentine
Department of Psychiatry, The University of Texas MD Anderson Cancer Center, 1515 Holcombe Blvd, Unit 1454, Houston, TX 77030, USA
e-mail: rlynn@mdanderson.org; avalenti@mdanderson.org

L. Grassi and M. Riba (eds.), *Psychopharmacology in Oncology and Palliative Care*, 317
DOI 10.1007/978-3-642-40134-3_17, © Springer-Verlag Berlin Heidelberg 2014

minimized by careful attention to drug–drug interactions and attempts to minimize polypharmacy as well as consideration of toxicity syndromes with similar presentations.

17.1   Introduction

Psychotropic drugs are mainstays of the management of many behavioral emergencies (e.g., hyperactive delirium, suicidal depression, catastrophic anxiety, combative behavior) and of symptom control in palliative care. The nature of oncology and palliative care practice is such that psychopharmacological drugs are often used in the setting of advanced disease or critical illness, multi-organ failure, and polypharmacy with associated problematic drug–drug interactions. It follows that, in the setting of these complex medical conditions, clinicians will encounter situations in which the drugs themselves are potential causes of urgent or emergent clinical problems.

A thorough discussion of psychiatric emergencies is beyond the scope of this text. The approach and response to such emergencies is generally based on appropriate psychiatric assessment and clinical decision making so as to minimize clinical risks and assure patient and staff safety. Here we focus on emergencies or dangers arising from pharmacologic management itself, including serotonin syndrome, neuroleptic malignant syndrome, and overdose of psychotropic drugs commonly utilized in oncology and palliative care. This is not simple in the setting of a medically complex patient population undergoing active chemotherapy, major surgical procedures, and palliative interventions carrying increased risk of polypharmacy and medication interactions. We hope to help define and identify these risks to help guide clinical management.

17.2   Serotonin Syndrome

Serotonin syndrome is a psychopharmacologic emergency both dangerous and difficult to diagnose. In the settings of oncology and palliative care where polypharmacy is common, increased vigilance for serotonin toxicity is prudent.

Serotonin toxicity is caused by excessive levels of circulating serotonin in the central nervous system and periphery. In conducting a comprehensive medication list review, it is important to be cognizant of all potential sources for increased circulating serotonin: increased serotonin synthesis, augmented serotonin release, blockade of serotonin reuptake from the synapse, inhibition of serotonin metabolism, direct antagonism of serotonin receptors, and increased postsynaptic response to serotonin (Woytowish and Maynor 2013) (see Table 17.1). Medication sources include traditional antidepressant medications (selective serotonin reuptake inhibitors (SSRIs), serotonin norepinephrine reuptake inhibitors (SNRIs,) bupropion, mirtazepine, etc.), herbal supplements (St. John's Wort, L-tryptophan), and opioid pain medications (methadone, fentanyl, codeine). Illicit drugs including

Table 17.1 Serotonergic agents organized by mechanism of increasing serotonin concentration and drug class [Woytowish and Maynor (2013), Quinn and Stern (2009)]

	Antidepressant/Anxiolytic/Stimulants	Analgesics	Herbal supplement	Illicit psychotropics	Other
Increased serotonin synthesis			L-Tryptophan		
Augmentation of serotonin release	Amphetamine and derivatives, Mirtazapine	Codeine		Cocaine, MDMA	Levodopa, Reserpine, Linezolid, Procarbazine
	MAOI Tranylcypromine, Phenelzine, Selegiline				
Blockade of serotonin reuptake	SSRI Citalopram, Escitalopram, Fluoxetine, Fluvoxamine, Sertraline, Paroxetine	Dextromethorphan, Fentanyl, Meperidine,[a] Methadone, Tramadol	St. John's wort		Sumitriptan and other triptans
	SNRI Venlafaxine, Duloxetine				
	TCA Amitriptyline, Clomipramine, Desipramine, Doxepin, Imipramine, Nortriptyline, Protriptyline				
	NRI Trazodone				
Inhibition of serotonin metabolism	MAOI Tranylcypromine, Phenelzine, Selegiline		St. John's wort	Cocaine	Linezolid, Procarbazine
Direct antagonism of seratonin receptors	Buspirone			Lysergic acid diethylamide	Bromocriptine, Carbamazepine, Lithium
Increased postsynaptic response	Trazdone				Lithium

[a]Meperidine is frequently used to block chills associated with antifugal infusions

cocaine, amphetamines, MDMA (3,4-methylenedioxymethamphetamine), and lysergic acid diethylamide (LSD) can influence circulating serotonin levels. There are other drugs with significantly different, nonpsychiatric active clinical purpose which are known to influence serotonin levels (linezolid, procarbazine, meperidine.) Additionally severe hepatic dysfunction will decrease CYP450 enzyme activity thereby increasing concentrations of SSRIs which are normally excreted/metabolized through this pathway (Woytowish and Maynor 2013).

Serotonin toxicity is protean in its clinical presentation and nature. As a toxicologic syndrome, it is a diagnosis of exclusion.

Despite diverse presentations, serotonin toxicity is classically described as a triad including mental status changes, autonomic hyperactivity, and neuromuscular abnormalities (Quinn and Stern 2009; Boyer and Shannon 2005). The impact of this toxicity can range in intensity from mild/nearly imperceptible to lethal. It is associated with current or recent administration of serotonergic agents and most often arises shortly after (6–12 h) initiation of or in change in such a medication (Quinn and Stern 2009; Boyer and Shannon 2005).

Due to the insidious and often occult nature of the presentation, community incidence is difficult to describe; it is thought to be rising with the increasing availability and use of pro-serotonergic agents in clinical practice (Boyer and Shannon 2005). In its mild from, serotonin toxicity presents as a series of minor symptoms easily attributable to other causes in a medically complicated patient: tachycardia, shivering, diaphoresis, restlessness/inability to sit still, intermittent myoclonus, and hyperreflexia (Quinn and Stern 2009; Boyer and Shannon 2005).

With moderate severity, additional signs and symptoms of serotonin toxicity are observed. Patients may present with moderate hypertension, hyperthermia, or hyperactive bowel sounds. They may have inducible clonus in their extremities or ocular clonus. They may appear slightly agitated, hypervigilant, or exhibit pressured speech (Quinn and Stern 2009). Overall, the presence of clonus is thought to be the most important clinical finding to support a diagnosis of serotonin toxicity (Woytowish and Maynor 2013; Quinn and Stern 2009).

In severe cases of serotonin toxicity, autonomic instability is observed, with resulting abrupt fluctuations from severe hypertension and tachycardia to hypotensive shock (Boyer and Shannon 2005). Patients experience delirium and extreme hypertonicity and muscle rigidity. It is often only in these severe cases that serotonin toxicity is accompanied by laboratory findings: metabolic acidosis, rhabdomyolysis and elevated serum creatinine and aminotransferase. Patients may go on to develop seizures, renal failure, and disseminated intravascular coagulopathy (Quinn and Stern 2009; Boyer and Shannon 2005).

Clinical Case

A 41-year-old white female with a history of Stage I Breast Cancer status post surgery and radiation therapy, with no current evidence of disease, presented to outpatient psychiatry clinic for exacerbation of chronic

(continued)

depression. She reported a greater than 10-year history of major depressive disorder and a history of difficulty tolerating many different trials of antidepressant medications due to severe side effects occurring at the time of medication introduction. Despite this, she was placed on citalopram and slowly titrated to a dose 60 mg/day with variable relief of depressive symptoms. Her residual symptoms included insomnia and intense pessimistic ruminations. Over several weeks, multiple different medications were added to treat her residual symptoms. Lorazepam was effective in reducing residual anxiety but not insomnia. Zolipdem and trazodone were of marginal benefit. Olanzapine resulted in mild tremor and morning drowsiness. Lastly, temazepam 15–30 mg was added to target her residual insomnia.

The patient subsequently presented to clinic complaining of severe nausea and light-headedness and vertigo. Her vital signs were stable. Citalopram was decreased to 40 mg/day. Within a few days, she represents now to the emergency room reporting worsening nausea, vomiting, tremor, and vertigo. She was noted to have stable blood pressure, with tachycardia ranging from 100–120 s. The patient was admitted for presumed serotonin toxicity. Citalopram was discontinued. Supportive measures were initiated, including intravenous hydration, intravenous lorazepam, and use of scopolamine and dexamethasone to treat her nausea. Over a 10-day course, her symptoms gradually improved. Following discharge home, she remained drowsy and fatigued for several weeks but was eventually able to return to activities of daily living. She continued treatment of her depression with buproprion and psychotherapy.

Given the protean nature of the presentations of this toxicologic syndrome, use of existing diagnostic criteria often helps clarify the diagnosis of serotonin toxicity. The first diagnostic criteria developed, Sternbach's criteria, required the presence of three serotonergic symptoms in the setting of serotonergic drug use and a clear absence of other potential causes, including the absence of neuroleptic use (Woytowish and Maynor 2013; Quinn and Stern 2009; Sternbach 1991) (see Table 17.2). In the setting of the oncology/palliative care patient, often with multiple possible complications, immune compromise, and possible organ toxicity, our ability to completely rule out other causes is impractical. Sternbach's criteria are now recognized to under-identify early, mild presentations of serotonin toxicity (Woytowish and Maynor 2013). The later devised Hunter Serotonin Toxicity Criteria (HSTC) describe five different signs/symptom pairs/trios diagnostic of serotonin toxicity when observed in association with recent use of a serotonergic agent (Woytowish and Maynor 2013; Dunkley et al. 2003) (see Table 17.2). These are noted to be both more sensitive (84 % vs. 75 %) and more specific (97 % vs. 96 %) than the Sternbach Criteria (Woytowish and Maynor 2013; Dunkley et al. 2003). Review of these criteria once again reminds us of the central role of clonus in establishing a diagnosis for serotonin toxicity.

When confronted with clinical suggestion by symptom cluster, it is important to closely review the patient's recent medication exposures looking for changes or

Table 17.2 Diagnostic criteria for serotonin toxicity

Sternbach criteria: Sternbach (1991)		
• Recent addition or increase of a serotonergic agent		
• No recent addition of a neuroleptic agent		
Absence of other potential etiologies		
≥3 of the following	• Mental status changes	• Agitation
	• Myoclonus	• Hyperreflexia
	• Diaphoresis	• Shivering
	• Tremor	• Diarrhea
	• Incoordination	• Fever
Hunter serotonin toxicity criteria: Dunkley et al. (2003)		
The presence of any of the following in association with use of a serotonergic agent in the last 5 weeks:		
	• Spontaneous clonus	
	• Inducible clonus and agitation or diaphoresis	
	• Ocular clonus and agitation or diaphoresis	
	• Tremor and hyperreflexia	
	Hypertonic and temperature >38 °C and ocular clonus	

additions of serotonergic agents. In the oncologic setting, there are certain medications which can cause an unintended rise in serotonin. Non-psychotropic MAOIs are increasingly common in the oncologic setting, leading to a more common concern for this interaction. Monoamine oxidase inhibitors act via either reversible or irreversible inhibition of the enzyme involved in serotonin metabolism. Thus, especially irreversible MAOIs (e.g., selegiline) are strongly associated with serotonin toxicity when administered with other serotoninergic agents (Boyer and Shannon 2005).

Procarbazine is an antineoplastic (chemotherapy) agent with monoamine oxidase inhibitor properties currently used in the treatment of central nervous system lymphoma. It is recommended that use of traditional serotonergic agents like SSRIs be held during the period of procarbazine treatment. Depending on the agent, a washout period of up to 5 weeks prior to initiation of procarbazine is recommended. The risks of potential serotonin syndrome must be weighed against the risks of decreased therapeutic effectiveness from withholding chemotherapeutic agents. This determination requires collaboration with the full treatment team.

Linezolid is an oxazolidinone antimicrobial agent widely used in the treatment of drug-resistant gram positive infections. It is also a weak, reversible nonselective monoamine oxidase inhibitor. While initial Phase III trials did not demonstrate occurrence of serotonin toxicity with concurrent SSRI use (Rubinstein et al. 2003), post-marketing studies suggested findings of linezolid-associated serotonin toxicity (Lawrence et al. 2006). In 2011, the Food and Drug Administration (FDA) officially issued a caution about coadministration of linezolid with serotonergic agents. A pooled retrospective analysis of data from 20 Phase III and IV comparison trials for linezolid reviewed all patients concomitantly taking a serotonergic agent with their antimicrobial therapy. It found similar rates of serotonin toxicity (by either

Sternbach or Hunter criteria) between those patients on linezolid and the comparator antimicrobial agents, with 9 of 2,208 linezolid patients (0.41 %) and 3 of the 2,057 comparator patients (0.15 %) meeting Sternbach criteria and 2 (0.14 %) of the linezolid and 1 (0.05 %) of the comparator patients meeting Hunter criteria (Butterfield et al. 2012). Recent small retrospective reviews have suggested slightly higher incidence rates (2–4 %) for serotonin toxicity in patients taking concomitant serotonergic agents with linezolid (Woytowish and Maynor 2013; Taylor et al. 2006).

Linezolid-associated serotonin toxicity is expected to present within 1 day to 3 weeks of coadministration (Quinn and Stern 2009). It has, however, been described in cases of nonoverlapping administration with washout periods of 3–18 days (Wigen and Goetz 2002; Morales and Vermette 2005). Given the low incidence, current recommendations urge careful risk–benefit analysis to determine the appropriate course for any patient in need of concurrent use of both seratonergic agents and linezolid (Woytowish and Maynor 2013; Quinn and Stern 2009).

Treatment of serotonin toxicity is defined primarily by removal of the identified offending agent and supportive care measures (Boyer and Shannon 2005). Supportive measures include the administration of intravenous fluids and correction of abnormal vital signs. As the hyperthermia of serotonin toxicity is resultant from muscular activity, rather than alteration of the hypothalamic set point, treatment of this alteration is approached through use of muscle relaxants rather than antipyretics. Benzodiazepines are the intervention of choice for mild to moderate cases, with full neuromuscular paralysis (with sedation and intubation) recommended for severely hyperthermic patients. Succinylcholine is contraindicated in these cases due to the risk of arrhythmias associated with likely hyperkalemia seen in patients with several rhabodomyolysis (Boyer and Shannon 2005). Use of physical restraints, potentially increasing isometric muscle contractions, is not recommended for patients with serotonin syndrome.

5-HT receptor antagonists can be considered for moderate to severe risk cases. Cyproheptadine, an antihistamine with 5-HT1A and 5-HT2A antagonist activity can quickly saturate the receptors with repeated administration. Chlorpromazine, a phenothiazine with antagonism at the 5-HT2A receptor has also been used successfully (Musselman and Saely 2013; Ramsey et al. 2013).

Other therapies, including propranolol, Bromocriptine, and dantroline, are not recommended (Boyer and Shannon 2005). While a 5-HT1A antagonist, propranolol use can result in hypotension and shock through beta blockade. Bronmocriptine may precipitate rather than treat serotonin toxicity and dantrolene has not been found to have survival benefits.

17.3 Neuroleptic Malignant Syndrome

Neuroleptic malignant syndrome (NMS) is another rare but potentially life-threatening psychopharmacologic emergency. It shares several properties with serotonin syndrome, occurring in the setting of recent or ongoing use of a

Table 17.3 Comparison of clinical presentation of serotonin toxicity and neuroleptic malignant syndrome

	Serotonin toxicity	Neuroleptic malignant syndrome
Time from exposure	<24 h	Within 72 h
Vital signs	Hypertension, tachycardia, tachypnea, hyperthermia	Hypertension, tachycardia, tachypnea, hyperthermia
Neuromuscular tone	Increased	"Lead pipe" rigidity
Reflexes	Hyperreflexia, clonus	Bradyreflexia
Mental status	Altered	Altered
Laboratory findings	None specific or suggestive	Elevated CK, WBC

predominately psychotropic medication, and can present with a complex collection of symptoms (Table 17.3).

NMS is most commonly linked to medications causing dopamine blockade, but can be similarly provoked by abrupt withdrawal of dopamine agonist medications (Perry and Wilborn 2012). Despite this link to dopamine, the underlying pathophysiology of NMS is not fully understood. Clinical and laboratory observations suggest a central role of dopaminergic hypofunction in the development of NMS, yet there is similar evidence to implicate sympathoadrenal dysfunction as well (Strawn et al. 2007). The frequency of NMS in the general population is low and thought to be decreased due to increased awareness (Strawn et al. 2007). Reports have described rates ranging from 0.01 to 2.2 % of at risk patients (Strawn et al. 2007; Hermesh et al. 1992; Keck et al. 1989a).

Many attempts have been made to clarify the potential risk factors for development of NMS. Limitations of studies have made it difficult to distinguish true independent risk factors from confounding variables or associations (Perry and Wilborn 2012). Rapidly escalating neuroleptic doses has been identified as potentially increasing a patient's risk of developing NMS (Perry and Wilborn 2012). Consideration for age, sex, external heat load, route of administration (INTRAMUSCULAR or depot), and level of agitation as potential risk factors have been proposed (Keck et al. 1989b). Strict review of the literature has failed to confirm strong evidence for these as predictive risk factors for the development of NMS (Perry and Wilborn 2012; Strawn et al. 2007).

Clinically, NMS mostly commonly presents with four cardinal symptoms: muscle rigidity, hyperpyrexia, mental status changes, and autonomic instability (Perry and Wilborn 2012). Within 72 h of initiation of dopaminergic medication, patients are observed to experience hyperthermia, profuse diaphoresis, and "lead pipe" rigidity. They are noted to have a change in mental status, often becoming confused, inattentive, or catatonic. Autonomic instability is encountered with elevated or fluctuating blood pressure, tachycardia, and tachypnea (American Psychiatric Association 2013). Laboratory findings may be associated with but not are specific for the diagnosis of NMS (Strawn et al. 2007). Associated laboratory values include marked elevation of creatine kinase, elevated white blood cell count, and decreased serum iron concentration. NMS is also associated with elevated catecholamines and elevated transaminases (Perry and Wilborn 2012; Strawn et al. 2007; American Psychiatric Association 2013). Several other neurologic signs or symptoms are described including tremor, sialorrhea, akinesia, dystonia, trismus, myoclonus, dysarthria, dysphagia, and urinary incontinence.

Unlike serotonin syndrome, there is no single, definitively accepted collection of diagnostic criteria for NMS. Several attempts have been made to define unified, validated diagnostic criteria (Keck et al. 1989a; Addonizio et al. 1987; Sachdev 2005; Gurrera et al. 2011). All agree on the central requirement of recent exposure to dopamine antagonists vs. withdrawal of dopamine agonists. "Recent" is commonly defined as within the last 72 h (American Psychiatric Association 2013; Gurrera et al. 2011) but has also been described as within the last 2 weeks or last 30 days (Perry and Wilborn 2012; Strawn et al. 2007). Recently organized collaboration of experts in the field resulted in the development of consensus criteria (Table 17.4). These have yet to be validated (Gurrera et al. 2011).

Given the central features of high fever, altered mental status, autonomic instability, and neurologic symptoms, the differential diagnosis for NMS could be extensive, including bacterial, fungal, or viral infections; antichlinergic delirium; serotonin toxicity, and malignant hyperthermia (Owen 2011). Appropriate work- up would involve full cultures including cerebrospinal fluid, neuroimaging, and other assays as indicated by the specifics of each patient's medical situation.

The mainstay treatment of NMS is similar to that of serotonin toxicity: remove the offending/causative agent and provide supportive care. Supportive measures often include fluid resuscitation, cooling measures, and cardiovascular support. Close attention to respiratory and renal function must also be paid.

Several agents have been considered as treatments for NMS. Dantrolene, a peripheral muscle relaxant, acting through inhibition of intracellular calcium release, is a treatment for malignant hyperthermia and has been used and is often listed as the main treatment for NMS. No prospective trials exist, and recent review of published case reports did not demonstrate clear benefit over current advanced supportive care approaches alone (Reulbach et al. 2007). Bromocriptine and amantadine have been proposed through their action as dopamine agonists for the treatment of NMS as well. However, some investigators have concluded that these agents have similarly failed to demonstrate benefit over supportive care alone (Sakkas et al. 1991).

In the setting of oncologic and palliative care, it is important to be aware that frequently used antiemetic drugs including metaclopromide and promethazine are dopaminergic agents, potentially causing NMS. Use of metaclopromide alone has resulted in cases of NMS (Nachreiner et al. 2006). Close attention must be paid when these agents are used with other dopamine agonists or antagonists.

Table 17.4 Proposed diagnostic criteria for neuroleptic malignant syndrome

• Exposure to dopamine antagonist or withdrawal of dopamine agonist in the last 72 h

• Hyperthermia (record of two prior temperatures >100.4 °F or >38.0 °C)

• Rigidity

• Alteration of mental status

• Elevation of creatinine kinase (>4× the upper limit of normal)

• Lability of the sympathetic nervous system, including two of the following:

  • Elevation of blood pressure (with systolic or diastolic ≥ 25 % above baseline)

  • Fluctuation of blood pressure (with ≥ 25 mmHg systolic or ≥20 mmHg diastolic change in 24 h)

  • Diaphoresis

  • Urinary incontinence

• Evidence of hypermetabolism (heart rate ≥25 % above baseline and respiratory rate ≥50 % above baseline)

• Negative work up for infectious, toxic, metabolic, or neurologic causes

Adapted from Guerra et al. (2011)

17.4 Overdose/Intoxication

Drugs that would be reasonably well tolerated in healthy individuals are potentially dangerous in high acuity and end stage disease settings. In our experience these situations are usually of accidental or idiosyncratic etiology as opposed to the result of deliberate actions (e.g., suicide).

17.4.1 Benzodiazepines

These drugs usually have a favorable safety profile. However, the therapeutic/toxic ratio of benzodiazepines (BZPs) is often much smaller than in other (ambulatory care) settings. Potential BZP-associated medical emergencies would include hypotension, decreased respiratory drive, or respiratory arrest. This risk is increased when the drugs are used with other central nervous system depressants (e.g., opioid analgesics, some antihypertensive agents, alcohol.) Especially in the critically ill and cognitively impaired, BZPs can cause or exacerbate delirium (Gaudreau et al. 2005; Rothberg et al. 2013).

While the risk of BZP-associated emergencies is decreased by avoiding or minimizing their use, when indicated, use of shorter-acting agents, such as lorazepam, is safer in the setting of critical illness and palliative care. There likely is a limited role for benzodiazepine antagonists and specifically of flumazenil in specific cases of acute BZP intoxication or overdose (Park et al. 1995; Weinbroum et al. 1996). However, the utility of flumazenil, has not been addressed in the oncology and palliative care literature.

17.4.2 Antipsychotics

Overdose of antipsychotic medications is common in the general population (Bronstein et al. 2011). In our experience in a tertiary care cancer center, intentional overdoses involving antipsychotics are rare. Given polypharmacy, the possibility of accidental overdose or poisoning must be anticipated.

There has been a substantial move to use of second generation or atypical antipsychotics in general psychiatric settings and a trend toward the same in medical psychiatric care (see Chap. 10). An exception is management of delirium, where the use of intravenous haloperidol predominates. Fatalities associated with second generation antipsychotic overdose are rare (Trenton et al. 2003). While a wide range of side effects are encountered, emergent toxicity of second generation antipsychotics will usually involve the cardiovascular and/or central nervous systems (Minns and Clark 2012). In elderly patient with dementia, second generation antipsychotics are associated with an approximate twofold increase of sudden cardiac death compared to nonusers of such drugs. A large retrospective review reveals the same risk for typical antipsychotics (Ray et al. 2009). The exact mechanisms of cardiac death in this and other studies could not be definitely determined, though dysrhythmias associated with cardiac conduction delays are implicated (Jolly et al. 2009). This data contributed to FDA requirements for black box warnings regarding the use of these drugs in this patient population.

A recent review found that significant hypotension is also an uncommon side effect of these medications, quetiapine being an exception (Tan et al. 2009). Antimuscarinic effects of second generation antipsychotics are such that they may be primary or contributing causes of anticholinergic delirium; this is especially true of clozapine, quetiapine, and olanzapine (Levine and Ruha 2012).

Prolongation of the QTc interval has been reported with many second generation antipsychotics but lethal dysrhythmias, including torsades de pointes (TdP), appear to be rare (Jolly et al. 2009). Ziprasidone appears to have the highest risk of QTc prolongation of the second generation antipsychotics (Beach et al. 2013).

Of the typical, or first generation, antipsychotics, thioridazine is most associated with QTc prolongation and TdP, resulting in less frequent use in consultation-liaison psychiatry settings. Other typical antipsychotics have also been linked to QTc prolongation. Of these, haloperidol, particularly in the intravenous formulation, is front-line (though off-label) therapy for management of delirium and a potential cause for concern (Beach et al. 2013). Though the risk of QTc prolongation and TdP associated with most typical and second generation antipsychotics is actually fairly modest, it should be remembered that in oncology and palliative care settings, these drugs will not be used in isolation. Patients may be at risk because of simultaneous use of other QTc-prolonging drugs. Additional contributing medical factors may include electrolyte disturbances, baseline cardiovascular disease, and other comorbid illnesses.

17.4.3 Antidepressants

Antidepressant medications are also frequently involved in suicidal ingestions (White et al. 2008). There is considerable variability of toxicity and lethality between and within classes of antidepressants. Monoamine oxidase inhibitors and tricyclic/tetracyclic antidepressants (excepting mirtazapine) are more frequently implicated in completed suicides and those with serious medical consequences, than are newer agents including SSRIs and SNRIs and others (White et al. 2008; Hawton et al. 2010).

The potential for serious or lethal side effects of MAOIs, including hypertensive crisis (due to ingestion of tyramine-rich foods and drug–drug interactions) and serotonin toxicity, is such that these antidepressants are rarely used in oncology and palliative care settings.

Tricyclic antidepressants (TCAs) are most often used in oncology and palliative care as adjuncts in treatment of neuropathic pain. This is typically at low doses which minimizes the risk of serious toxicity in the absence of drug–drug interactions or intentional overdose. Common side effects of TCAs include anticholinergic effects and hypotension, to which oncology and palliative care patients may be quite vulnerable. At high doses, TCAs can be associated with seizures. TCAs are potentially lethal in overdose secondary to cardiac conduction delays and non-recoverable cardiac dysrhythmias. These drugs should be used cautiously, if at all, in individuals at high risk for suicide and in patients with histories of cardiac disease, including chemotherapy-associated cardiomyopathy (Torta and Ieraci 2013).

Selective serotonin reuptake inhibitors are relatively safe in intentional overdose. They are associated with little risk of cardiac conduction delays or dysrhythmias, citalopram being a possible exception (Beach et al. 2013). Used alone or in combination with other serotonergic drugs (see Case), SSRIs are associated with serotonin toxicity.

Mixed action and "atypical" antidepressants (serotonin–norepinephrine reuptake inhibitors, bupropion, trazodone) are also relatively safe in overdose. As with other antidepressants, risk of serotonin toxicity increases in the setting of polypharmacy. Bupropion is associated with increased risk of seizures in predisposed individuals.

Conclusion

Psychopharmacologic emergencies in oncology and palliative care are most often a function of acuity of illness and polypharmacy. Given these complexities, frequent consideration of the differential diagnosis of possible drug toxicity is critical to maintain safety and meet goals of care. Close collaboration with other providers (oncology, infectious disease, neurology, pharmacy, critical care) and other members of the full psychosocial team is essential to safe pharmacologic management of these patients.

▶ **Key Points**

Use of psychotropic drugs in the setting of oncology and palliative care is associated with several possible serious complications.

Close attention must be paid to mild/moderate serotonin toxicity to avoid progression to potential emergent complications.

Clinicians should be vigilant in monitoring for polypharmacy so as to minimize potential toxicities.

References

Addonizio G, Susman VL, Roth SD. Neuroleptic malignant syndrome: review and analysis of 115 cases. Biol Psychiatry. 1987;22(8):1004–20.

American Psychiatric Association. Diagnostic and statistical manual of mental disorders. 5th ed. Arlington, VA: American Psychiatric Association; 2013.

Beach SR, et al. QTc prolongation, torsades de pointes, and psychotropic medications. Psychosomatics. 2013;54(1):1–13.

Boyer EW, Shannon M. The serotonin syndrome. N Engl J Med. 2005;352(11):1112–20.

Bronstein AC, et al. 2010 Annual Report of the American Association of Poison Control Centers' National Poison Data System (NPDS): 28th annual report. Clin Toxicol (Phila). 2011;49(10):910–41.

Butterfield JM, et al. Comparison of serotonin toxicity with concomitant use of either linezolid or comparators and serotonergic agents: an analysis of Phase III and IV randomized clinical trial data. J Antimicrob Chemother. 2012;67(2):494–502.

Dunkley EJ, et al. The hunter serotonin toxicity criteria: simple and accurate diagnostic decision rules for serotonin toxicity. QJM. 2003;96(9):635–42.

Gaudreau JD, et al. Psychoactive medications and risk of delirium in hospitalized cancer patients. J Clin Oncol. 2005;23(27):6712–8.

Gurrera RJ, et al. An international consensus study of neuroleptic malignant syndrome diagnostic criteria using the Delphi method. J Clin Psychiatry. 2011;72(9):1222–8.

Hawton K, et al. Toxicity of antidepressants: rates of suicide relative to prescribing and non-fatal overdose. Br J Psychiatry. 2010;196(5):354–8.

Hermesh H, et al. Risk for definite neuroleptic malignant syndrome. A prospective study in 223 consecutive in-patients. Br J Psychiatry. 1992;161:254–7.

Jolly K, et al. Sudden death in patients receiving drugs tending to prolong the QT interval. Br J Clin Pharmacol. 2009;68(5):743–51.

Keck Jr PE, et al. Frequency and presentation of neuroleptic malignant syndrome in a state psychiatric hospital. J Clin Psychiatry. 1989a;50(9):352–5.

Keck Jr PE, et al. Risk factors for neuroleptic malignant syndrome. A case-control study. Arch Gen Psychiatry. 1989b;46(10):914–8.

Lawrence KR, Adra M, Gillman PK. Serotonin toxicity associated with the use of linezolid: a review of postmarketing data. Clin Infect Dis. 2006;42(11):1578–83.

Levine M, Ruha AM. Overdose of atypical antipsychotics: clinical presentation, mechanisms of toxicity and management. CNS Drugs. 2012;26(7):601–11.

Minns AB, Clark RF. Toxicology and overdose of atypical antipsychotics. J Emerg Med. 2012;43(5):906–13.

Morales N, Vermette H. Serotonin syndrome associated with linezolid treatment after discontinuation of fluoxetine. Psychosomatics. 2005;46(3):274–5.

Musselman ME, Saely S. Diagnosis and treatment of drug-induced hyperthermia. Am J Health Syst Pharm. 2013;70(1):34–42.

Nachreiner R, et al. Neuroleptic malignant syndrome associated with metoclopramide in a burn patient. J Burn Care Res. 2006;27(2):237–41.

Owen JA. Psychopharmacology. In: Levenson JL, editor. The American Psychiatric Publishing textbook of psychosomatic medicine: psychiatric care of the medically ill. Washington, DC: American Psychiatric Publishing; 2011. p. 241–59.

Park GR, Navapurkar V, Ferenci P. The role of flumazenil in the critically ill. Acta Anaesthesiol Scand. 1995;39:23–34.

Perry PJ, Wilborn CA. Serotonin syndrome vs neuroleptic malignant syndrome: a contrast of causes, diagnoses, and management. Ann Clin Psychiatry. 2012;24(2):155–62.

Quinn DK, Stern TA. Linezolid and serotonin syndrome. Prim Care Companion J Clin Psychiatry. 2009;11(6):353–6.

Ramsey TD, Lau TT, Ensom MH. Serotonergic and adrenergic drug interactions associated with linezolid: a critical review and practical management approach. Ann Pharmacother. 2013; 47(4):543–60.

Ray WA, et al. Atypical antipsychotic drugs and the risk of sudden cardiac death. N Engl J Med. 2009;360(3):225–35.

Reulbach U, et al. Managing an effective treatment for neuroleptic malignant syndrome. Crit Care. 2007;11(1):R4.

Rothberg MB, et al. Association between sedating medications and delirium in older inpatients. J Am Geriatr Soc. 2013;61(6):923–30.

Rubinstein E, et al. Worldwide assessment of linezolid's clinical safety and tolerability: comparator-controlled phase III studies. Antimicrob Agents Chemother. 2003;47(6):1824–31.

Sachdev PS. A rating scale for neuroleptic malignant syndrome. Psychiatry Res. 2005;135(3): 249–56.

Sakkas P, et al. Drug treatment of the neuroleptic malignant syndrome. Psychopharmacol Bull. 1991;27(3):381–4.

Sternbach H. The serotonin syndrome. Am J Psychiatry. 1991;148(6):705–13.

Strawn JR, Keck Jr PE, Caroff SN. Neuroleptic malignant syndrome. Am J Psychiatry. 2007; 164(6):870–6.

Tan HH, Hoppe J, Heard K. A systematic review of cardiovascular effects after atypical antipsychotic medication overdose. Am J Emerg Med. 2009;27(5):607–16.

Taylor JJ, Wilson JW, Estes LL. Linezolid and serotonergic drug interactions: a retrospective survey. Clin Infect Dis. 2006;43(2):180–7.

Torta RG, Ieraci V. Pharmacological management of depression in patients with cancer: practical considerations. Drugs. 2013;73(11):1131–45.

Trenton A, Currier G, Zwemer F. Fatalities associated with therapeutic use and overdose of atypical antipsychotics. CNS Drugs. 2003;17(5):307–24.

Weinbroum A, et al. Use of flumazenil in the treatment of drug overdose: a double-blind and open clinical study in 110 patients. Crit Care Med. 1996;24(2):199–206.

White N, Litovitz T, Clancy C. Suicidal antidepressant overdoses: a comparative analysis by antidepressant type. J Med Toxicol. 2008;4(4):238–50.

Wigen CL, Goetz MB. Serotonin syndrome and linezolid. Clin Infect Dis. 2002;34(12):1651–2.

Woytowish MR, Maynor LM. Clinical relevance of linezolid-associated serotonin toxicity. Ann Pharmacother. 2013;47(3):388–97.

Psychopharmacology in Palliative Care and Oncology: Childhood and Adolescence

18

Marcy Forgey and Brenda Bursch

Abstract

A diagnosis of childhood cancer is an unexpected event that can interrupt a child's developmental trajectory. Palliative symptom management can improve quality of life as well as psychological, functional, and medical outcomes for a child who is coping with cancer. Within a larger framework of behavioral and family-based interventions, this chapter focuses on palliative psychopharmacological treatment recommendations for children with cancer. Sertraline, citalopram, or escitalopram should be considered first line for anxiety, PTSD, or depression. Risperidone or quetiapine can be an effective second-line adjunct for children with severe anxiety or trauma symptoms. Aggressive pain management with opiates can prevent iatrogenic trauma symptoms. Sleep problems may respond to melatonin, diphenhydramine, or trazodone. A low dose of quetiapine may treat insomnia due to delirium or severe anxiety. Risperidone is recommended for hypoactive/mixed delirium and haloperidol for hyperactive delirium.

M. Forgey (✉)
Pediatric C/L Psychiatry Service Division of Child Psychiatry, Department of Psychiatry and Biobehavioral Sciences, UCLA Semel Institute for Neuroscience and Human Behavior, David Geffen School of Medicine at UCLA, 760 Westwood Plaza, Semel 58-242C, Los Angeles, CA 90024, USA
e-mail: mforgey@mednet.ucla.edu

B. Bursch
Pediatric C/L Psychiatry Service Division of Child Psychiatry, Department of Psychiatry and Biobehavioral Sciences, UCLA Semel Institute for Neuroscience and Human Behavior, David Geffen School of Medicine at UCLA, 760 Westwood Plaza, Semel 58-242C, Los Angeles, CA 90024, USA

Department of Pediatrics, UCLA Semel Institute for Neuroscience and Human Behavior, David Geffen School of Medicine at UCLA, 760 Westwood Plaza, Semel 48-253C, Los Angeles, CA 90024, USA
e-mail: bbursch@mednet.ucla.edu

L. Grassi and M. Riba (eds.), *Psychopharmacology in Oncology and Palliative Care*,
DOI 10.1007/978-3-642-40134-3_18, © Springer-Verlag Berlin Heidelberg 2014

331

18.1   Introduction

Despite numerous stressors, pediatric cancer patients report relatively few psychological symptoms (Erickson and Steiner 2000; Phipps and Srivastava 1999). Nevertheless, some children fare less well than the majority, with significant psychological and/or physical sequelae from their cancer experience. Over time, the need for intervention during acute treatment to improve quality of life and minimize negative outcomes has been increasingly recognized. This chapter focuses on assessment and treatment of common psychological and physical symptoms in pediatric oncology.

18.2   Treatment of Psychiatric Symptoms

18.2.1 Anxiety

Children with cancer are at risk for anxiety. Contributing factors include noxious physical symptoms, distressing procedures, medications, hospital environment, separation from parents, parents' emotional response, fear of pain or death, or lack of consistent, accurate, age-appropriate information. Those at the end of life may experience significant restlessness as a result of unrelieved physical symptoms such as pain or hypoxia (Stuber and Bursch 2009).

Behavioral interventions should target underlying causes. Children benefit from age-appropriate explanations, having personal belongings with them in the hospital, a predictable schedule, familiar activities, and parent support (Kersun and Shemesh 2007). Cognitive behavioral therapy is effective for anxiety symptoms and exposure, and systematic desensitization is helpful to treat food aversion or needle phobia (Piacentini and Bergman 2001).

For persistent distressing or disabling anxiety symptoms, selective serotonin reuptake inhibitors (SSRIs) should be considered. Fluvoxamine, fluoxetine, and sertraline are superior to placebo in treating youth with separation anxiety, social anxiety, or generalized anxiety disorder (RUPP 2001; Walkup et al. 2008). Fluvoxamine is safe, effective, and well tolerated in children with cancer and anxiety (Gothelf et al. 2005). Consideration must be given to potential medication interactions as well as SSRI effects on bodily systems. Sertraline, citalopram, and escitalopram have minimal drug/drug interactions (Bursch and Forgey 2013).

Since platelet serotonin reuptake inhibition may result in reduced platelet function, platelet levels should be over 100,000 before starting an SSRI (Meijer et al. 2004; Bursch and Forgey 2013). Use of linezolid, a weak monoamine oxidase inhibitor, in combination with an SSRI increases risk of serotonin toxicity. This combination should only be used if benefits outweigh risks (Ramsey et al. 2013). Optimally, SSRIs should be started 2 weeks after linezolid has been discontinued. If a child already taking an SSRI must be started on linezolid, observation for signs of serotonin toxicity should occur for a minimum of 3 weeks (Quinn and Stern 2009).

Children with cancer frequently undergo treatment with cardiotoxic chemotherapy drugs and may be on QTc prolonging medications like methadone (Simbre et al. 2005; Mercadante et al. 2013). Since high doses of citalopram may cause QTc prolongation, the FDA recommends a 20 mg maximum dose for patients with liver dysfunction, poor CYP 219 metabolizers, and those taking cimetidine. Children with congenital long QT syndrome should not take citalopram (FDA 2013). Evidence suggests that escitalopram has potentially similar concerns (Hayes et al. 2010).

Despite little data for use of benzodiazepines as a primary childhood anxiety treatment, they are often used in the hospital for sedation since they have an IV route of administration. However, children are at potential risk of a paradoxical, agitated reaction to benzodiazepines that can worsen anxiety. Some youth also dislike the sedative effects and find it difficult to use coping skills while under their influence. Additional risks include dependence, decreased slow wave (most restorative) sleep, anterograde amnesia, and delirium (Owens 2009; Smith et al. 2011a, b). If IV administration is not required, antipsychotics such as low dose risperidone or quetiapine can be helpful to treat acute anxiety. Benzodiazepines may be effectively used in children with cancer who have seizures, catatonia, air hunger, or severe treatment-resistant nausea, assuming there is no adverse reaction (Bursch and Forgey 2013).

Since pain is often comorbid with anxiety, effective pain management may alleviate anxiety. For example, morphine is analgesic, euphoriant, and anxiolytic (Stuber and Bursch 2009). If anxiety is comorbid with insomnia, neuropathic pain, diarrhea, and/or weight loss, tricyclic antidepressants may be beneficial (Pao and Bosk 2011).

18.2.2 Pediatric Iatrogenic Medical Trauma

Trauma- and stress-related disorders commonly seen in children with cancer include posttraumatic stress disorder (PTSD), acute stress disorder, and adjustment disorders. Pediatric iatrogenic medical trauma, the subject of this section, is defined as illness- or treatment-related trauma symptoms (Forgey and Bursch 2013).

Between 8 and 19 % of youth with cancer develop PTSD and many more develop subthreshold trauma symptoms. One study of 48 babies and toddlers with cancer (ages 8–48 months) revealed that 15 months after diagnosis, 18.8 % met the age-appropriate criteria for full PTSD, and 41.7 % met criteria for partial PTSD. In a study of 209 children 5–6 weeks after an accident, or new diagnosis of cancer or diabetes, 11 % had moderate to severe trauma symptoms (guilt, intrusive memories, distress in response to trauma triggers, re-experiencing) (Landolt et al. 2003).

If inadequately or untreated, childhood trauma can become a chronic illness (Laor et al. 1997; Scheeringa et al. 2005). A longitudinal study of 6,542 childhood cancer survivors found that 9 % continued to meet criteria for PTSD and another 23.7 % had partial PTSD many years later (Stuber et al. 2011). Exposure to invasive procedures is the strongest predictor of posttraumatic stress symptoms 6 weeks after hospital discharge (Rennick et al. 2004). Pediatric inpatients who experienced delirium with frightening delusional memories are also at high risk (Colville et al. 2008). Young children are vulnerable due to limited coping skills, dependence on primary caregivers to protect them, and the rapid development that occurs during early childhood. Teens who are at higher risk for PTSD are female, have endured multiple or repeated traumas, have less social support, and/or have serious physical health problems.

Family functioning can be a protective or risk factor for children. In a study of 144 adolescent cancer survivors 1–12 years post–cancer treatment (M = 5.3 years) and their parents, the cancer survivors who had PTSD (8 %) were more than five times more likely to come from a poorly functioning family (in the areas of problem solving, affective responsiveness, and affective involvement) than a well-functioning one (Alderfer et al. 2009).

Adequate pain control (pharmacological and behavioral), child and family support, and clear communication using a team approach can be useful to prevent posttraumatic stress (Stuber and Shemesh 2006). Opiates may help prevent PTSD development in patients with significant pain. Morphine inhibits norepinephrine production in the locus coeruleus and decreases fear conditioning by reducing norepinephrine turnover in the amygdala, reducing hyperarousal symptoms (Pao and Bosk 2011). Preventative interventions provided within a psychological resiliency framework promote adaptive coping behavior use. Psycho-education should include typical child development, children's expected emotional/behavioral reactions to stressful situations, and mitigators of medical trauma effects. Emotional regulation skills (including traumatic reminder management techniques), goal setting/problem solving skills, and family communication skills are also important. A family timeline of illness symptoms, diagnostic process, and treatment experiences in a narrative framework can be used to increase family understanding, communication, support, and cohesion. Goals of family-based treatment include developing or strengthening skills that support parent leadership and positive parent–child interactions during times of high medical stress (Lester et al. 2010, 2011).

Trauma symptoms require treatment if they are severe, persist beyond several weeks, or lead to non-adherence. To assist with rapport development, mental health clinicians should avoid wearing white medical coats and explain to children that they will not be physically touched during the clinical encounter. Trauma-focused cognitive-behavioral therapy, an evidence-based intervention, should be utilized as first-line treatment. Clinicians should consider use of an SSRI in addition to therapy for PTSD treatment (Cohen et al. 2010), especially for hyperarousal symptoms (Robb et al. 2010; Cohen et al. 2007). Citalopram, escitalopram, or sertraline can be helpful as described above for anxiety, with attention to the same safety concerns (Forgey and Bursch 2013).

Dopamine has been implicated in the fear response associated with PTSD (De Bellis et al. 1999). Children with severe trauma symptoms may benefit from a dopamine antagonist, such as low dose risperidone (Reich et al. 2004; Hamner et al. 2003). 0.25–0.5 mg may be effective (Forgey and Bursch 2013). Although data for its use for PTSD in children is limited (Stathis et al. 2005), low doses of quetiapine (12.5–50 mg) can be useful for pre-procedure anxiety symptoms (Forgey and Bursch 2013).

Adult and animal studies have raised concern that using benzodiazepines during acute trauma (as in a medical setting) can exacerbate trauma symptoms and lead to the development of PTSD due to heightened emotional memories which prevent spontaneous trauma recovery. As a result, benzodiazepines should be avoided if at all possible in the treatment of children with cancer who are experiencing ongoing trauma (Forgey and Bursch 2013).

Open-label studies have shown that clonidine and propranolol may reduce hyperarousal and should be considered a third-line treatment (Harmon and Riggs 1996; Famularo et al 1988). Comorbid symptoms/medication side effect profiles may guide medication choices. A child with hypertension, anxiety, and sleep disturbance who cannot take oral medications may benefit from a clonidine patch. While initial studies of carbamazapine and divalproex show promise, current evidence does not support routine use in this population (Forgey and Bursch 2013).

18.2.3 Depression

Prevalence rates for Major Depressive Disorder vary from 7 to 17 % in children with cancer (Fritz and Williams 1988; Kashani and Hakami 1982). Rait et al. (1988) found a prevalence rate of 52 % of adjustment disorder in pediatric cancer patients, with mainly depression. Of 319 pediatric brain tumor survivors, 12 % had experienced suicidal ideation and 1.5 % had made a suicide attempt (Brinkman et al 2013).

Diagnosing depression in children with cancer is challenging due to the overlap between symptoms of cancer itself and depression. Symptoms suggestive of depression may be caused by medications, withdrawal from recreational substances, infections, neurological conditions, endocrine dysfunction, and other medical disorders (Rey and Birmaher 2009). While the DSM-5 diagnostic criteria for Major Depressive Disorder note that one should not include symptoms that are clearly attributable to another medical condition, clinicians are advised to consider a diagnosis of depression in a person who has experienced disability or loss due to a medical condition (APA 2013). Since medically ill children typically are able to distract themselves with enjoyable activities despite significant physical symptoms, anhedonia may be a more reliable indicator of depression for children who remain functional. New impairments in functioning, including a cessation of play, typically indicate an exacerbation of illness or the presence of depression or delirium. Measures such as the Children's Depression Inventory (CDI) or Memorial Symptom Assessment Scale (MSAS) can augment the evaluation of depression in medically ill children (Kersun and Shemesh 2007).

Risk factors for suicide attempts include adolescence, comorbid psychiatric disorders, suicidal intent and/or plan, completed suicide in a family member, minimal social supports, poor coping skills, impulsivity, recent improvement in depressive symptoms, symptoms of intractable pain, persistent insomnia, or seizures. While it has been theorized that a dying child may commit suicide to control the death process, current research does not support this hypothesis (Brinkman et al. 2013). Evaluation includes assessment of suicidal fantasies or actions, beliefs about what would happen if suicide was achieved, past suicide attempts, circumstances surrounding and motivations for suicide, understanding of and experiences with death, depression, family, and other social stressors (Birmaher et al. 2007; Stuber and Bursch 2009). Pain management should be evaluated as well as any other medications which may be responsible for mood symptoms, such as steroids (Bischoff et al. 2013; Ularntinon et al. 2010).

Cognitive behavioral therapy (CBT) and interpersonal psychotherapy (IPT) are evidence-based treatments for childhood depression. In children who do not respond adequately to therapy or who have severe symptoms, antidepressant medication is indicated (Birmaher et al. 2007; Rey and Birmaher 2009). SSRIs should be considered first line. FDA approvals for depression include fluoxetine (≥ 8 years) and escitalopram (≥ 12 years). Fluoxetine's drug interactions are a significant barrier to use. Small studies in pediatric oncology suggest that citalopram and fluvoxamine are safe and effective (Dejong and Fombonne 2007). Citalopram, escitalopram, and sertraline have the fewest drug interactions (Bursch and Forgey 2013). Potential cautions for use of SSRIs in pediatric cancer/palliative care were discussed in the section on anxiety.

If SSRIs are not tolerated or are ineffective, bupropion can be considered. Bupropion has been shown to be effective in open-label trials of childhood depression and can increase energy and improve attention (Daviss et al. 2001; Glod et al. 2003). Due to potential risk of seizure with high doses, history of seizures, abnormal EEG, cerebrovascular disease, head trauma, and multiple concomitant medications, a risk/benefit analysis is needed (Tripp 2010).

While mirtazapine may beneficially increase appetite and improve sleep, randomized controlled trials in youth have shown no benefit over placebo for childhood depression. Venlafaxine research has had similar outcomes (Cheung et al. 2005; Emslie et al. 2007). While case reports show some promise for the use of duloxetine in pediatric patients with chronic pain comorbid with depression (Meigen 2007), there is not sufficient evidence for its use.

While helpful in low doses for pain, sleep, or nausea, tricyclic antidepressants are no more efficacious than placebo in randomized controlled trials and meta-analysis for adolescent depression. When used at antidepressant doses, these medications can have significant cardiovascular side effects, have uncomfortable effects such as dry mouth, constipation, sedation, or difficulties with urination, and are fatal in overdose (Hazell and Mirzaie 2013), Monoamine oxidase inhibitors should be avoided due to their adverse interactions with foods and medications (Stuber and Bursch 2009).

Antidepressants can increase the short-term risk of suicidal thinking and behavior in youth (Bridge et al. 2007; Hammad et al. 2006; Mosholder and Willy 2006). Youth should be closely monitored for worsening of symptoms, suicidal ideation, or unusual behavior changes. Additional caution should be exercised in individuals with the suicide risks factors described above. Addressing a lack of perceived control, isolation, and distressing physical symptoms should be a high priority as these may lead to suicidal risk (Birmaher et al. 2007).

18.2.4 Delirium

Delirium is an acute disturbance of consciousness that presents with a fluctuating course of inattention and an impaired ability to receive, process, store, or recall information. ICU literature describes delirium as "ICU psychosis, ICU syndrome, acute confusional state, encephalopathy, and acute brain failure." Delirium develops over a short period of time (usually hours to a few days), reflects a change from baseline attention, cognition, and awareness, normally fluctuates in severity during the course of a day, and is often worse in the evening hours.

A study of 819 children with cancer over a 6-year period demonstrated a prevalence of acute mental status changes of 11 %. Of this group, 27 % were diagnosed with encephalopathy. The most common causes were coagulopathies, medication effects, systemic shock, and central nervous system infections. The death rate was an alarming 29 % within the first week (Dimario and Packer 1990). This is consistent with other small, prospective studies which estimate the prevalence of delirium in critically ill children to be 30 % (Smith et al. 2013). This is higher than the 20 % rate in a large sample of critically ill children (Turkel and Tavare 2003).

Critically ill pediatric patients can develop delirium with a hyperactive, hypoactive, mixed, or veiled presentation. The hyperactive subtype is most frequently identified and treated since these patients demonstrate agitation, mood lability, non-adherence, and/or psychosis (Karnik et al. 2007; Schieveld et al. 2007). Hypoactive delirium in children may present with mutism, lethargy, sluggishness, and/or regressive behavior and is often missed or misidentified as illness or treatment side effects, depression, or trauma. Validated assessment tools for pediatric delirium are the Pediatric Confusion Assessment Method for the Intensive Care Unit (pCAM-ICU) (Smith et al. 2011a) and the Cornell Assessment of Pediatric Delirium (Traube et al. 2014). Signs and symptoms of delirium are listed in Table 18.1.

Interventions for delirium may be targeted if a known etiology exists (Stern et al. 2013). Family education is important to enable family members to soothe the delirious child as opposed to becoming fearful or annoyed with the unusual behaviors they are witnessing. Familiar objects, photographs, and people can be helpful as can clocks, calendars, and signs posted on the wall for support and reorientation.

Pharmacological intervention may be indicated if the child is distressed by the delirium, if there are safety concerns due to agitation, or if treatment non-adherence is a problem. Karnik et al. (2007) describe an algorithm for treatment based on hypothesized neurotransmitter disturbances for the subtypes of delirium. Hyperactive delirium is hypothesized to be an elevated dopaminergic state of agitation/

Table 18.1 Signs and symptoms of delirium

• Child is easily distracted by irrelevant stimuli. Questions must be repeated
• The child perseverates; has difficulty shifting attention
• There is a change in at least one other area of cognition, such as recent memory, learning, orientation to time and place, alteration in language, perceptual distortions, or a perceptual-motor disturbance
• Perceptual disturbances include misinterpretations, paranoid thoughts, illusions, or hallucinations; visual disturbances are most common; perceptual disturbances can be simple or complex
• An inability to engage with the clinician should be considered severe inattention; an acute onset of a low-arousal state indicates severe inattention and cognitive change, and therefore, should be considered delirium
• Sleep–wake cycle disturbances are very commonly associated with delirium; ask about daytime sleepiness, nighttime agitation, difficulty falling asleep, excessive sleepiness throughout the day, and wakefulness throughout the night
• Anxiety, fear, depression, irritability, anger, euphoria, and/or apathy may be present and may shift in brief periods of time
• Yelling, screaming, cursing, muttering, moaning, or vocalizations may be present, especially at night

aggression, with relief through treatment with D2 blockade from haloperidol. Hypoactive/mixed delirium is hypothesized to be due to a dopaminergic/cholinergic imbalance in the medial prefrontal cortex, benefiting from the mixed receptor effects of risperidone on both the D2 and 5HT2A receptors there. Turkel et al. (2012) describe successful treatment of delirium with olanzapine, quetiapine, and risperidone. Response was comparable across all three medications at average daily doses of 10 mg for olanzapine, 1.3 mg for risperidone, and 56 mg of quetiapine.

Correcting electrolyte disturbances and monitoring of electrocardiographic QTc intervals to prevent arrhythmia are important in treating medically ill children with antipsychotics, especially when using IV haloperidol. Benzodiazepines are contraindicated, as they can exacerbate the confusional state by sedating or disinhibiting the child and are a common contributor to delirium in this population (Bursch and Forgey 2013).

18.2.5 Primary Psychiatric Disorders

Treatment of preexisting primary psychiatric disorders in youth with cancer should follow the same evidence-based treatments as for those without medical comorbidity. Stable medications should be continued unless symptoms change, side effects develop, or potential drug/drug interactions become evident. Examples include hypotension in a patient taking a blood pressure lowering medication for ADHD such as guanfacine or clonidine or significant QTc prolongation in a patient taking a neuroleptic when taking multiple QTc prolonging medications such as methadone.

18.3 Treatment of Cancer-Related Symptoms

Theunissen et al. (2007) found that children in the end stage of cancer reported a mean of 6.3 (SD 2.7) physical symptoms. Most common were pain, poor appetite, fatigue, lack of mobility, and vomiting. Another study of 185 children (aged 4–19) who died of cancer concurred with these findings (Goldman et al. 2006).

18.3.1 Pain

Pain is one of the most common and feared experiences for children. Pain may be illness related, treatment/procedure related, or unrelated to illness. A pain assessment includes factors such as etiology, location, intensity, duration, and prior treatment of pain and is measured by self-report, observational, and/or physiological measures. Pain-related distress and fear-related distress can be difficult to differentiate. Although pain is best assessed by asking the child about his or her pain, a number of barriers can limit the assessment. These may include worries related to talking to clinicians, taking medications, getting injections, being viewed as weak or demanding, or distressing others. Other barriers are limited language, sedation, cognitive impairment, or new knowledge that their condition is worsening. Some children have heard their parents worry they will become a "drug addict" if they take pain medication. Additionally, some children are adept at using distraction or dissociation to cope with pain and might appear comfortable even though they are in substantial pain. It is confusing for a clinician to see a child with extreme pain behaviors alternating with normal play or sleep. Structured pain assessment tools have been developed for use with medically ill children (Cohen et al. 2008; Stinson et al. 2008; von Baeyer and Spagrud 2007). Measures should be developmentally appropriate and pain prospectively rated (in the moment) if possible.

Since anxiety can exacerbate pain, soothing techniques are helpful for pain reduction. Examples include increasing the child's sense of control, holding the child, encouraging the child to use behavioral activation or distraction techniques, providing the child with familiar belongings, arranging predictable time to be spent with parents, and communicating with the child in a developmentally appropriate manner.

Procedural pain may be reduced with modeling/rehearsing the procedure, performing breathing or imagery/distraction exercises, and offering positive incentive (Jay et al. 1987). Providing the child a choice of injection locations and the use of a topical anesthetic, ice, or another skin coolant is helpful for needle sticks.

For cancer pain, postoperative pain, posttraumatic pain, and other acute pain, an analgesic ladder is the standard of care (See Fig. 18.1). Nonopioid analgesics such as acetaminophen and ibuprofen are recommended for mild pain. An opioid such as morphine is recommended for moderate to severe pain. For children with persistent pain, pain medication should be given on a regular schedule with breakthrough medication available as needed (WHO 2012). Oral medications can be made to

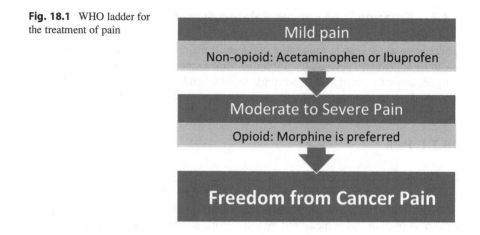

taste better if mixed with something sweet, such as honey, or when preceded by
something cold, such as ice (Gyulay 1989). Commercial flavoring is also available
and can be added at a pharmacy for most medicines. Medication for chronic pain
should be titrated to an effective dose schedule and then provided around the clock,
at regular intervals, rather than on an "as needed" basis. Long-acting medications
result in better patient adherence (Bursch and Zeltzer 2004). Acute or procedural
pain may require breakthrough medication, given as needed. It is important to
remember that there are significant variations in pain sensitivity and the consequent
need for analgesics.

18.3.2 Nausea/Vomiting

The *American Society of Clinical Oncology* recommends the use of two-drug
therapy for children undergoing chemotherapy of high emetogenic potential. This
combination includes a 5HT-3 antagonist such as ondansetron or granisetron
combined with a steroid, preferably dexamethasone. Dopamine antagonists (including metoclopramide and prochlorperazine) are not recommended as first line in
children due to potential dystonic reactions. Although there is no recommendation
for children, lorazepam and diphenhydramine are recommended in adults (ASCO
et al. 2006). Intractable nausea/vomiting is a symptom for which the benefits of
benzodiazepines may outweigh the risks (Table 18.2).

A Cochrane Review of 28 randomized control trials for chemotherapy-induced
nausea/vomiting in pediatric cancer concurred with the ASCO recommendation.
5HT-3 antagonists were more effective than metoclopramine or chlorpromazine.
Granisetron was the most effective if used in high doses and adding dexamethasone
doubled the likelihood of complete control. Cannabanoids were noted to be likely to
be effective, but produce many side effects which may be patient specific. Finally,
there was not enough evidence on newer agents such as substance P antagonists and
neurokinin receptor antagonists to recommend their use in children (Philips
et al. 2010).

Table 18.2 Recommended medications for psychiatric symptoms for children/adolescents with cancer

Symptom	Medication
Anxiety	Citalopram
Depression and/or	Escitalopram
Trauma symptoms/Posttraumatic stress disorder (first line)	Sertraline
Depression (second line if ADHD or SSRI failure)	Bupropion
Trauma symptoms/PTSD (severe/second line)	Risperidone
	Quetiapine
Trauma symptoms (third line)	Propranolol
	Clonidine
Pre-procedure anxiety (PRN)	Quetiapine
Hyperactive delirium	Haloperidol
Hypoactive/mixed delirium	Risperidone
Insomnia	Diphenhydramine
	Melatonin
	Trazodone
Insomnia with anxiety/delirium	Quetiapine

18.3.3 Anorexia

Changes in taste, pain, oral thrush, swallowing problems, constipation, bland food, noxious odors, nausea, vomiting, medication, depression, metabolic issues, sensation of fullness, and radiation therapy may all contribute to anorexia in children with cancer (Stuber and Bursch 2009). Food-related issues may also be an expression of independence or aggression by the child. Children with developmental disorders may have preexisting food challenges.

Treatment includes addressing any underlying causes and physical/emotional symptoms. A child should have access to food at all times if not medically contraindicated. Mealtime should be fun and noxious odors should be eliminated. Food preferences may change at the end of life with a cold food preference (Stuber and Bursch 2009). Clinicians should educate parents about appropriate intake expectations to reduce parents' frustration or guilt over the child's reduced consumption. Parents may be coached on ways to help their child express anger and independence in developmentally appropriate ways not involving food. Appetite stimulation may be helpful; cyproheptadine hydrocholoride and megestrol acetate may help to increase weight in children with cancer (Couluris et al. 2008).

18.3.4 Fatigue

Causes of fatigue include disease effects, deconditioning, poor nutrition, impaired sleep, depression, chemotherapeutic agents, and other drugs and radiation treatment. Physical therapy can also help to maintain functioning by increasing activity and reducing muscular atrophy (Stuber and Bursch 2009). Exercise training can improve physical fitness and reduce fatigue in children with cancer (Braam et al. 2013; Chang et al. 2013). Fatigue may decrease in early phases of treatment as physical symptoms resolve (Hooke et al. 2011). With more extensive treatment and in the terminal phase of cancer, ongoing fatigue may be addressed by treating physical and emotional symptoms; insuring adequate sleep, nutrition, and hydration; and controlling medication side effects (Stuber and Bursch 2009).

Psychostimulant use in children with cancer is reportedly rare (Pao et al. 2006). Modafanil shows promise for use in cancer-related fatigue in adults (Jean-Pierre et al. 2010). Case reports note the benefit of psychostimulants to treat secondary narcolepsy in children with brain tumors (Marcus et al. 2002). Sung et al. (2013) are currently studying the use of modafanil to improve neurocognitive functioning in children with brain tumors. Rosen and Brand (2011) report improved daytime sleepiness in children with cancer treated with psychostimulants (methylphenidate, modafanil, mixed amphetamine salts). Blood transfusions may also help to increase energy levels in those with low platelets (Munzer 2010), which may be especially important to allow the child to achieve important end of life goals.

With reduced functioning at end of life, children should be given supports such as a stroller, wagon, walker, or wheelchair to help conserve energy for special events, while maximizing their independence. To avoid a disappointing moment of misplaced hope that their child is unexpectedly improving, parents should be made aware that end of life may bring with it a temporary energy increase which may last for several hours (Stuber and Bursch 2009).

18.3.5 Sleep Disturbance

Excessive daytime sleepiness has been reported in 60–80 % of children with cancer. Sleep disturbance in children with cancer may include the full spectrum of sleep disorders (hypersomnia, sleep-disordered breathing, insomnia, parasomnias, circadian rhythm, disorders) (Rosen and Brand 2011). Physical symptoms (pain, bladder/bowel distention, urination, night sweats), anxiety and mood symptoms, or sleep pattern reversal are often to blame. Problems with light, noise, activating electronic toys or video games, and temperature may also be significant contributors (Stuber and Bursch 2009). Some medications (such as steroids), medication withdrawal (such as from benzodiazepines), or other substances (such as caffeine) can also contribute.

Sleep disturbance treatment in children with cancer should address the cause, including physical/emotional contributors and primary sleep disorders. Earplugs, eye masks, noise reduction, and lighting optimization may reduce environmental contributors (Kudchadkar et al. 2014). Sleep hygiene education and relaxation strategies can be helpful. At the end of life, sleep phase reversal may not need to be corrected as long as the family is reassured.

Research into medication treatment of childhood insomnia is limited. Melatonin and diphenhydramine have some evidence for this use in children (Andrade et al. 2001; Pelayo and Dubik 2008). Diphenhydramine has the benefit of an IV formulation. Low-dose trazodone may also be useful in this setting (Bursch and Forgey 2013).

If sleep disturbance is present with anxiety or delirium, one may use low dose of a sedating neuroleptic such as quetiapine (12.5–25 mg). If pain is a significant contributor, a low dose of a tricyclic antidepressant may be used. Benzodiazepines should be avoided unless the child is experiencing intractable nausea/air hunger or requires IV medication and is nonresponsive to diphenhydramine (Bursch and Forgey 2013).

Conclusion

A diagnosis of cancer is an unexpected and highly distressing event for most children and their family members. The main goal of pediatric palliative care is to allow a seriously ill child to grow and develop despite his or her serious illness. This is accomplished by a team approach to provide developmentally tailored symptom management, communication, and support. Although palliative care services may not be necessary for all pediatric cancer patients, it is an essential service for some. The careful use of psychopharmacological medications can vastly improve the quality of life and improve outcomes for children with cancer.

Clinical Vignette

A child psychiatry consult was requested to evaluate Grace, a previously healthy 6-year-old girl with a new diagnosis of leukemia, because she was having extreme agitation related to minor procedures. It was taking several adults to hold Grace down for blood draws and physical exams. She would bite, spit, kick, hit, and scream the entire time. One nurse said Grace looked like a feral cat who had been caught. She would cry whenever a staff would enter her room and yell "no, no, no." The nurses felt her mom was an ineffective parent and Grace was used to getting her way. However, the nurses' attempts at setting firmer limits with Grace were not effective in reducing her aggression. Likewise, traditional child life preparations for procedures did not appear to help Grace either. Psychiatric evaluation revealed a history of severe domestic violence between the parents, witnessed by Grace. This pasttraumatic experience placed Grace at increased risk for experiencing a trauma reaction when she feared she would be physically harmed. Also traumatized, her mother was incapable of providing Grace the support she needed.

Due to Grace's significant distress from trauma symptoms, citalopram 5 mg was started. She was initially started on quetiapine 12.5 mg prior to procedures, which was increased at 12.5 mg increments until an effective dose of 25 mg was reached. The quetiapine brought her much needed relief pre-procedure. After 1 week on the citalopram, Grace was feeling

(continued)

significantly better. She was able to tolerate staff entering the room and was able to cooperate with routine interventions such as blood draws and exams without agitation. She was also now able to engage in distraction, use relaxation skills, and learn other pre-procedure psychosocial skills much more effectively. As a result, she was no longer requiring quetiapine for minor procedures. For more significant interventions, she continued to require pre-procedure quetiapine, which was automatically ordered each time she returned to the hospital.

References

Alderfer MA, Navsaria N, Kazak AE. Family functioning and posttraumatic stress disorder in adolescent survivors of childhood cancer. J Fam Psychol. 2009;23(5):717–25.

American Psychiatric Association. Diagnostic and statistical manual of mental disorders. Arlington, VA: American Psychiatric Publishing; 2013.

American Society of Clinical Oncology, Kris MG, Hesketh PJ, et al. American Society of Clinical Oncology guidelines for antiemetics in oncology: update 2006. J Clin Oncol. 2006;24 (18):2932–47.

Andrade C, Srihari BS, Reddy KP, et al. Melatonin in medically ill patients with insomnia: a double-blind, placebo-controlled study. J Clin Psychiatry. 2001;62(1):41–5.

Birmaher B, Brent D, AACAP Workgroup on Quality Issues, et al. Practice parameter for the assessment and treatment of children and adolescents with depressive disorders. J Am Acad Child Adolesc Psychiatry. 2007;46(11):1502–26.

Bischoff K, Weinberg V, Rabow MW. Palliative and oncologic co-management: symptom management for outpatients with cancer. Support Care Cancer. 2013;21(11):3031–7.

Braam KI, van der Torre P, Takken T, et al. Physical exercise training interventions for children and young adults during their treatment for childhood cancer. Cochrane Database Syst Rev. 2013;4, CD008796.

Bridge JA, Iyengar S, Salary CB, et al. Clinical response and risk for reported suicidal ideation and suicide attempts in pediatric antidepressant treatment: a meta-analysis of randomized controlled trials. JAMA. 2007;297(15):1683–96.

Brinkman TM, Liptak CC, Delaney BL, et al. Suicide ideation in pediatric and adult survivors of childhood brain tumors. J Neurooncol. 2013;113(3):425–32.

Bursch B, Forgey M. Psychopharmacology for medically ill adolescents. Curr Psychiatry Rep. 2013;15:395.

Bursch B, Zeltzer LK. Pediatric pain management. In: Behrman RE, Kliegman RM, Jenson HB, editors. Nelson textbook of pediatrics. 17th ed. Philadelphia, PA: Saunders; 2004. p. p519–30.

Chang CW, Mu PF, Jou ST, et al. Systemic review and meta-analysis of nonpharmacological interventions for fatigue in children and adolescents with cancer. Worldviews Evid Based Nurs. 2013;10:208–17.

Cheung AH, Emslie GH, Mayes TL. Review of the efficacy and safety of antidepressants in youth depression. J Child Psychol Psychiatry. 2005;46:735–54.

Cohen JA, Mannarino AP, Perel JM, et al. A pilot randomized controlled trial of combined trauma-focused CBT and sertraline for childhood PTSD symptoms. J Am Acad Child Adolesc Psychiatr. 2007;46(7):811–9.

Cohen LL, Lemanek K, Blount RL, et al. Evidence-based assessment of pediatric pain. J Pediatr Psychol. 2008;33(9):939–55.

Cohen JA, Bukstein O, Walter H, et al. Practice parameter for the assessment and treatment of children and adolescents with posttraumatic stress disorder. J Am Acad Child Adolesc Psychiatr. 2010;49(4):414–30.

Colville G, Kerry S, Pierce C. Children's factual and delusional memories of intensive care. Am J Respir Crit Care Med. 2008;177(9):976–82.

Couluris M, Mayer JLR, Freyer DR, et al. The effect of cyproheptadine hydrochloride (Periactin) and megestrol acetate (Megace) on weight in children with cancer/treatment-related cachexia. J Pediatr Hematol Oncol. 2008;30(11):791–7.

Daviss WB, Bentivoglio P, Racusin R, et al. Bupropion sustained release in adolescents with comorbid attention-deficit/hyperactivity disorder and depression. J Am Acad Child Adolesc Psychiatry. 2001;40(3):307–14.

De Bellis MD, Keshevan MS, Clark DB, et al. Developmental traumatology, part II: brain development. Biol Psychiatry. 1999;45(10):1271–84.

Dejong M, Fombonne E. Citalopram to treat depression in pediatric oncology. J Child Adolesc Psychopharmacol. 2007;17(3):371–7.

Dimario FJ, Packer RJ. Acute mental status changes in children with systemic cancer. Pediatrics. 1990;85:353–60.

Emslie GJ, Findling RL, Yeung PP, et al. Venlafaxine ER for the treatment of pediatric subjects with depression: results of two placebo-controlled trials. J Am Acad Child Adolesc Psychiatry. 2007;41:1190–6.

Erickson SJ, Steiner H. Trauma spectrum adaptation: somatic symptoms in long-term pediatric cancer survivors. Psychosomatics. 2000;41:339–46.

Famularo R, Kinscherff R, Fenton T. Propranolol treatment for childhood posttraumatic stress disorder, acute type. A pilot study. Am J Dis Child. 1988;142(11):1244–7.

FDA drug safety communication: Revised recommendations for Celexa (citalopram hydrobromide) related to a potential risk of abnormal heart rhythms with high doses. http://www.fda.gov/Drugs/DrugSafety/ucm269068.htm#data. Accessed Oct 2013

Forgey M, Bursch B. Assessment and management of pediatric iatrogenic medical trauma. Curr Psychiatry Rep. 2013;15(2):340.

Fritz GK, Williams JR. Issues of adolescent development for survivors of childhood cancer. J Am Acad Child Adolesc Psychiatry. 1988;27:712–5.

Glod CA, Lynch A, Flynn E, et al. Open trail of bupropion SR in adolescent major depression. J Child Adolesc Psychiatr Nurs. 2003;16(3):123–30.

Goldman A, Hewitt M, Collins GS, et al. Symptoms in children/young people with progressive malignant disease: United Kingdom Children's Cancer Study Group/Paediatric Oncology Nurses Forum Survey. Pediatrics. 2006;117(6):e1179–86.

Gothelf D, Rubinstein M, Shemesh E, et al. Pilot study: fluvoxamine treatment for depression and anxiety disorders in children and adolescents with cancer. J Am Acad Child Adolesc Psychiatry. 2005;44(12):1258–62.

Gyulay J. Home care for the dying child. Issues Compr Pediatr Nurs. 1989;12:33–69.

Hammad TA, Laughren T, Racoosin J. Suicidality in pediatric patients treated with antidepressant drugs. Arch Gen Psychiatry. 2006;63(3):332–9.

Hamner MB, Faldowski RA, Ulmer HG, et al. Adjunctive risperidone treatment in post-traumatic stress disorder: a preliminary controlled trial of effects on comorbid psychotic symptoms. Int Clin Psychopharmacol. 2003;18:1–8.

Harmon RJ, Riggs PD. Clinical perspectives: clonidine for post traumatic stress disorder in preschool children. J Am Acad Child Adolesc Psychiatry. 1996;35:1247–9.

Hayes BD, Klein-Schwartz W, Clark RF, et al. Comparison of toxicity of overdoses with citalopram and escitalopram. J Emerg Med. 2010;39(1):44–8.

Hazell P, Mirzaie M. Tricyclic drugs for depression in children and adolescents. Cochrane Database Syst Rev. 2013;6, CD002317.

Hooke MC, Garwick AW, Gross CR. Fatigue and physical performance in children and adolescents receiving chemotherapy. Onc Nurs Forum. 2011;38(6):649–57.

Jay SM, Elliot CH, Katz E, et al. Cognitive-behavioral and pharmacologic interventions for children's distress during painful medical procedures. J Consult Clin Psychol. 1987;55 (6):860–5.

Jean-Pierre P, Morrow GR, Roscoe JA, et al. A phase 3 randomized, placebo-controlled, double blind, clinical trial of the effect of modafanil on cancer-related fatigue among 631 patients receiving chemotherapy: a University of Rochester Cancer Center Community Clinical Oncology Program Research Base Study. Cancer. 2010;116(14):3513–20.

Karnik NS, Joshi SV, Paterno C, et al. Subtypes of pediatric delirium: a treatment algorithm. Psychosomatics. 2007;48(3):253–7.

Kashani J, Hakami N. Depression in children and adolescents with malignancy. Can J Psychiatry. 1982;27:474–7.

Kersun LS, Shemesh E. Depression and anxiety in children at the end of life. Pediatr Clin North Am. 2007;254(5):691–708. xi.

Kudchadkar SR, Aljohani OA, Punjabi NM. Sleep of critically ill children in the pediatric intensive care unit: a systematic review. Sleep Med Rev. 2014;18:103–10.

Landolt MA, Vollrath M, Ribi K, et al. Incidence and association of parental and child posttraumatic stress symptoms in pediatric patients. J Child Psychol Psychiatry. 2003;44:1199–207.

Laor N, Wolmer L, Mayes LC, et al. Israeli preschool children under scuds: a 30-month follow-up. J Am Child Adolesc Psychiatry. 1997;36(3):349–56.

Lester P, Stein J, Bursch B, et al. Family-based processes associated with adolescent distress, substance use, and risky sexual behavior in families affected by maternal HIV. J Clin Child Adolesc Psychol. 2010;39(3):328–40.

Lester P, Saltzman W, Woodward K, et al. Evaluation of a family-centered prevention intervention for military children and families facing wartime deployments. Am J Public Health. 2011;102 (S1):S48–54.

Marcus C, Trescher WH, Halbower AC, et al. Secondary narcolepsy in children with brain tumors. Sleep. 2002;25(4):435–9.

Meigen KG. Duloxetine treatment of pediatric chronic pain and co-morbid major depressive disorder. J Child Adolesc Psychopharmacol. 2007;17(1):121–7.

Meijer WEE, Heerdink ER, Nolen WA, et al. Association of risk of abnormal bleeding with degree of serotonin reuptake inhibition by antidepressants. Arch Intern Med. 2004;164(21):2367–70.

Mercadante S, Prestia G, Adile C, et al. Changes of QTc interval after opioid switching to oral methadone. Support Care Cancer. 2013;21:3421–4.

Mosholder AD, Willy M. Suicidal adverse events in pediatric randomized, controlled clinical trials of antidepressant drugs are associated with active drug treatment: a meta-analysis. J Child Adolesc Psychopharmacol. 2006;16(1–2):25–32.

Munzer M. Transfusion in palliative care in child with malignant disease. Transfus Clin Biol. 2010;17(5–6):353–6.

Owens J. Pharmacotherapy of pediatric insomnia. J Am Acad Child Adolesc Psychiatry. 2009;48 (2):99–107.

Pao M, Bosk A. Anxiety in medically ill children/adolescents. Depress Anxiety. 2011;28(1):40–9.

Pao M, Ballard ED, Rosenstein D, et al. Psychotropic medication use in pediatric patients with cancer. Arch Pediatr Adolesc Med. 2006;160:818–22.

Pelayo R, Dubik M. Pediatric sleep pharmacology. Semin Pediatr Neurol. 2008;15:79–90.

Philips RS, Gopaul S, Gibson F, et al. Antiemetic medication for prevention and treatment of chemotherapy-induced nausea and vomiting in childhood. Cochrane Database Syst Rev. 2010;9, CD007786.

Phipps S, Srivastava DK. Approaches to the measurement of depressive symptomatology in children with cancer: attempting to circumvent the effects of defensiveness. J Dev Behav Pediatr. 1999;20:150–6.

Piacentini J, Bergman RL. Developmental issues in cognitive therapy for childhood anxiety disorders. J Cogn Psychother. 2001;15:165–82.

Quinn DK, Stern TA. Linezolid and serotonin syndrome. J Clin Psychiatry. 2009;11(6):353–6.

Rait DS, Jacobsen PB, Lederberg MS, et al. Characteristics of psychiatric consultations in a pediatric cancer center. Am J Psychiatry. 1988;145(3):363–4.

Ramsey TD, Lau TT, Ensom MH. Serotonergic and adrenergic drug interactions associated with linezolid: a critical review and practical management approach. Ann Pharmacother. 2013;47 (4):543–60.

Reich DB, Winternitz S, Hennen J, et al. A preliminary study of risperidone in the treatment of posttraumatic stress disorder related to childhood abuse in women. J Clin Psychiatry. 2004;65:1601–6.

Rennick JE, Morin I, Kim D, et al. Identifying children at high risk for psychological sequelae after pediatric intensive care unit hospitalization. Pediatr Crit Care Med. 2004;5(4):358–63.

Rey J, Birmaher B. Treating child and adolescent depression. Baltimore, MD: Lippincott Williams & Wilkins; 2009.

Robb AS, Cueva JE, Sporn J, et al. Sertraline treatment of children and adolescents with posttraumatic stress disorder: a double-blind, placebo-controlled trial. J Child Adolesc Psychopharmacol. 2010;20(6):463–71.

Rosen G, Brand SR. Sleep in children with cancer evaluated in a comprehensive pediatric sleep center. Support Care Cancer. 2011;19:985–94.

Scheeringa MS, Zeanah CH, Myers L, et al. Predictive validity in a prospective follow-up of PTSD in preschool children. J Am Acad Child Adolesc Psychiatry. 2005;44(9):899–906.

Schieveld JN, Leroy PL, van Os J, et al. Pediatric delirium in critical illness: phenomenology, clinical correlates and treatment response in 40 cases in the pediatric intensive care unit. Intensive Care Med. 2007;33(6):1033–40.

Simbre VC, Duffy SA, Dadlani GH, et al. Cardiotoxicity of cancer chemotherapy: implications for children. Paediatr Drugs. 2005;7(3):187–202.

Smith HA, Boyd J, Fuchs DC, et al. Diagnosing delirium in critically ill children: validity and reliability of the Pediatric Confusion Assessment Method for the Intensive Care Unit. Crit Care Med. 2011a;39(1):150–7.

Smith HA, Fuchs DC, Pandharipande PP, et al. Delirium: an emerging frontier in the management of critically ill children. Anesthesiol Clin. 2011b;29(4):729–50.

Smith HA, Berutti T, Brink E, et al. Pediatric critical care perceptions on analgesia, sedation, and delirium. Semin Respir Crit Care Med. 2013;34(2):244–61.

Stathis S, Martin G, McKenna JG. A preliminary case series on the use of quetiapine for posttraumatic stress disorder in juveniles within a youth detention center. J Clin Psychopharmacol. 2005;26(6):539–44.

Stern TA, Fricchione GL, Cassem NH, et al., editors. Massachusetts general handbook of general hospital psychiatry. 5th ed. Philadelphia, PA: Mosby Inc.; 2013.

Stinson J, Yamada J, Dickson A, et al. Review of systematic reviews on acute procedural pain in children in the hospital setting. Pain Res Manag. 2008;13(1):51–7.

Stuber ML, Bursch B. Psychiatric care of the terminally ill child. In: Chochinov HM, Breitbart W, editors. Psychiatric dimensions of palliative medicine. 2nd ed. New York: Oxford University Press; 2009. p. 519–30.

Stuber ML, Shemesh E. Post-traumatic stress response to life-threatening illnesses in children and their parents. Child Adolesc Psychiatr Clin N Am. 2006;15(3):597–609.

Stuber ML, Meeske KA, Leisenring W, et al. Defining medical posttraumatic stress among young adult survivors in the Childhood Cancer Survivor Study. Gen Hosp Psychiatr. 2011;33 (4):347–53.

Sung L, Zaoutis T, Ullrich NJ, et al. Children's Oncology Group's 2013 blueprint for research: cancer control and supportive care. Pediatr Blood Cancer. 2013;60(6):1027–30.

The Research Unit on Pediatric Psychopharmacology Anxiety Study Group. Fluvoxamine for the treatment of anxiety disorders in children and adolescents. N Engl J Med. 2001;344(17):1279–85.

Theunissen JM, Hoogerbrugge PM, van Achterberg T, et al. Symptoms in the palliative phase of children with cancer. Pediatr Blood Cancer. 2007;49(2):160–5.

Traube C, Silver G, Kearney J, et al. Cornell assessment of pediatric delirium: a valid, rapid, observational tool for screening delirium in the ICU. Crit Care Med. 2014;42:656–63.

Tripp A. Bupropion, a brief history of seizure risk. Gen Hosp Psychiatry. 2010;32(2):216–7.

Turkel SB, Tavare CJ. Delirium in children and adolescents. J Neuropsychiatry Clin Neurosci. 2003;15:431–5.

Turkel SB, Jacobson J, Munzig E, et al. Atypical antipsychotic medications to control symptoms of delirium in children and adolescents. J Child Adolesc Psychopharmacol. 2012;22(2):1–5.

Ularntinon S, Tzuang D, Dahl G, et al. Concurrent treatment of steroid-related mood and psychotic symptoms with risperidone. Pediatrics. 2010;125:e1241.

von Baeyer CL, Spagrud LJ. Systematic review of observational (behavioral) measures of pain for children and adolescents aged 3 to 18 years. Pain. 2007;127(1–2):140–50.

Walkup JT, Albano AM, Piacentini J, et al. Cognitive behavioral therapy, sertraline, or a combination in childhood anxiety. N Engl J Med. 2008;359(26):2753–66.

World Health Organization. Persisting pain in children package: WHO guidelines on the pharmacological treatment of children with medical illnesses. Geneva: World Health Organization; 2012.

Special Issues in Psychopharmacology: The Elderly

19

Andrea Iaboni, Peter Fitzgerald, and Gary Rodin

Abstract

Pharmacotherapy of the elderly cancer patient requires attention to changes in the absorption, metabolism, distribution, and excretion of medication in the elderly, as well as to increased end-organ sensitivity. Polypharmacy, errors in the administration of medication, medical comorbidity, and cognitive impairment are more common in the elderly and may all contribute to the increased likelihood of adverse effects with antidepressants, anxiolytics, and neuroleptics. Psychotropic medication with fewer active metabolites, less accumulation, shorter duration of action, and fewer side effects are most suitable in the elderly. The medication should be initiated at a lower dose in this population and the dose should be increased more slowly. More research is needed to better establish the efficacy and safety of psychopharmacotherapy in elderly cancer patients.

A. Iaboni (✉)
Department of Psychiatry, Toronto Rehabilitation Institute, University Health Network, 550 University Avenue, 5-105-3, Toronto, ON, Canada M5G 2A2
e-mail: andrea.iaboni@uhn.ca

P. Fitzgerald
Department of Psychosocial Oncology and Palliative Care, Princess Margaret Cancer Centre, University Health Network, 610 University Avenue, Toronto, ON, Canada M5G 2M9
e-mail: Peter.Fitzgerald@uhn.ca

G. Rodin
Department of Psychosocial Oncology and Palliative Care, Princess Margaret Cancer Centre, University Health Network, 16-724, 610 University Avenue, Toronto, ON, Canada M5G 2M9
e-mail: Gary.Rodin@uhn.ca

L. Grassi and M. Riba (eds.), *Psychopharmacology in Oncology and Palliative Care*,
DOI 10.1007/978-3-642-40134-3_19, © Springer-Verlag Berlin Heidelberg 2014

19.1   Introduction

The risk of cancer rises progressively with age, as does other medical comorbidity and the potential for adverse effects from pharmacological agents (Cresswell et al. 2007). This chapter will address the age-related physiological changes that may affect the response to psychotropic medication and their clinical implications for the use of psychopharmacologic treatments in elderly patients with cancer. We have regarded age as a continuous variable, without specifying a specific chronological threshold by which to define the elderly. This is consistent with the approach commonly adopted in the recent geriatric literature, in which frailty (Clegg et al. 2013) and life stage (Fitzgerald et al. 2012) have replaced chronological age in the demarcation of this population. We have also assumed in this chapter that psychological, social, and environmental interventions, which may be the first-line and primary treatment of psychological distress and of many psychiatric disorders in elderly cancer patients, have been introduced as needed. Similarly, we have assumed that the alleviation of pain and other physical distress and the treatment of underlying or contributing medical conditions have been undertaken, which may alleviate psychological distress and psychiatric illness.

In the following sections, we first discuss the general pharmacokinetic and pharmacodynamic factors that are important to consider in the context of pharmacotherapy for the older cancer patient, along with clinical implications relevant to this population such as risk of adverse events, polypharmacy, non-adherence, and under-treatment (Sect. 19.2). Subsequent sections discuss specific considerations in relation to psychopharmacotherapy of the older cancer patient regarding the treatment of depression (Sect. 19.3), anxiety (Sect. 19.4) and delirium (Sect. 19.5).

19.2   Drugs and Aging

This section addresses the effects of biological aging on the way that drugs move through and are processed by the body (pharmacokinetic changes), as well as on the pharmacologic effects of the drugs (pharmacodynamic changes). Although we have generalized about these effects in older individuals, there is enormous interindividual variability in both pharmacokinetics and pharmacodynamics in older adults due to such factors as medical illness, organ damage or failure, and use of prescription and over-the-counter medication.

19.2.1 Aging and Pharmacokinetics

Many adverse drug events (ADEs) in the elderly are related to pharmacokinetic changes that result in the accumulation of toxic drug concentrations. The domains in which these changes tend to occur are described below, of which metabolism and excretion are the most likely to be clinically significant.

Absorption

Physiological changes in the elderly, particularly a decrease in gastric acid secretion (either primary or secondary to the widespread use of proton pump inhibitors) and decreased gastrointestinal (GI) blood flow, may diminish drug absorption and therefore bioavailability. Slowing of gastric motility has the opposite effect and can increase the bioavailability of poorly permeable drugs. The overall effect is thus variable and dependent upon the characteristics of the drug (i.e., whether it requires an acidic environment for absorption, the permeability of the drug, and the degree of first-pass metabolism, in which the bioavailability of the drug is decreased before it reaches the systemic circulation). There is little evidence about age-related changes that specifically affect the absorption of psychotropic drugs.

Distribution

There are three principal age-related changes in body composition that can impact the bioavailability of drugs that are extensively protein bound or highly lipid soluble. First, progressive reduction of albumin levels occurs with advancing age, resulting in an increase in the unbound fraction of many drugs, most notably phenytoin, diazepam, and valproate. For valproate, the difference is dramatic— 6.4 % free in young adults vs. 10.7 % in the elderly (Perucca et al. 1984)—and is likely clinically significant. The second notable age-related change that affects distribution is a 20–40 % increase in body fat, resulting in an increase in the half-life of those drugs stored in fat. Finally, the 10–15 % decrease in body water that is concomitant with old age leads to an increased concentration of water-soluble drugs, most notably lithium.

Metabolism

The liver is the principal organ involved in metabolizing drugs. Its capacity to do so is influenced by hepatic blood flow and by enzymes in the liver. Aging is known to reduce hepatic blood flow in the order of 40 %. Since most drugs are "blood flow limited" in their metabolism, the rate of metabolism of these agents is decreased in the elderly. The metabolism of a small number of drugs is limited by the capacity of the drug-metabolizing enzymes. The age-related decrease in the size of the liver, and perhaps in the expression of enzyme genes, results in reduced enzyme capacity. This intensifies the effect of drug-induced enzyme inhibition, primarily for drugs metabolized through the cytochrome P450-mediated phase I metabolic pathways. These effects may be present even when liver function tests, which are not a clinically sensitive predictor of hepatic metabolic function, are normal. By contrast, phase II metabolism, including acetylation, sulfation, methylation, and glucuronidation, is well preserved in aging.

Excretion

Decreased renal blood flow in aging has a significant impact on the excretion of many drugs. Glomerular filtration rate also decreases with age, but this change is small in healthy older adults, and in the absence of hypertension, diabetes, or renal disease. The elimination of many drugs is dependent upon renal function, but this is most critical with drugs, such as lithium, that are almost exclusively excreted by the kidney and that have narrow therapeutic indices.

19.2.2 Aging and Pharmacodynamics

Changes to the aging brain result in an increased sensitivity to the effects of psychotropic medication at lower doses in the elderly compared to younger adults. The classic study by Reidenberg (Reidenberg et al. 1978) showed that older adults were more sedated at lowered serum levels of diazepam than were younger adults. The biological basis for this increased sensitivity has been postulated to include the effects of brain atrophy, altered neurotransmitter receptor sensitivities, reduced levels of neurotransmitters, such as dopamine and acetylcholine, increased blood–brain barrier permeability, and neurodegenerative changes, such as plaques and tangles. As a result of these brain changes, the elderly are also at increased risk for cognitive, sedative, parkinsonian, and anticholinergic side effects of psychotropic medication.

Age-related physiological changes in other organ systems also contribute to an increase in risk of a variety of ADEs, including some geriatric-specific toxicities that are only rarely seen in younger adults. An important example is the increased risk of QT prolongation and sudden cardiac death that occurs with the use of psychotropic medication in older adults. Alterations in the cardiovascular response to postural changes also increase the susceptibility of older adults to orthostatic hypotension with such medication as antidepressants and antipsychotics. Hyponatraemia with the use of selective serotonin reuptake inhibitors (SSRIs) is rarely observed outside of the geriatric population but occurs in about 10 % of older adults within 1–4 weeks after onset of the medication. Most cases are mild and asymptomatic and do not necessitate treatment discontinuation. However, moderate to severe hyponatraemia occurs in about 0.5 % of older SSRI users and is associated with concomitant use of diuretics and lower baseline serum sodium concentration (Jacob and Spinler 2006).

Example: Anticholinergic delirium

Anticholinergic delirium is a common complication of drugs in older adults, particularly those with preexisting cognitive impairment. Common psychotropic medications with significant anticholinergicity are shown in Table 19.1. This toxicity is likely related to a central cholinergic deficit that is produced by these medications. The cumulative effect of several of these drugs can be measured using a serum anticholinergicity assay. Higher serum anticholinergicity is associated with impaired cognitive and functional performance, and most dramatically, with the development of delirium (Flacker

(continued)

Table 19.1 Psychotropic drugs with significant anticholinergicity

Drug class	Notable examples
Tricyclic antidepressants	Amitriptyline, Doxepin, Clomipramine, Imipramine
SSRI antidepressants	Paroxetine
Typical antipsychotics	Chlorpromazine, Fluphenazine, Loxapine
Atypical antipsychotics	Clozapine, Olanzapine
Other commonly prescribed or over-the-counter medications	Diphenhydramine, Dimenhydrinate, Diphenhydramine, Hydroxyzine, Oxybutynin, Tolterodine, Amantadine, Benztropine

et al. 1998). Whenever possible in the treatment of older adults, it is best to select a drug with minimal anticholinergicity. It is also crucial to be aware of the central and peripheral (e.g., constipation, blurry vision, dry mouth, urinary retention) anticholinergic effects of medications to prevent the addition of further medications to treat the side effects (commonly termed the prescribing cascade). A tool such as the "Anticholinergic Burden List" (Boustani et al. 2008) can be used to identify problematic medications.

Case Example

Mrs. G is an 81-year-old retired teacher who has a diagnosis of locally advanced breast cancer for which she underwent neoadjuvant chemotherapy followed by mastectomy and radiotherapy. She presents with ongoing neuropathic chest pain post-completion of treatment. There is no evidence of breast cancer recurrence. Her medical history is notable for dyslipidemia, hypertension, insomnia, and urge urinary incontinence. Her medications are simvastatin, amlodipine, enteric coated aspirin, tolterodine, and clonazepam 0.5 mg as needed for sleep. She lives independently in her own home and has the support of a daughter who lives nearby.

At first, acetaminophen and ibuprofen offer some relief, but Mrs. G reports the pain is increasingly distressing and uncomfortable. She is started on amitriptyline 10 mg at bedtime by her oncologist, which is increased to 25 mg a few weeks later by the family doctor. Over the course of several weeks, her daughter observes her to be progressively more confused and anxious. She has episodes of waking disoriented in the night and believing it to be daytime. She begins switching between English and her native language in her speech. She reports to her family doctor that she is terrified that the cancer has recurred and that she is taking large doses of acetaminophen and ibuprofen to manage the pain. He prescribes diazepam 5 mg twice daily as needed for anxiety and agitation.

(continued)

Several days later, she is admitted to hospital after a fall and is diagnosed with an acute delirium related to the effects of the benzodiazepine and the anticholinergic medication. The delirium improves over the next few weeks with discontinuation of diazepam and the anticholinergic medications amitriptyline and tolterodine. She is initiated on pregabalin with some improvement in pain, along with acetaminophen and, as needed, low-dose hydromorphone. She also obtains some relief with a topical lidocaine patch and massage and is able to discontinue the hydromorphone a few weeks after going home. She is switched from clonazepam to zopiclone 5 mg as needed for insomnia. She is referred to a program for non-pharmacological management of urge incontinence.

19.2.3 Other Factors Related to Drugs and Aging

Polypharmacy

Polypharmacy is common in older adults, with 35 % of American community-dwelling adults >65 years of age found to be taking more than three prescription drugs (National Center for Health Statistics 2012). Psychotropic medications account for a substantial portion of this, with 15 % of older adults in the USA found to be on an antidepressant and 10 % on a hypnotic/sedative (National Center for Health Statistics 2012). There is a strong association between the number of drugs taken and the risk of having an ADE reaction, both because the number of medications is a marker of medical comorbidity and disease burden, and because risk of pharmacokinetic and pharmacodynamic drug interactions is proportional to the number of drugs prescribed. Psychotropic drugs with the worst profile for drug–drug interactions (such as fluoxetine, with its potent inhibition of cytochrome P450 enzymes) are generally considered to be inappropriate in the elderly.

Medication Administration Errors or Non-adherence

Errors in medication administration and noncompliance are common across all ages and for all prescribed medications. Age per se does not appear to be a risk factor for non-adherence, except through its association with an increase in the number of prescribed medications and age-related factors, such as cognitive impairment (Vik et al. 2004). However, the consequences of non-adherence and medication administration errors are more serious in older adults, compounded by medical comorbidities and frailty.

Patient-related factors limiting adherence in the elderly include cognitive deficits, increased frequency of side effects, and beliefs about their illness and the likely effects of medications. Depression itself has also been implicated in non-adherence to medications, particularly antidepressants (Gehi et al. 2005; Zivin and Kales 2008). The prescribing of psychotropic medication in the elderly should thus involve an assessment of their ability and willingness to take the medication safely. This is particularly important with medications, such as tricyclic antidepressants (TCAs), that have a narrow therapeutic range and highly toxic effects in overdose.

There are also many drug-related factors in non-adherence to prescribed treatments. The number of medications, the complexity of their administration, and even such factors as the ease of swallowing them can impact on willingness or ability to comply with a treatment. Medications that require strict adherence to a specific diet (such as monoamine oxidase (MAO) inhibitors) or have otherwise burdensome dosing regimens should generally be avoided, except when their administration is supervised. However, unintentional causes of non-adherence (such as forgetting a dose or to refill a prescription) are outstripped by intentional non-adherence (such as non-persistence with therapy due to concern about side effects or lack of efficacy) (Vik et al. 2004). Further, as many as 20–30 % of psychotropic prescriptions are never filled (Fischer et al. 2010). The prevention of intentional non-adherence is largely contingent on the prescriber–patient relationship and patient education. Frank discussions about the expected benefits and side effects, timeline for improvement, and plans for reevaluation of the drug are invaluable in supporting adherence.

19.2.4 Clinical Implications

Adverse Drug Events and Their Prevention

Injuries related to the use of medications occur at higher rates in the elderly (Gurwitz et al. 2003). One study found that 30 % of hospitalizations in those over age 75 are secondary to ADEs (Chan et al. 2001). ADEs in the elderly are largely preventable in nature (Beijer and De Blaey 2002) (Table 19.2).

There are many different approaches to preventing ADEs, including pharmacist-led reviews of medications, computerized systems, and educational outreach to patients and carers. However, ADEs can occur even when there is careful and appropriate medication prescription, with some 10–20 % of ADEs being idiosyncratic in nature (Beijer and De Blaey 2002). Many ADEs involve multiple factors, including comorbid illness, interactions with co-prescribed medications, and altered pharmacokinetic and pharmacodynamic interactions. Unfortunately, even with the most sophisticated surveillance, ADEs are an inevitable complication of medication in the elderly.

Example: SSRIs and upper gastrointestinal bleeding

SSRIs have been shown to affect platelet aggregation, resulting in some impairment of their haemostatic function. A rare but notable consequence of this is upper GI bleeding. Upper GI bleeds are more common in older

(continued)

Table 19.2 General guidelines for prescribing psychotropic medications in the elderly

1. Complete a thorough assessment of target symptom or illness
2. Review side effects of current medications to prevent prescribing cascade
3. Have a clear goal of therapy with plan for reevaluation of medication effectiveness
4. Review the patient's medical history and status, with special attention to renal, hepatic, cardiovascular, and cognitive function
5. Review current medications for pharmacokinetic and pharmacodynamic drug interactions
6. Assess patient medication safety (appropriate use, cognitive capacity to manage medications independently)
7. Avoid making more than one medication change at a time
8. Avoid potentially inappropriate drugs if possible. Select a drug with:
(a) Fewer active metabolites
(b) Less accumulation
(c) Shorter action
(d) Less prone to side effects
9. Initiate drug at low dose and increase dose slowly
10. Evaluate response to medication and consider adjustment of dose, and substitution or discontinuation if there is no evidence of a meaningful treatment effect

adults, and a history of this complication is the most significant risk factor for an SSRI-related GI bleed. Concurrent use of nonsteroidal anti-inflammatory drugs (NSAID's), anticoagulants, and antiplatelet agents also increase the risk of bleeding, while the use of proton pump inhibitors appears to decrease the risk (De Abajo 2011).

Maintaining an index of suspicion for ADEs is also an important component of prescribing psychotropic medication in the elderly, since drug-induced symptoms and signs, such as confusion or gait instability, may be mistakenly attributed to the aging process itself. Monitoring for ADEs can take many forms. For example, a baseline cognitive screen allows changes in cognitive functioning due to medications to be identified. Similarly, documenting abnormalities in tone or gait facilitates the detection of new or intensified Parkinsonism or other movement-related disorders. Regular examination for abnormal movements is necessary to detect the emergence of tardive dyskinesia related to the use of antipsychotics. Ideally, the benefits of drugs should also be monitored at baseline and follow-up with validated measures to assess depression, anxiety, and other symptoms. Regular review of the drug effects allows for dose adjustment, discontinuation or substitution if no benefit is observed or if there are serious side effects. The "prescribing cascade," in which the side effect of one medication is treated by the addition of further medications (Rochon and Gurwitz 1997) is a trap that should be avoided (see example below).

Example: Drug-induced movement disorders
Older adults are at increased risk of developing extrapyramidal symptoms and tardive dyskinesia in response to antipsychotic treatment. There is a 5 % annual incidence of tardive dyskinesia with atypical antipsychotics, and a 30 % annual incidence with typical antipsychotics (Caligiuri et al. 2000). Antipsychotic-induced parkinsonism is even more common, seen in 30–60 % of those treated with typical antipsychotics. This complication can take months to years to resolve after discontinuation of the offending agent. If the etiology of such symptoms is not recognized, they may be mistakenly treated with additional psychoactive medications, producing a prescribing cascade. An example of this is treating drug-induced parkinsonism with the addition of dopaminergic agents. Similarly, akathisia or tardive movements can be misdiagnosed as agitation and treated with escalating doses of sedative or antipsychotic medications.

Under-treatment

Although the risks of prescribing psychotropic medications in the elderly are clear, there is also a risk of under-prescribing. Both patient and clinician factors may contribute to such under-treatment of conditions such as depression (Barry et al. 2012). Patients are sometimes reluctant to take medication because they fear the side effects, are pessimistic about the possible benefits, or feel stigmatized by taking it. Clinicians must also examine their own judgments about the value of interventions such as antidepressant treatment.

19.3 Pharmacotherapy of Depression in the Elderly Cancer Patient

In general, the medications used to treat depression in younger cancer patients are as effective in the elderly. Therefore, the choice of medication in this circumstance is influenced by careful consideration of the pharmacokinetic and pharmacodynamic factors in the context of each individual case. Important factors to take into account in order to maximize the potential for effective treatment and minimize the potential for detrimental side effects or harmful drug interactions include the presence of polypharmacy, medical comorbidity, and cognitive impairment or physical frailty. Characteristics of an "ideal" antidepressant for the elderly cancer patient are outlined in Table 19.3. These include a safe and tolerable medication that is effective in treating depression, has a once daily dosing regimen to aid compliance, a minimal potential for interactions with concurrent drugs, and is inexpensive for the patient.

Table 19.3 General characteristics of an "ideal" antidepressant for the older patient with cancer

• Effective, with a side effect profile that is safe with coexisting medical morbidity (e.g., little effect on cardiovascular system) and tolerable (e.g., low anticholinergic or sedative effects)
• A reasonably short half-life to avoid potential drug accumulation and toxicity
• Once daily dosing to minimize compliance problems
• Low protein-binding capacity to reduce risk of displacement of other highly protein bound medications (e.g., digoxin or warfarin)
• Minimal effect on hepatic P450 enzymes to reduce potential effect on the metabolism of concurrent medications
• Inexpensive, with a satisfactory cost–benefit ratio
• Availability in multiple formulations (i.e., tablet, liquid, orodispersible forms)

19.3.1 Classes of Antidepressants

Selective Serotonin Reuptake Inhibitors

SSRIs are usually the first choice for the pharmacological treatment of major depression in the elderly cancer patient (Roth and Modi 2003; Roose and Schatzberg 2005). These agents are as effective as other classes of antidepressants but are more tolerable and safer in case of overdose. Furthermore, many of the SSRIs are now available in elixir formulations that are more acceptable to elderly patients who have an impaired ability to swallow tablets.

Although all SSRIs are hepatically metabolized, the degree to which they inhibit the P450 isoenzyme system varies within class from one SSRI to another (see Table 19.4). This is an important consideration in the selection of an antidepressant, since most elderly cancer patients take several concurrent medications and are therefore at increased risk for drug–drug interactions (see above). Medications, such as fluoxetine, that have a long half-life and strong P450 effects, should generally be avoided in this population for this reason. In addition, fluoxetine is highly protein bound and therefore carries a further risk of interactions with other common medications such as warfarin or the chemotherapeutic agent, cisplatin. Of the SSRIs, citalopram and escitalopram have the least effect on the P450 isoenzyme system, reasonably low protein-binding properties, and relatively short half-lives. In general, these qualities make them good first-line choices in the elderly cancer patient. However, there have been recent regulatory warnings of a possible dose-related risk of QT prolongation and arrhythmias with these medications, with increased risk in the elderly for this complication. This has led some to suggest lower maximum dose restrictions of these SSRIs in this population.

SSRI medications are associated with an increased risk of falls in the elderly, similar to that with the tricyclic antidepressants. However, the former are associated with an increased risk of bone fracture rate due to the detrimental effect of prolonged SSRI use on bone mineral density (Coupland et al. 2011). There is also evidence that SSRIs are associated with a greater risk of GI bleeding, a result of blockade of platelet serotonin reuptake. Older age is also an important risk factor for the development of hyponatraemia associated with antidepressant use,

Table 19.4 Important considerations of the commonly used antidepressants in the context of the older cancer patient

Medication	Drug half-life	Protein-binding	Common side-effects	Comments/considerations
SSRIs				
Escitalopram	27–32 h	56 %	GI disturbance, restlessness, sexual dysfunction	At higher doses, risk of QT prolongation
				Little hepatic P450 effects
Citalopram	~35 h	80 %	As above	As above
Sertraline	~26 h	98 %	Fatigue, dizziness, headache	Moderate P450 effects; short-half life
Fluoxetine	1–6 days	95 %	Stimulating; weight loss	Strong hepatic P450 effects; once weekly dosing possible; long washout period needed
Paroxetine	~24 h	95 %	More sedating; more anticholinergic effects	Strong P450 effects; discontinuation symptoms more likely
Atypical antidepressants				
Mirtazapine	20–40 h	85 %	Sedating; appetite stimulation less GI side effects; less sexual dysfunction	Also antiemetic properties; available in an orodispersible tablet; little hepatic P450 effects
Venlafaxine	5–10 h	27 %	Discontinuation symptoms; nausea; headache; sleep disturbance	Little hepatic P450 effects; potential blood pressure elevation; useful in reducing hot flash symptoms
Duloxetine	~12 h	95 %	Nausea, dizziness, fatigue	Used for neuropathic pain also; rarely hepatic insufficiency
Buproprion	~20 h	84 %	Minimal effect on weight; increased seizure risk	Stimulating; smoking cessation aid also
TCAs				
Amitriptyline	~15 h	>90 %	Sedating; hypotensive; anticholinergic effects	Pro-arrhythmogenic; efficacy in neuropathic pain
Nortriptyline	16–90 h	95 %	Less sedative; anticholinergic	
Lofepramine	~23 h	99 %	Less cardiotoxic	Best tolerated and safest TCA
Psychostimulants				
Methylphenidate	2–12 h	30 %	Anxiety, tremor, insomnia, hypertension/ tachycardia, tolerance can develop	Rapid onset of action may improve fatigue and attention/concentration
Dextroamphetamine	10–12 h	15–40 %		
Modafinil	12–15 h	60 %	No seizure risk	Atypical stimulant: less potential for dependence or tolerance

particularly with the SSRIs (Giorlando et al. 2013). This complication tends to develop within the first few weeks of treatment or after dosage adjustments, and therefore sodium levels should be monitored closely during these periods in the elderly.

Serotonin–Norepinephrine Reuptake Inhibitors (SNRIs) and Newer-Generation Antidepressants

Venlafaxine and duloxetine are both serotonin- and norepinephrine reuptake inhibitors (SNRIs). The SNRIs are often used when patients do not respond to SSRI antidepressants, although they can also be used as first-line treatments for depression. Venlafaxine has very low protein binding and so is unlikely to result in clinically significant displacement of any co-prescribed highly protein-bound medications. There is evidence that SNRIs are efficacious in treating neuropathic pain and also in reducing hot flash symptoms that may arise from androgen ablation therapy in prostate cancer or tamoxifen-induced hot flashes in breast cancer (Stearns 2004). Venlafaxine is associated with a risk of GI bleeding similar to that with the SSRIs and can elevate blood pressure at higher doses, which requires monitoring.

Mirtazapine is a sedating dual acting noradrenergic and serotonergic antidepressant. It is less likely to cause GI distress and has appetite stimulating and mild antiemetic properties. These side effects tend to be beneficial in the cancer population, in whom insomnia, GI distress, and weight loss are prominent concerns. Mirtazapine is also the only antidepressant available in an orally disintegrating tablet form that dissolves on the tongue, which can aid compliance in some elderly with swallowing difficulties.

Bupropion is an antidepressant that appears to work through its effects on the noradrenergic and dopamine system. It tends to be weight neutral, but can have a stimulating effect. This may be helpful for elderly cancer patients with significant fatigue, although it may cause or worsen anxiety or restlessness in some patients. Buproprion lowers the seizure threshold in a dose-dependent manner and therefore should be avoided in patients with a history of seizure disorders or head injury, or current brain tumors or malnutrition. It also has efficacy as a smoking cessation aid through its dopaminergic effects.

The Tricyclic Antidepressants

TCAs are generally not appropriate medications for the treatment of depression in the elderly oncology population. Their overall use has declined significantly over the past 30 years, as equally efficacious but safer and better tolerated medications have been developed. Peripheral anticholinergic side effects, such as urinary retention, and central anticholinergic effects, such as confusion, agitation, and memory disturbance, are more common in the elderly and can lead to poor tolerance or serious ADEs. The tricyclics also carry risks of cardiac arrhythmias, hypotension, sedation, falls, and lowering of the seizure threshold. Because of these toxicities, the use of tricyclic antidepressants diminished overall, although they retain a significant role in the treatment of neuropathic pain syndromes, for which lower doses are efficacious and better tolerated (Dharmshaktu et al. 2012). When TCAs are deemed appropriate for treatment of depression, then second-generation tricyclics, such as desipramine or lofepramine, should be considered first as these have less anticholinergic effects, less cardiotoxicity, and are safer in overdose than their predecessors.

Psychostimulants

Psychostimulants, such as methylphenidate, dextroamphetamine, and modafinil, have been used to treat depressive symptoms in the elderly cancer patient, especially when these symptoms are accompanied by psychomotor slowing, significant fatigue, and/or apathy. Due to the reported quicker onset of action of psychostimulants in comparison to other classes of antidepressants, they are often used in a palliative care or hospice setting where there may be more urgency for a rapid therapeutic response. However, the efficacy of psychostimulants to treat depression in cancer patients has not yet been clearly established (Li et al. 2012; Kerr et al. 2012). In relatively low doses the stimulant medications have been shown to decrease feelings of fatigue in cancer patients and they are often also helpful to counter the sedating side effects of opioid medications. There are no age-related considerations regarding dosage regimes in adults, though caution should be employed in those with a comorbid dementia who may experience worsening agitation or confusion. Symptomatic cardiovascular disease or moderate to severe hypertension are contraindications.

19.3.2 Antidepressant Treatment Response in the Elderly

Knowledge regarding the response to pharmacotherapy in the elderly comes from the general psychiatry and psycho-geriatric literature rather than from oncology or general medicine. Two studies from The Sequenced Treatment Alternatives to Relieve Depression Trial (STAR_D) demonstrated that elderly patients with late onset major depression treated with citalopram showed no difference in treatment response, remission rates, and time to remission compared with younger depressed patients (Zisook et al. 2007; Kozel et al. 2008). However, the presence of cognitive deficits, in particular executive dysfunction, has been shown to be associated with worse antidepressant treatment response (Baldwin et al. 2004). There is also evidence that suggests that SSRI treatment is associated with worsening of cognitive impairment in depressed individuals older than 75 years (Culang et al. 2009; Sneed et al. 2010). In these studies, the antidepressant treatment worsened cognitive decline, particularly in treatment of nonresponders. Therefore, it is valuable to monitor cognitive functioning in this group of patients taking SSRIs. There is some evidence that donepezil (a cholinesterase inhibitor) add-on treatment to standard antidepressant therapy may provide cognitive enhancement in elderly depressed patients with comorbid cognitive impairment, although it might also increase the subsequent risk of depressive episode recurrence (Reynolds et al. 2011).

19.4   Pharmacotherapy of Anxiety in the Elderly Cancer Patient

The presentation of significant anxiety in the elderly cancer patient must prompt a thorough bio-psycho-social assessment to determine the causative factors. These may include inadequate pain control, respiratory distress secondary to underlying lung disease, sepsis, or underlying biochemical abnormalities. It may be appropriate to use anxiolytic medication in the short term in such cases, but accurate identification of the underlying medical problem and the application of a specific medical intervention are needed. When the primary diagnosis of an anxiety disorder is established, pharmacotherapy can play a primary or secondary role. In these patients, the treatment response is similar to that of the younger population, though specific considerations relevant to the elderly must be taken into account. These include the choice of medication used and the expected benefit–risk ratio of treatment, which are discussed below.

19.4.1 Classes of Antianxiety Medications

Antidepressants

Many antidepressants (e.g., SSRIs and SNRIs, see above) are effective first-line pharmacological treatments of anxiety disorders in elderly patients. The selection and monitoring of an antidepressant in this circumstance is guided by the same principles that apply to treatment of depression. If anxiety is severe, it may be appropriate to consider the short-term co-prescription of a more immediate-acting anxiolytic medication in the weeks prior to the onset of action of antidepressants. The latter should then be phased out as the anxiolytic effect of the antidepressant takes effect. In general, stimulating antidepressants (e.g., bupropion) should be avoided in elderly patients with severe anxiety, as these medications may worsen this symptom. Antidepressant treatment should begin with low doses initially to minimize the potential to exacerbate anxiety during initial phase of treatment.

Benzodiazepines

Pharmacotherapy to treat anxiety symptoms in the elderly cancer population should be approached carefully and with a clear rationale and treatment plan. While short-term use of benzodiazepines may be one of the first lines of treatment of anxiety in a younger cancer patient, alternative medications may be more appropriate to try initially in the elderly. Benzodiazepines should be reserved for those who fail to respond to these measures. When used, they should be prescribed in lower doses than in the younger adult, with careful monitoring of tolerance and response.

The elderly are particularly vulnerable to develop adverse effects from benzodiazepines, with excessive sedation and confusion being the most common side effects experienced. The benzodiazepines that are longer acting (e.g., clonazepam, diazepam) or those which undergo phase I hepatic metabolism (e.g., alprazolam, diazepam, clonazepam) are at greatest risk of accumulation in the older patient and of causing adverse effects. Benzodiazepines that are metabolized by

Table 19.5 Important properties of common benzodiazepines in relation to elderly cancer patients

Medication	Half-life (h)	Protein binding	Hepatic metabolism	Adverse effects in the elderly
Diazepam	20–100	95 %	Phase I and II	**Common**: Sedation
Alprazolam	6–16	80 %	Phase I and II	Psychomotor impairment, dizziness
Lorazepam	10–20	85–90 %	Phase II only	**Occasional**: Ataxia
Clonazepam	16–50	85 %	Phase I and II	Blurred vision, low blood pressure
Oxazepam	4–15	86–99 %	Phase II only	**Rare**: Memory disturbance, agitation

conjugation (e.g., lorazepam, oxazepam) are preferable, because their clearance is unaffected by aging and, therefore, their active ingredients are less likely to accumulate and cause toxicity (see Table 19.5).

One of the most problematic adverse effects of these medications in the elderly patient is their potential to impair balance, leading to falls that cause significant morbidity and mortality. Benzodiazepines can also have synergistic central nervous system (CNS) depressant effects when used in combination with opioids and require careful monitoring in this context. A paradoxical disinhibiting or agitating effect can occur in patients with dementia or brain injury who are treated with benzodiazepines, and a similar worsening of confusion and agitation can occur in the setting of delirium (see below).

Pregabalin

This is an anticonvulsant that has been shown to have modest efficacy as an anxiolytic, especially in relation to generalized anxiety. It is generally well tolerated in the elderly with no specific age-related dose adjustments necessary and has an onset of action within a few weeks of commencing treatment. The most problematic potential side effect is dizziness, which is relatively common, and which may require discontinuation of the drug because of the risk of falls. Other common side effects include somnolence and weight gain, although these can be advantageous for patients with insomnia and cancer-related weight loss.

Buspirone

This is a non-benzodiazepine medication that can be a helpful anxiolytic in the elderly with generalized anxiety (Mokhber et al. 2010). Buspirone has several advantages over benzodiazepines in terms of safety and tolerability. It produces little or no sedation, and causes no serious cognitive or psychomotor impairment, respiratory depression, or withdrawal symptoms following its discontinuation. However, similar to antidepressant medication, the onset of therapeutic effect can take several weeks. This delay may limit its usefulness in patients with severe anxiety that require rapid relief of symptoms. The need for twice or three times a day dosing can also hinder compliance. It is usually well tolerated by patients, though can be pro-convulsant and therefore is contraindicated in patients with a history of seizures.

Antipsychotic Medications

Clinical experience suggests that antipsychotic medications can alleviate acute anxiety in some elderly cancer patients, although their efficacy has not been systemically studied in the literature. Atypical antipsychotics have several advantages over benzodiazepines in the elderly due to their lesser effect on respiration and cognitive functioning. This may be clinically beneficial for some anxious elderly patients, such as in those with significant lung disease, those on high dose opioids, or at risk of delirium. The atypical antipsychotics, such as quetiapine, olanzapine, and risperidone, are preferred to the older typical antipsychotics, such as haloperidol or chlorpromazine, because they are better tolerated and associated with fewer extrapyramidal side effects (EPSE). However, these agents may be associated with adverse metabolic effects, such as hyperglycemia, hyperlipidemia, and weight gain. In addition, antipsychotics are associated with an increased risk of mortality and cerebrovascular disease in the elderly, especially in the context of dementia, where they should generally be avoided. However, in the setting of advanced cancer and comorbid dementia, antipsychotics may still play a useful role in the alleviation of distress and agitation after a careful consideration of the aims, risks, and benefits of such treatment.

19.5 Pharmacotherapy of Delirium in the Elderly Cancer Patient

Older age is a strong risk factor for the development of delirium due to the impact of comorbid medical illness, polypharmacy, reduced cerebral reserve due to age and preexisting neurocognitive impairment, and physical frailty. While more research is needed on the pathophysiology of delirium, underactivity of the cholinergic system is thought to play a prominent role. This may explain why anticholinergic medications may precipitate or worsen an episode of delirium, particularly in the elderly who are more sensitive to adverse drug effects. The cholinergic hypothesis also explains the efficacy of dopamine antagonists in the treatment of delirium, since the central dopaminergic and cholinergic systems are intimately and reciprocally related.

Management of delirium involves a careful assessment and identification of the syndrome, followed by correction of underlying medical causes. In the older cancer patient, this commonly includes an evaluation of polypharmacy and discontinuation or dose adjustment of offending medications identifying environmental contributors and introducing both non-pharmacological and pharmacological strategies. Non-pharmacologic interventions include the provision of a structured and consistent environment, such as a quiet, well-lit room with a visible clock or calendar, and the presence of family or other caregivers who can provide reassurance and regular reorientation. Often these supportive interventions are insufficient on their own to relieve distress and symptomatic treatment with antipsychotic medications is necessary. However, careful consideration of the potential risks and benefits from such treatment should be made prior to initiation of pharmacotherapy and on its continuation. This is important in view of the possibility that such medications may lead to further ADEs (e.g., falls) in an already vulnerable population. Once pharmacotherapy has been commenced, it must be monitored closely for treatment response, and emerging side effects or poor tolerability, with attention to the need for dose reductions, substitution with other agents, or discontinuation of pharmacotherapy.

19.5.1 Antipsychotic Medications

Current evidence is supportive of the short-term use of antipsychotics in the treatment of symptoms of delirium, with close monitoring for possible adverse effects (Breitbart and Alici 2012). Haloperidol remains the first-line treatment of choice, due to its efficacy at low doses and good safety profile (e.g., lack of active metabolites, minimal anticholinergic effects, low risk of extrapyramidal side effects at doses under 3.5 mg daily, and several possible routes of administration). It is usually effective in divided doses of between 1 and 3 mg daily. However, there is growing evidence for the efficacy of atypical antipsychotics in the management of delirium (see Table 19.6).

Monitoring the Effects of Antipsychotic Medications

It is recommended that elderly patients with delirium should be monitored daily for adverse effects of antipsychotics. This should include a baseline ECG, which should be repeated after dose increases or more frequently if high doses of antipsychotics (e.g., haloperidol >5 mg daily) or other QT-prolonging medications are administered or if ongoing electrolyte disturbances or unstable cardiac disease are present. A QTc interval of >500 ms or an increase of more than 20 % from baseline indicates an increased risk of torsades de pointes and merits discontinuation of the antipsychotic and consultation with a cardiac specialist. In addition, it is important to evaluate on a daily basis the emergence of medication-induced extrapyramidal effects including akathisia, dystonia, and neuroleptic malignant syndrome. These complications may occur with all antipsychotics, though less often with the atypicals and when the haloperidol daily dose is low.

Benzodiazepines and Delirium

Benzodiazepines alone are generally ineffective for managing symptoms of delirium and indeed may worsen the confusion and agitation, particularly in the elderly. An exception is delirium associated with alcohol or benzodiazepine withdrawal, for which benzodiazepines are indicated. Benzodiazepine withdrawal should be considered in the differential diagnosis of acute confusion that occurs within 3 days of hospital admission. Benzodiazepines also have a role in some other cases of delirium, in combination with antipsychotic medications, when rapid sedation of

Table 19.6 Antipsychotic medications that may be useful in the management of delirium in the older cancer patient

Name	Daily dose range and route	Considerations
Typical antipsychotics		
Haloperidol	0.5–2.5 mg, q2-12 h po/im/iv	First-line agent with less EPSE or anticholinergic effects at low doses; ECG monitoring advised
Chlorpromazine	12.5–50 mg, q4-12 h po/im	Greater anticholinergic and sedative effects; can be hypotensive
Atypical antipsychotics		
Quetiapine	12.5–100 mg, q12h po	Prominent sedating effects
Olanzapine	2.5–5 mg, q12h po/sublingual/im	Orodisperisble tablet available
Risperidone	0.25–2 mg, q12h po/sublingual	Risk of EPSE at higher doses
Aripiprazole	5–30 mg q24h po/im	Can be activating; some evidence of benefit in hypoactive delirium

po = oral; im = intramuscular; iv = intravenous; ECG = electrocardiogram

a highly agitated patient is required to ensure safety. A useful strategy in this regard is to add low-dose parenteral lorazepam to a regimen of haloperidol.

Summary and Conclusions

The use of psychotropic medications to treat psychiatric and cancer-related symptoms in the older cancer patient presents a major challenge to the clinician. Psychiatric symptoms can be disturbing and disabling in the elderly but these individuals are at higher risk to develop ADEs from the use of antidepressants, anxiolytics, and neuroleptics. This risk is due to age-related changes that affect the way these medications are absorbed, distributed, and metabolized and because of the frequency of preexisting cognitive deficits, medical comorbidity, and polypharmacy. A careful and systematic assessment of the indications, expected benefits, and potential adverse effects should be carried out prior to any pharmacological treatment, and a plan of care should be established to ensure ongoing assessment and follow-up. This medication can be initiated by psychiatric specialists or by oncologists who are aware of their indications, potential adverse effects and drug interactions, and how to liaise with expert psychiatric/psycho-oncology services for advice as needed. Finally, more psycho-oncological intervention research is needed, specifically in elderly cancer patients, to better establish the efficacy and safety of psychopharmacotherapy in this population. Such research will allow for the individual tailoring of treatment strategies that may improve tolerability and outcomes.

References

Baldwin R, Jeffries S, Jackson A, Sutcliffe C, Thacker N, Scott M, Burns A. Treatment response in late-onset depression: relationship to neuropsychological, neuroradiological and vascular risk factors. Psychol Med. 2004;34(1):125–36.

Barry LC, Abou JJ, Simen AA, Gill TM. Under-treatment of depression in older persons. J Affect Disord. 2012;136(3):789–96.

Beijer HJ, De Blaey CJ. Hospitalisations caused by adverse drug reactions (ADR): a meta-analysis of observational studies. Pharm World Sci. 2002;24(2):46–54.

Boustani M, Campbell N, Munger S, Maidment I, Fox C. Impact of anticholinergics on the aging brain: a review and practical application. Aging Health. 2008;4(3):311–20.

Breitbart W, Alici Y. Evidence-based treatment of delirium in patients with cancer. J Clin Oncol. 2012;30(11):1206–14.

Caligiuri MR, Jeste DV, Lacro JP. Antipsychotic-induced movement disorders in the elderly: epidemiology and treatment recommendations. Drugs Aging. 2000;17(5):363–84.

Chan M, Nicklason F, Vial JH. Adverse drug events as a cause of hospital admission in the elderly. Intern Med J. 2001;31(4):199–205.

Clegg A, Young J, Iliffe S, Rikkert MO, Rockwood K. Frailty in elderly people. Lancet. 2013;381 (9868):752–62.

Coupland C, Dhiman P, Morriss R, Arthur A, Barton G, Hippisley-Cox J. Antidepressant use and risk of adverse outcomes in older people: population based cohort study. BMJ. 2011;343: d4551.

Cresswell KM, Fernando B, McKinstry B, Sheikh A. Adverse drug events in the elderly. Br Med Bull. 2007;83:259–74.

Culang ME, Sneed JR, Keilp JG, Rutherford BR, Pelton GH, Devanand DP, Roose SP. Change in cognitive functioning following acute antidepressant treatment in late-life depression. Am J Geriatr Psychiatry. 2009;17(10):881–8.

De Abajo FJ. Effects of selective serotonin reuptake inhibitors on platelet function: mechanisms, clinical outcomes and implications for use in elderly patients. Drugs Aging. 2011;28 (5):345–67.

Dharmshaktu P, Tayal V, Kalra BS. Efficacy of antidepressants as analgesics: a review. J Clin Pharmacol. 2012;52(1):6–17.

Fischer MA, Stedman MR, Lii J, Vogeli C, Shrank WH, Brookhart MA, Weissman JS. Primary medication non-adherence: analysis of 195,930 electronic prescriptions. J Gen Intern Med. 2010;25(4):284–90.

Fitzgerald P, Nissim R, Rodin G. A life-stage approach to psycho-oncology. In: Grassi L, Riba M, editors. Clinical psycho-oncology: an international perspective. Chichester: Wiley; 2012. p. 155–63.

Flacker JM, Cummings V, Mach Jr JR, Bettin K, Kiely DK, Wei J. The association of serum anticholinergic activity with delirium in elderly medical patients. Am J Geriatr Psychiatry. 1998;6(1):31–41.

Gehi A, Haas D, Pipkin S, Whooley MA. Depression and medication adherence in outpatients with coronary heart disease: findings from the Heart and Soul study. Arch Intern Med. 2005;165 (21):2508–13.

Giorlando F, Teister J, Dodd S, Udina M, Berk M. Hyponatraemia: an audit of aged psychiatry patients taking SSRIs and SNRIs. Curr Drug Saf. 2013;8(3):175–80.

Gurwitz JH, Field TS, Harrold LR, Rothschild J, Debellis K, Seger AC, Cadoret C, Fish LS, Garber L, Kelleher M, Bates DW. Incidence and preventability of adverse drug events among older persons in the ambulatory setting. JAMA. 2003;289(9):1107–16.

Jacob S, Spinler SA. Hyponatremia associated with selective serotonin-reuptake inhibitors in older adults. Ann Pharmacother. 2006;40(9):1618–22.

Kerr CW, Drake J, Milch RA, Brazeau DA, Skretny JA, Brazeau GA, Donnelly JP. Effects of methylphenidate on fatigue and depression: a randomized, double-blind, placebo-controlled trial. J Pain Symptom Manage. 2012;43(1):68–77.

Kozel FA, Trivedi MH, Wisniewski SR, Miyahara S, Husain MM, Fava M, Lebowitz B, Zisook S, Rush AJ. Treatment outcomes for older depressed patients with early versus late onset of first depressive episode: a Sequenced Treatment Alternatives to Relieve Depression Trial (STAR*D) report. Am J Geriatr Psychiatry. 2008;16(1):58–64.

Li M, Fitzgerald P, Rodin G. Evidence-based treatment of depression in patients with cancer. J Clin Oncol. 2012;30(11):1187–96.

Mokhber N, Azarpazhooh MR, Khajehdaluee M, Velayati A, Hopwood M. Randomized, single-blind, trial of sertraline and buspirone for treatment of elderly patients with generalized anxiety disorder. Psychiatry Clin Neurosci. 2010;64(2):128–33.

National Center for Health Statistics. Health, United States, 2011: with special feature on socioeconomic status and health. Table 99. Hyattsville, MD: National Center for Health Statistics; 2012.

Perucca E, Grimaldi R, Gatti G, Pirracchio S, Crema F, Frigo GM. Pharmacokinetics of valproic acid in the elderly. Br J Clin Pharmacol. 1984;17(6):665–9.

Reidenberg MM, Levy M, Warner H, Coutinho CB, Schwartz MA, Yu G, Cheripko J. Relationship between diazepam dose, plasma level, age, and central nervous system depression. Clin Pharmacol Ther. 1978;23(4):371–4.

Reynolds 3rd CF, Butters MA, Lopez O, Pollock BG, Dew MA, Mulsant BH, Lenze EJ, Holm M, Rogers JC, Mazumdar S, Houck PR, Begley A, Anderson S, Karp JF, Miller MD, Whyte EM, Stack J, Gildengers A, Szanto K, Bensasi S, Kaufer DI, Kamboh MI, DeKosky ST. Maintenance treatment of depression in old age: a randomized, double-blind, placebo-controlled evaluation of the efficacy and safety of donepezil combined with antidepressant pharmacotherapy. Arch Gen Psychiatry. 2011;68(1):51–60.

Rochon PA, Gurwitz JH. Optimising drug treatment for elderly people: the prescribing cascade. BMJ. 1997;315(7115):1096–9.

Roose S, Schatzberg AF. The efficacy of antidepressants in the treatment of late-life depression. J Clin Psychopharmacol. 2005;25(4 Suppl 1):S1–7.

Roth AJ, Modi R. Psychiatric issues in older cancer patients. Crit Rev Oncol Hematol. 2003;48(2):185–97.

Sneed JR, Culang ME, Keilp JG, Rutherford BR, Devanand DP, Roose SP. Antidepressant medication and executive dysfunction: a deleterious interaction in late-life depression. Am J Geriatr Psychiatry. 2010;18(2):128–35.

Stearns V. Management of hot flashes in breast cancer survivors and men with prostate cancer. Curr Oncol Rep. 2004;6(4):285–90.

Vik SA, Maxwell CJ, Hogan DB. Measurement, correlates, and health outcomes of medication adherence among seniors. Ann Pharmacother. 2004;38(2):303–12.

Zisook S, Lesser I, Stewart JW, Wisniewski SR, Balasubramani GK, Fava M, Gilmer WS, Dresselhaus TR, Thase ME, Nierenberg AA, Trivedi MH, Rush AJ. Effect of age at onset on the course of major depressive disorder. Am J Psychiatry. 2007;164(10):1539–46.

Zivin K, Kales HC. Adherence to depression treatment in older adults: a narrative review. Drugs Aging. 2008;25(7):559–71.

Sedation for Psychological Distress at the End of Life

20

Laura Ferrari and Augusto Caraceni

Abstract

Terminally ill patients sometimes experience intolerable suffering and, in case of refractory symptoms (e.g. delirium, dyspnoea, pain, nausea and vomiting, psychological distress and existential suffering) at the end of life, palliative sedation therapy (PST) is an important option. Although there is no international consensus on the definition of PST, its main aim is to deliberately induce a temporary or permanent light-to-deep sleep, in patients with terminal illness and refractory symptoms, in order to mitigate the experience of suffering, but not to hasten the end of life. The aims of the chapter are to offer an in-depth insight regarding PST when dealing with suffering at the end of life. The type of PST (in terms of depth and duration), the indication and clinical practice for psychological/existential suffering, the difference between PST and euthanasia, the most important guidelines and the types of drugs (e.g. antipsychotics, benzodiazepines, sedative antiepileptic drugs, general anaesthetics) commonly used in PST are described.

20.1 Introduction

Terminally ill patients sometimes experience intolerable suffering and, in case of refractory symptoms at the end of life, palliative sedation is an important therapeutic option.

A symptom is considered refractory if (1) none of the conventional treatments are effective, (2) the treatments might cause important morbidity and/or (3) the treatments are not effective within an acceptable time frame. By contrast, a difficult symptom could possibly respond, within a tolerable time frame, to interventions

L. Ferrari (✉) • A. Caraceni
Palliative Care, Pain Therapy and Rehabilitation Fondazione IRCCS Istituto Nazionale dei Tumori, Milan, Italy
e-mail: laura.ferrari.1987@gmail.com; Augusto.Caraceni@istitutotumori.mi.it

L. Grassi and M. Riba (eds.), *Psychopharmacology in Oncology and Palliative Care*,
DOI 10.1007/978-3-642-40134-3_20, © Springer-Verlag Berlin Heidelberg 2014

that yield adequate relief and preserve consciousness, without excessive adverse effects. It is therefore of paramount importance distinguishing between refractory and difficult symptoms.

The most common refractory symptoms at the end of life are delirium, dyspnea, pain, nausea and vomiting (Maltoni et al. 2012). However, psychological distress and existential suffering are also considered among the indications for palliative sedation. Palliative sedation for existential distress is a controversial issue because, by its very nature, psychological suffering is difficult to define, assess, and treat and is not be limited to the terminal phase of the disease.

Aim of this chapter is offering a more in-depth insight regarding palliative sedation when dealing with this type of suffering.

20.2   Major Issues

20.2.1 Definition

There is no international consensus on the definition of palliative sedation therapy (PST). The European Association for Palliative Care (EAPC) defines PST as "the monitored use of medications intended to induce a state of decreased or absent awareness (unconsciousness) in order to relieve the burden of otherwise intractable suffering, in a manner that is ethically acceptable to the patient, family and healthcare providers" (Cherny et al. 2009). Similarly, De Graeff and Dean describe PST as "the use of sedative medications to relieve intolerable suffering from refractory symptoms by a reduction in patient's consciousness" (de Graeff and Dean 2007). The American Association of Hospice and Palliative Medicine forgoes a definition but implies that the use of sedatives is intended to decrease a patient's level of consciousness to mitigate the experience of suffering, but not to hasten the end of life. The primary intention is to deliberately induce a temporary or permanent light-to-deep sleep, in patients with terminal illness and refractory symptoms.

When talking about sedation, some authors distinguish between *natural, consequential*, and *palliative* sedation (Fraser Health hospice palliative care program 2011; Morita et al. 2005). Natural sedation, or drowsiness, occurs as part of the dying process, due to a combination of pathophysiological mechanisms causing various degrees of encephalopathy. Consequential sedation is the unintended but predictable side effect of many drugs used for symptom control, also in patients who are not dying. This type of sedation might be transient and may be modified or eliminated by adjusting the dose or by tolerance development. Brief periods of sedation may also be induced when managing delirium, pain or dyspnoea, but this does not constitute PST, as it is not limited to terminally ill patients.

20.2.2 Classification

PST is classified according to duration and depth of sedation. Most of the time, both criteria are used to describe the type of sedation (e.g. Continuous-deep sedation).

Duration of Sedation

Intermittent sedation, also known as respite sedation, is intended to be temporary. The patient is sedated and then awakened, by downwardly titrating the sedative dose, after a predetermined interval, to reassess the situation and to evaluate whether or not the symptoms remain refractory and intolerable (Rousseau 2004).

Continuous sedation refers to the use of sedatives intended specifically for lowering consciousness continuously until the patient dies.

A recent systematic review by Maltoni and colleagues revealed that the mean duration of PST ranged from 0.8 to 12.6 days (Maltoni et al. 2012). However, even shorter duration periods have been reported (1–3.5 days) in a home care setting (Mercadante et al. 2011). An observational study of patients referred to a tertiary cancer centre resulted in a median duration of sedation till death of 45 h (range 6–96 h) (Caraceni et al. 2012).

Depth of Sedation

Deep sedation causes complete unconsciousness, with the primary aim to relieve the patient from suffering.

Mild sedation is the administration of sedatives to the point where the patient is somnolent and doesn't experience suffering but can still communicate.

Objective measures of the depth of sedation are considered for clinical practice in some guidelines (SICP Italian Society for palliative care 2007; Royal Dutch Medical Association 2009).

20.2.3 Indication and Clinical Practice for Psychological/Existential Suffering

At the end of life, hopelessness, anxiety, remorse, loneliness, and loss of meaning also cause suffering (Chochinov et al. 2009; Chochinov et al. 2008). Suffering, meant as "a sense of helplessness or loss in the face of a seemingly relentless and unendurable threat to quality of life or integrity of self" (Cassell and Rich 2010), involves the whole person in physical, psychological, and spiritual ways. Existential suffering describes the experience of patients facing terminal illness, who may or may not have physical symptoms but report distress. It arises as a result of facing one's own mortality and may be expressed as feelings of pointlessness, emptiness, anguish, a desire not to experience death or the dying process consciously, or to preserve one's dignity or sometimes also to hasten death (Fraser Health hospice palliative care program 2011; Royal Dutch Medical Association 2009).

Sedation in the management of refractory psychological symptoms, and existential distress is different from other situations and still controversial for various reasons. First of all, when dealing with existential suffering, it is difficult to establish which symptoms are indeed refractory, by virtue of their dynamic and idiosyncratic nature. Second, ordinary treatments usually have low intrinsic morbidity and should be preferred and always used as first-line therapy. And last but not least, the presence of these symptoms does not necessarily correlate with an advanced physical deterioration.

According to the EAPC framework, palliative sedation for existential distress should be reserved for patients in advanced stages of a terminal illness. Furthermore, the designation of this condition as refractory should only be performed after repeated assessments by clinicians skilled in psychological care and after routine approaches for depression, anxiety and existential distress.

A multidisciplinary case evaluation is mandatory, to be performed not only by the clinicians providing bedside care but also including representatives from psychiatry and/or psychology, and, if necessary, from chaplaincy and ethics, because of the complexity and multifactorial nature of this situation (SICP Italian Society for palliative care).

20.2.4 Guidelines for Palliative Sedation

In 2005 the Royal Dutch Medical Association (RDMA), drawing from previous local guidelines, published a national guideline for palliative sedation, later updated in 2009. The guideline restricts the application of continuous sedation to patients who experience refractory symptoms and who are expected to die within 1 or 2 weeks. It also regards PST as common medical practice and is the first and only guideline which is mandatory for all physicians within a country in this field.

The untreatable nature of a symptom is to be proven beyond reasonable doubt. This means that reversible causes of suffering must be meticulously excluded before a decision of starting PST is taken. For example, in case of agitation there might be underlying treatable causes, such as pain, constipation or urine retention, withdrawal symptoms, side effects of medications, hypoglycaemia or electrolyte disorders (in advanced stages of various diseases, the patient reduces his intake of food and liquid); psychological causes for agitation should also be addressed: coming to term with and accepting the situation, might determine agitation, anxiety, and suchlike.

If PST is indeed deemed appropriate and proportionate to the situation, it should be initiated on a respite basis for 6–24 h, with planned downward titration to reassess the patient's condition. Continuous-deep sedation should be adopted when intermittent or mild sedation has been effective after repeated trials.

Nonetheless, continuous-deep sedation might be selected as first choice if (Morita et al. 2005):

- The suffering is intense and definitely refractory: as previously stated, the difficulty lays in recognizing and evaluating a refractory psycho-existential symptom; however, we must not forget that the refractory nature of a symptom is best evaluated by the patient himself, and so the clinician has to consider the patient's reports and wishes.

- Death is to occur within several hours to days: in practice it is not always easy to predict how long a patient is going to live. Once a number of characteristics of the dying phase have been observed, it can be assumed that the patient is approaching the stage where death is imminent.
- Suffering will not be palliated by respite sedation.

The Italian guidelines on PST state that, although psychological distress can be difficult to define, sometimes a therapeutic approach may be necessary, including sedation. However, PST should not be adopted for those patients who have no refractory symptoms: again, diagnosing refractory existential symptoms requires a multidisciplinary evaluation, as suggested by all guidelines.

20.2.5 Exceptional Situations

Sometimes a patient exhibits refractory symptoms, but death is not expected to occur in the near future (within 1 or 2 weeks). This situation is quite common with conditions such as amyotrophic lateral sclerosis (ALS), muscular dystrophy, or respiratory or cardiac insufficiency. In some cases of this kind, it is difficult to ascertain whether or not a patient is in the final stages of his disease, but it is nonetheless important to avoid premature continuous-deep sedation until the time of death.

In such situations, respite or mild sedation might be initiated as a first step, and this provides an opportunity to establish the permanent refractory nature of the symptom. Respite sedation also gives the physician the opportunity to reevaluate the situation with the patient and/or the family and, if necessary, to review the management of the case.

20.2.6 Palliative Sedation and Euthanasia

Part of the controversy regarding PST and euthanasia stems from the confusion, present at both policy and practice levels, about the distinction between deep-continuous sedation till the time of death and euthanasia.

The RDMA's guidelines offer a thorough and poignant evaluation of the situation, considering that both interventions are legal in the Netherlands.

Continuous-deep sedation differs from euthanasia in that its aim is to relieve severe refractory suffering and not to shorten life. In fact, there is evidence that PST, if carried out accordingly with good medical practice, does not hasten death (Maltoni et al. 2012).

In the case of euthanasia, the physician intends the death of the patient and selects types of drugs and dosages that are lethal by all objective measures. After administering them, the physician makes sure that the patient not only loses consciousness but also next ceases to breath, and eventually undergoes complete cardiac arrest.

In the case of palliative sedation, the intent is very different: it is to relieve otherwise unmanageable symptoms, not to cause death. This intent is implicit in the drugs selected, which have been proven to safely achieve sedation in other settings. The dosage is carefully titrated to reach the intended level of consciousness, opposite to euthanasia, where barbiturates and muscle relaxants are administered in rapid overdosing. Death occurs at some point after symptom relief has been achieved, as a result of the underlying condition, not of the physician's intervention.

Lack of honest and open communication between clinician and patient and/or family also tends to exacerbate the controversy. Claessens et al. (2008) have reported that 25 % of families experience high levels of distress over the decision to initiate palliative sedation for a loved one. They also complain about insufficient information about the process and lack of compassion shown by physicians and nurses. Moreover, they fear their decision has shortened the life of the family member, as he or she was sedated and later died.

Whenever possible, PST should be initiated with the consent of the patient, which should be ensured while the patient is still lucid. This means that the possibility of PST should be addressed, if possible, long before the stage where it is the only remaining option. The process of exchanging information and dissipating doubts and concerns might help both the patient and the family understanding the situation and reduce the level of distress (SICP Italian Society for palliative care; Royal Dutch Medical Association 2009).

20.2.7 Pharmacology of Sedation

The medications used to initiate and maintain PST are primarily guided by the patient's care location (home, hospice, acute medical unit, tertiary palliative unit, critical care unit) and the availability of medication administration routes such as intravenous.

Ideal medications have a rapid onset and a short duration of action that facilitate titration to the desired effect.

If a patient is already being treated with opioids and/or antipsychotics, these medications should be continued during sedation, in accordance with the patient's needs.

Anxiolytic Sedatives

The most common choice of PST medication is a benzodiazepine, such as midazolam or lorazepam. Benzodiazepines reduce anxiety and cause amnesia; they also have a synergistic sedative effect with opioids and antipsychotics, are anticonvulsants and may help prevent the development of seizures. At sedative doses, the risk of respiratory depression is low, thus providing a safety margin: however, caution is of paramount importance, since they can cause paradoxical agitation, withdrawal, if the dose is rapidly reduced after continual infusion, and tolerance.

The use of midazolam by continuous subcutaneous infusion (CSCI) can be preferable in the home setting. Intravenous administration allows a more accurate dose titration and prompt adaptation to different patient's needs.

Midazolam is the most commonly used agent because of its more immediate titration responsiveness (brief duration of action due to rapid redistribution, opposed to lorazepam's slower pharmacokinetics). Initiation dose is a 2.5–5 mg bolus (0.05–0.07 mg/kg) or 0.2–1 mg/h CSCI (plus supplementary doses of 1.25–2.5 mg, if needed). Usual effective dose is 10–120 mg/day, yet range is broad from 3 to 1,200 mg/day. There is no standard dose and individualized titration is required: at high dosages or if tolerance develops, it might be useful adding, or switching to, second-line treatment. This can be particularly helpful if sedation is prolonged and significant increases of midazolam doses are required. Midazolam is compatible with morphine and hydromorphone and can be combined in a single infusion.

Lorazepam is a second choice benzodiazepine because it is less amenable than midazolam to rapid up or down titration. It has a peak effect approximately 30 min after intravenous administration. Starting dose is 2–5 mg in slow bolus. Maintaining dose is 0.04–0.08 mg/kg every 2–4 h.

Neuroleptics

Neuroleptics are particularly indicated if the patient is manifesting signs and symptoms of delirium. Delirium is an acute confusional state that might be difficult to distinguish from extreme anxiety, and the administration of opioids or benzodiazepines as initial treatment for delirium can worsen the symptom. Neuroleptics with a more sedative profile should be chosen and their side effects also considered. Most common adverse effects are orthostatic hypotension, paradoxical agitation, extrapyramidal symptoms and anticholinergic effects (prostatic hypertrophy patients may be more sensitive to these effects and suffer additional discomfort).

Methotrimeprazine (Levomepromazine) is an antipsychotic phenothiazine and a useful second-line choice for PST. It has a rapid onset, acts on multiple receptors and has some antiemetic and analgesic effects. It provides significant sedation, can be used in combination with midazolam and can be administered orally or parenterally (intravenously, subcutaneously or intramuscularly), continuously or intermittently. Starting dose is 12.5–25 mg s.c. or 50–75 mg continual infusion. Dose range is up to 300 mg/day.

In alternative, chlorpromazine might be used. It is a widely available antipsychotic that can be administered orally, parenterally (IV or IM) and rectally. The SICP (Italian Society of Palliative Care) recommends it as first choice. Starting dose in a IV or IM bolus of 25–50 mg; maintenance dose 1–12.5 mg/h.

Haloperidol does not provide the degree of sedation necessary for PST; however, it remains useful for delirious patients. In addition to the aforementioned side effects, it can cause QT prolongation.

Sedative Antiepileptics

Some clinicians consider Phenobarbital a first-line PST drug, while others use it as a third-line option in case of inadequate response to midazolam and/or antipsychotic. It reliably and rapidly causes unconsciousness and may be useful in patients who have developed tolerance to opioids and benzodiazepines, since its mechanism of action differs from theirs. Starting dose is 100–200 mg s.c. and maintenance dose is 10–25 mg/h (600–1,200 mg/die).

General Anaesthetics

Propofol is generally considered a third- or even fourth-line PST medication (Fraser Health hospice palliative care program 2011; Royal Dutch Medical Association 2009), when symptom relief has not been achieved by other drugs. However, in a hospital setting, where intravenous access is easily attainable and anaesthesiologists are available, sometimes it becomes a second-line agent. It provides quick onset of sedation, ability to rapidly titrate and wash out, due to an ultrashort duration of action, and antiemetic activity. Initiation dose is 20–100 mg or 0.5 mg/kg/h; maintenance dose 0.5–2 mg/kg/h (usually 30–70 mg/h).

Other Drugs

Alpha-2-Adrenergics Agonists

Clonidine and dexmedetomidine are used in patients in intensive care for their central sedative activity. They are also devoid of major respiratory depressant effects and can be combined with other neuroleptics (Caraceni and Simonetti 2009). Clonidine is administered intravenously in boluses (50–150 µg 8-hourly in intensive care) or by continuous infusion. In our experience, infusions of 150 mcg/day, in adults, can be useful as a starting dose, in combinations with other sedative drugs. The onset of action after an intravenous dose is within 10 min and lasts for 3–7 h (Martin and Susan 2003). It produces dose-related sedation, analgesia, anxiolysis, and a reduction in the requirements of other anaesthetic agents and opioids. Dexmedetomidine is a newer Alpha-2 adrenoceptor agonist and shares a similar pharmacodynamics to that of clonidine.

Antihistamines

Antihistamines are sedative drugs without respiratory depressant effects and, especially promethazine (50 mg every 6–8 h), can increase benzodiazepines and/or neuroleptics effects (Caraceni and Simonetti 2009).

Medication	Initiation dose	Maintenance dose	Route of administration
Benzodiazepines			
First choice: Midazolam	Bolus: 2.5–5 mg (0.05–0.07 mg/kg) CSCI: 0.2–1 mg/h	10–120 mg/die (0.03–0.05 mg/kg/h or 0.5–5 mg/h)	s.c.—IV—IM—rectal
Lorazepam	Slow bolus: 2–5 mg		s.c.—IV

(continued)

Medication	Initiation dose	Maintenance dose	Route of administration
		0.04–0.08 mg/kg every 2–4 h or 0.25–1 mg/h	
Neuroleptics			
First choice: methotrimeprazine	s.c.: 12.5–25 mg CI: 50–75 mg	Up to 300 mg/die	s.c.—IV—IM
Chlorpromazine	IV or IM Bolus: 25–50 mg	1–12.5 mg/h	IV—IM—rectal
Haloperidol	s.c. bolus: 2–5 mg	5–100 mg/die	s.c.—IV
Sedative antiepiletics			
Phenobarbital	Bolus: 100–200 mg	10–25 mg/h 600–1,200 mg/die	s.c.—IV—rectal
General anaesthetics			
Propofol	Bolus: 20–100 mg or 0.5 mg/kg/h (titration with increases of 0.5 mg/kg/10–15 min)	0.5–2 mg/kg/h (30–70 mg/h)	IV
Other drugs			
Promethazine	Bolus: 50 mg	50 mg every 8 h	IV—IM
Clonidine	Boluses: 50–150 mcg 8-hourly (IV over 15 min, in ICU. See text)	IV: 0.1–2 mcg/kg/h	s.c.—IV

Conclusion

The recognition of intractable suffering at the end of life is a very delicate and sensitive clinical commitment. While the role of psychopharmacology and targeted multidisciplinary interventions cannot by underestimated to control psychological suffering in the final stages of incurable illnesses, the compassionate and careful use of sedation cannot be disregarded as a therapeutic option. Careful understanding of the clinical situation, specific palliative care skills, and resources with the contribution of competency from psychology and psychiatry are necessary to best serve complex patient needs in addressing this difficult clinical situation.

Clinical Case

C.C. was a young woman aged 37. She was married and mother to a small child.

She had a diagnosis of breast cancer; 2 years after the initial diagnosis and surgery, the disease progressed rapidly, several cycles of chemotherapy notwithstanding, and reached the end-stage phase with multiple metastases to

(continued)

pleura, lungs, meninges, and brain. She suffered from meningeal and radicular pain involving the lower extremities, progressive neurological involvement of cranial nerves and lumbo-sacral roots. The rapid progression did not allow enough time to adapt, at least gradually, in practical and psychological terms to the disease trajectory.

The patient manifested strong anxiety due to her family situation (difficult relationship with her parents and overwhelming anguish about leaving her child motherless) and, even though her pain was well controlled by PCI morphine infusions, she wasn't able to tolerate being awake when her husband was not at her bedside.

It was therefore decided to start intermittent sedation with boluses of lorazepam (4 mg IV) during night-time and, during the day, when the husband was not available. This regimen was maintained for 14 days; in the last 3 days she developed delirium and sedation was deepened and maintained till death.

Drug regimen during the time when intermittent sedation was provided; dosages are given in mg/day where appropriate

	16 August	23 August	30 August	2 September
IV Morphine	96 mg	240 mg	432 mg	480 mg
Morphine bol.	2	6	2	2
Bolus dose	15 mg	15 mg	20 mg	20 mg
Total morphine	126 mg	330 mg	472 mg	520 mg
Lorazepam	8 mg	8 mg	8 mg	8 mg
Haloperidol	2 mg	8 mg	8 mg	8 mg
Clorphenamine			10 mg	10 mg

Glasgow Coma Scale during the time when intermittent sedation was provided. GCS scores ranges from 15 that is a normal level of consciousness to 3 which is coma.

(continued)

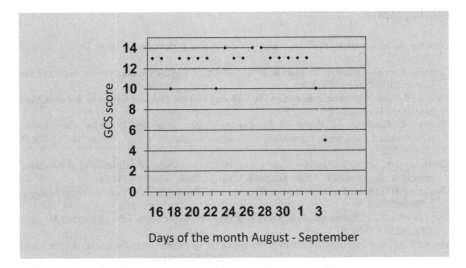

Days of the month August - September

▶ **Key Points**

- PST is an important practice in controlling suffering in the last days of life
- PST for existential/psychological distress is controversial
- Existential suffering evaluation requires psychological competencies
- Intermittent sedation should be preferred
- The advice of palliative care specialists should be required

Acknowledgements This work was partially funded by The Floriani Foundation of Milan

Key References

- Maltoni M. Palliative sedation in end-of-life care and survival: a systematic review. J Clin Oncol. 2012;30(12):1378–83.
- Cherny NI, Radbruch L, Board of the European Association for Palliative Care. EAPC recommended framework for the use of sedation in palliative care. Palliat Med. 2009b;23(7):581–93. doi:10.1177/0269216309107024.
- Rousseau P. Palliative sedation in the management of refractory symptoms. J Support Oncol. 2004b;2(2):181–6. Review.

Suggested Further Reading

- The Royal Dutch Medical Association's Guideline on palliative sedation. 2009 Update.

Bibliography

Caraceni A, Simonetti F. Palliating delirium in patients with cancer. Lancet Oncol. 2009;10 (2):164–72.

Caraceni A, et al. Palliative sedation at the end of life at a tertiary cancer center. Support Care Cancer. 2012;20(6):1299–307.

Cassell EJ, Rich BA. Intractable end-of-life suffering and the ethics of palliative sedation. Pain Med. 2010;11(3):435–8.

Cherny NI, Radbruch L, Board of the European Association for Palliative Care. EAPC recommended framework for the use of sedation in palliative care. Palliat Med. 2009;23 (7):581–93.

Chochinov HM, et al. The patient dignity inventory: a novel way of measuring dignity-related distress in palliative care. J Pain Symptom Manage. 2008;36(6):559–71.

Chochinov HM, et al. The landscape of distress in the terminally ill. J Pain Symptom Manage. 2009;38(5):641–9.

Claessens P, et al. Palliative sedation: a review of the research literature. J Pain Symptom Manage. 2008;36(3):310–33.

de Graeff A, Dean M. Palliative sedation therapy in the last weeks of life: a literature review and recommendations for standards. J Palliat Med. 2007;10(1):67–85.

Fraser Health Hospice Palliative Care Program: Refractory Symptoms and Palliative Sedation Therapy Guideline. 2011. http://www.fraserhealth.ca/EN/hospice_palliative_care_symptom_guidelines

Maltoni M, et al. Palliative sedation in end-of-life care and survival: a systematic review. J Clin Oncol. 2012;30(12):1378–83.

Martin S, Susan S. Drugs in anaesthesia and intensive care. 3rd ed. Oxford: Oxford University Press; 2003. p. 76–7.

Mercadante S, et al. Palliative sedation in patients with advanced cancer followed at home: a systematic review. J Pain Symptom Manage. 2011;41:754–60.

Morita T, et al. Development of a clinical guideline for palliative sedation therapy using the Delphi method. J Palliat Med. 2005;8(4):716–29.

Rousseau P. Palliative sedation in the management of refractory symptoms. J Support Oncol. 2004;2(2):181–6.

Royal Dutch Medical Association. Guideline for palliative sedation. 2009 http://knmg.artsennet.nl/home.htm

SICP (Italian Society for palliative care). Raccomandazioni della SICP sulla sedazione terminale/ sedazione palliative, 2007 http://www.sicp.it

Research Issues in Psychopharmacology in Oncology and Palliative Care Settings

21

Yesne Alici and Laura B. Dunn

Abstract

Psychopharmacologic interventions are commonly used in oncology and palliative care settings. However, there have been relatively few rigorously designed and conducted psychopharmacologic studies in these patient populations. Given a growing recognition of the importance of identifying and treating varied forms of distress in cancer patients and survivors, there is an urgent need to develop a more robust evidence base to guide psychopharmacologic treatment decisions. Such an evidence base would help address stigma regarding psychopharmacologic treatments as well as help clinicians working in psycho-oncology to educate their oncology colleagues. In addition to reviewing the rationale for psychopharmacologic research in psycho-oncology, this chapter describes a number of areas that are ripe for psychopharmacologic research in psycho-oncology, for example: efficacy and tolerability of antipsychotics for mood, anxiety, or insomnia; antipsychotic use in delirium; and psychostimulant use for fatigue and cognitive effects of cancer treatments. This chapter also reviews limitations of existing research on psychopharmacologic treatments in psycho-oncology. Suggestions for future research are provided, in the interest of providing "real-world" effectiveness data for the management of the numerous common symptoms and syndromes that occur in cancer patients and survivors. Examples include the study of co-occurring symptoms (e.g., depression and fatigue), research on the treatment of so-called subsyndromal levels of depressive or anxiety symptoms, and studies of specific treatments in specific cancer populations.

Y. Alici (✉)
Department of Psychiatry and Behavioral Sciences, Memorial Sloan Kettering Cancer Center, 641 Lexington Avenue, 7th Floor, New York, NY 10022, USA
e-mail: Aliciy@mskcc.org

L.B. Dunn
Department of Psychiatry, University of California, San Francisco, 401 Parnassus Avenue, Box 0984-F, San Francisco, CA 94002, USA
e-mail: Laura.Dunn@ucsf.edu

L. Grassi and M. Riba (eds.), *Psychopharmacology in Oncology and Palliative Care*, DOI 10.1007/978-3-642-40134-3_21, © Springer-Verlag Berlin Heidelberg 2014

21.1   Introduction

The need for research on psychopharmacologic interventions in psycho-oncology and palliative care is urgent and growing. There are a number of different factors that point to the need for a robust evidence base to guide treatment decisions: the epidemiology of cancer, demographic forces, burgeoning numbers of cancer survivors, and an increased awareness among cancer providers of the importance of providing comprehensive care to cancer patients—including aggressive treatment of all forms of distress. However, the research database has not kept pace with this demand for evidence. Therefore, the goals of this chapter are (1) to describe the rationale for psychopharmacologic research in psycho-oncology and palliative care and (2) to provide a series of recommendations for future research topics and methods.

21.2   Rationale for Psychopharmacologic Research in Psycho-oncology and Palliative Care

Although estimates vary widely depending on population studied, ascertainment (measurement) method, definition of "caseness," and study design, approximately 25–50 % of patients with cancer experience clinically significant symptoms of distress (Jacobsen and Ransom 2007; Zabora et al. 2001; Massie 2004; Chochinov 2001). Psychotropic medications—antidepressants, antipsychotics, mood stabilizers, sedative-hypnotics, and psychostimulants—are commonly used in oncology and palliative care settings (Rayner et al. 2011). However, there remains a relative paucity of rigorously designed and conducted studies in these patient populations (Jacobsen et al. 2006; Traeger et al. 2012; Li et al. 2012; Candy et al. 2012). For example, a recent meta-analysis identified only nine randomized controlled trials (RCTs) of antidepressants for the treatment of depression and depressive symptoms in cancer patients (Laoutidis and Mathiak 2013). Another recent meta-analysis that used stricter inclusion criteria identified only four trials that met the authors' criteria (Hart et al. 2012). Another systematic review found no studies meeting the inclusion criteria for prospective randomized trials of pharmacologic therapies for anxiety in palliative care patients (Candy et al. 2012). Most of the evidence for treatment has therefore been derived from studies on the use of these medications, in general medical populations or mentally ill patients in psychiatric settings.

Despite this paucity of research in these specific patient populations, a number of clinical practice guidelines have been developed worldwide that include recommendations for psychosocial care in oncology settings. In the United States, the National Comprehensive Cancer Network (NCCN) proposed clinical guidelines for the recognition and management of distress in patients with cancer in 1999. The guidelines are updated regularly to incorporate the most recent evidence, including psychopharmacologic intervention trials (Holland et al. 2007). However, most of the recommendations represent a uniform consensus among experts from the

NCCN member institutions that are based on clinical experience as opposed to higher-level evidence, such as randomized controlled trials (RCTs). Similarly, most other guidelines are consensus guidelines rather than evidence-based practice guidelines. In 2012, the Journal of Clinical Oncology published a series of comprehensive review articles on evidence-based management of psychiatric syndromes and symptoms in oncology settings to guide providers in treating cancer patients with these syndromes (Fann et al. 2012; Pirl et al. 2012; Hoffman et al. 2012; Jacobsen et al. 2012; Li et al. 2012; Carlson et al. 2012; Breitbart et al. 2012; Sheinfeld Gorin et al. 2012; Phelps et al. 2012; Northouse et al. 2012; Traeger et al. 2012). This series of review articles represents the growing body of research in psycho-oncology and palliative care, while illustrating numerous areas where there is a great need for further research. Prominent among these is the area of psychopharmacology.

One important aspect of treatment for psychiatric disorders in cancer patients that remains underexplored is the issue of stigma (Holland 2002). Stigma surrounds the use of psychotropic medications, perhaps primarily as a secondary effect of the continuing stigma of mental illness. When psychotropic medications are recommended for medically ill patients, patients and families may decline the medication. Some oncologists or other healthcare professionals also may harbor stigma (consciously or not) toward these medications, for a variety of reasons. Myths around the use of psychotropic medications are many and can interfere with effective management of mood, anxiety symptoms, and confusional states—to name a few. Therefore, psychopharmacologic research in psycho-oncology is of utmost importance to dispel myths regarding use of psychotropic medications for cancer patients and in the terminally ill.

This research could be very helpful in the same way that research on the benefits of palliative care has helped dispel myths about this important aspect of comprehensive cancer care. While many patients, families, and clinicians have long-held beliefs that palliative care hastens death (Irwin et al. 2013)—or signals defeat or loss of hope—a highly cited study by Temel and colleagues demonstrated that palliative care among patients with metastatic non-small-cell lung cancer was associated with significant improvements in quality of life, mood, and symptom burden—as well as with longer survival (Temel et al. 2010). This study and others support the benefits of palliative care early in the course of metastatic disease treatment. Based on these studies and other evidence, clinicians can confidently inform patients and families that palliative care has important symptom and quality of life benefits and does not hasten death. This work highlights the importance of conducting well-controlled studies for demonstrating the effects of interventions that may carry some degree of stigma or that may challenge beliefs in oncology.

A further rationale for research into the effectiveness of psychopharmacologic interventions for cancer patients is the need to educate our colleagues. Many oncologists are well aware of the potential benefits of psychopharmacologic interventions for their patients. Others, however, may lack an adequate understanding of the nature, causes, and harms of psychiatric symptoms and syndromes, and may lack awareness or understanding of how medications may help their patients better cope and even thrive despite their cancer diagnosis and treatment. A stronger evidence base would therefore bolster the continuing efforts of psycho-oncology and palliative care clinicians and investigators to "make the case" for the value of their work. Moreover, a more robust evidence base would help us educate our colleagues about how best to assess, manage, and refer their oncology patients in order to address more optimally their psycho-oncology and palliative care symptoms.

Another rationale for psychopharmcologic research is the manner in which these medications are currently prescribed. Psycho-oncology and palliative care providers often find themselves managing patients by focusing on symptoms rather than specific syndromes (e.g., antidepressants for neuropathic pain, insomnia, or appetite; low dose antipsychotics for insomnia, nausea, anxiety, or appetite). In the presence of identifiable specific syndromes such as depressive or anxiety disorders, psychotropic medications can be used to target the syndrome itself. There are well-known challenges, however, in making definitive syndromal diagnoses.

The effects of cancer itself, treatment-related side effects, overlapping symptoms, or an underlying psychiatric disorder could all present with similar symptom constellations. Regardless of the etiology of the symptoms, however, psychopharmacologic management often plays an essential role for symptom relief. Choice of psychotropic medication is therefore largely affected by the side effect profile of the medication, onset of action, and effects on sleep, appetite, fatigue, and energy. Thus, clinicians find themselves frequently conducting empirical "n of 1" trials with medications in order to relieve patients' symptoms and suffering. The balance between creative psychopharmacology and the principle of "first do no harm" is a fine one, however, underscoring the need for well-designed, randomized controlled trials testing the efficacy and safety of psychotropic medications.

Psycho-oncologists frequently encounter patients who would be excluded from many if not all of the randomized controlled psychopharmacologic studies due to their medical disease burden or the number of medications these patients are on. Lack of evidence may lead to under-treatment of those patients due to concerns for side effects, reluctance to increase the dose, or concerns about using a medication with better efficacy but a worse side effect profile. Following are several examples of area of psychopharmacologic management of cancer patients that remain challenging due to the paucity of well-designed studies:

- Use of antipsychotics for mood disturbance, anxiety symptoms, or insomnia: Antipsychotics are commonly prescribed for treatment of mood and anxiety symptoms and for symptoms such as insomnia or anorexia. Rapid onset of action, effectiveness for possible subsyndromal delirium, and sedating effects that may help treat insomnia or improve the sleep–wake cycle make antipsychotics particularly useful in cancer patients. These medications, however, have specific challenges, including (depending on the medication) risks of extrapyramidal side effects, hypotension, oversedation, QTc prolongation, and concern for increased mortality and increased risk of cardiovascular and cerebrovascular morbidity in elderly patients with dementia. In the absence of well-designed studies, clinicians find themselves in a difficult position when discussing the risk–benefit profile of antipsychotics for off-label indications with patients, families, and other clinicians.

- Use of antipsychotics for delirium: Delirium is the most common neuropsychiatric syndrome encountered among hospitalized cancer patients. Despite an increasing number of randomized controlled trials on the use of antipsychotics for treatment of delirium, only a small number of those studies have focused on cancer patients and the terminally ill (Breitbart and Alici 2012). Moreover, most delirium studies include small sample sizes and heterogeneous samples, and most lack systematic assessment of side effects with valid side effect rating scales. Delirium is a medical emergency; therefore, patients treated are at higher risk of experiencing side effects compared to more medically stable patients. Psycho-oncologists encounter many patients and families who refuse the use of antipsychotics for treatment of delirium symptoms due to concerns about side effects. The safe dose ranges of each antipsychotic medication, as well as the optimal duration of antipsychotic use for the treatment of delirium, are only a few of the questions that remain to be explored in well-designed trials in cancer populations.

- Use of psychostimulants for fatigue and cognitive effects of cancer treatment: An increasing number of patients at risk for functional and cognitive impairment (e.g., due to older age) receive cancer treatments with curative or palliative intent. Placebo-controlled, randomized studies are required to study the efficacy and safety of psychostimulants (and other pharmacologic therapies) for both treatment of fatigue and improvement of treatment-related cognitive impairment (primarily attentional deficits). The current evidence base falls far short of what would be necessary for recommending psychostimulants in the treatment of cancer-related fatigue or in patients with cancer or cancer treatment-related cognitive impairments (Bruera et al. 2006; Sood et al. 2006). This gap also leaves clinicians between a rock and a hard place when seeking to ameliorate patients' symptoms, some of which can be debilitating.

21.3 Limitations of the Current Body of Psychopharmacologic Research

A number of limitations of the currently available research-driven evidence base are outlined in Table 21.1. There are numerous methodological limitations of existing studies that require attention from investigators to improve the quality of evidence-based management guidelines. One of the most significant challenges is that of diagnosis. The diagnosis of psychiatric syndromes in cancer patients can be extremely challenging. For example, no fewer than five different approaches have been proposed and utilized in the psycho-oncology literature for diagnosing depression among advanced cancer patients (Trask 2004). A critical challenge in diagnosing depression in medically ill patients is the interpretation of physical/somatic symptoms of depression. Therefore, when conducting psychopharmacologic studies among depressed cancer patients, investigators must consider a

Table 21.1 Limitations of current research base

• Limited **number** of pharmacologic treatments in cancer patients and among the terminally ill

• **Methodological** limitations of existing studies

  – Open label vs. randomized controlled trials

  – Cross-sectional vs. longitudinal

  – Diagnostic challenges in establishing syndromes in cancer patients

  – Inclusion and exclusion criteria

    Examples of challenges: Other comorbidities, age, stage of disease, overly heterogeneous vs. overly homogeneous samples

  – Validity of measures and instruments used as outcome measures

  – Recruitment and retention

    Challenges in recruiting medically ill and terminally ill patients

    Attrition may be higher in medically ill populations (need extra efforts to retain participants; consider more frequent telephone or other contact)

• Limited **research training in psychopharmacology among psycho-oncologists**

• Minimal use of quality metrics in psychopharmacology research

• Meta-analyses are scant and due to the limitations with current research noted above quantitative meta-analytic techniques cannot be used

number of important design issues that may seriously affect the sample and outcomes of the study, including, for example, whether to utilize screening scales or a structured clinical interview, and how to handle comorbid conditions (e.g., anxiety disorders).

The study design, in and of itself, is a critical question for any researcher who wants to study psychopharmacologic interventions. While open-label and cross-sectional studies have limited value in informing evidence-based practices, prospective longitudinal studies are difficult to conduct among cancer patients, especially among the terminally ill, due to high attrition rates and low survival rates. Randomized controlled trials are sparse, yet these are the most valuable studies for establishing tolerability and effectiveness of psychotropic agent. As medical comorbidities play an important role in symptoms and symptom clusters, a determination of whether it is the psychotropic medication or the improvement of the underlying medical condition that abates the psychiatric symptoms can be best determined if a placebo arm is included in the study.

While a full review of methodological considerations for psychopharmacology research is beyond the scope of this chapter, the reader is referred to the section on "Suggested further reading" for helpful books and articles.

21.4   Recommendations for Future Research Agenda

Psycho-oncology and palliative care clinicians, and more importantly, their patients, would be well-served by a number of types of research studies. These are "ideal" scenarios, given with the awareness of the difficulties of securing funding as well as of conducting large-scale studies. Nevertheless, the paucity of studies represents a major gap in the evidence base needed to provide comprehensive care for the whole cancer patient—the ultimate goal (Institute of Medicine 2007).

Larger-scale, adequately powered, prospective RCTs are needed to establish effectiveness of every drug class in cancer patients and for multiple symptoms. This will likely require multisite trials—e.g., the equivalent of cooperative group studies for psycho-oncology. These studies need to be carefully designed, with close attention to the methodological issues discussed above, as well as to adherence to quality metrics for clinical trials.

Because most patients with cancer are taking multiple medications for various symptoms, it will be important in such trials to be more inclusive than exclusive, which in turn requires larger samples in order to have the power to control for possible confounding variables. For example, it will be next to impossible to conduct a trial in cancer populations in which patients are not also being prescribed benzodiazepines for nausea, anxiety, or insomnia. The key point of conducting such larger-scale studies will be to provide "real-world" effectiveness data regarding how psychopharmacologic medications work in samples of patients who are as representative as possible of the cancer populations under consideration. Careful consideration of all of the variables that may be associated with outcomes of interest is required in the design stage of any psychopharmacologic trial. These then need to be factored into considerations of recruitment, inclusion and exclusion criteria, and analytic strategy.

At a more advanced stage, psycho-oncology and palliative care researchers will need to move to studies of drug treatment algorithms, combinations (including with psychotherapy), and more advanced psychopharmacology. Trials of some agents, such as ketamine [an N-methyl-D-aspartate receptor antagonist with rapid-acting antidepressant effects; Krystal et al. (2013)], also appear to be warranted for the treatment of depression in some well-defined categories of cancer patients (Zarate et al. 2006). Given that many patients with depression do not respond to the first drug they are prescribed (Rush et al. 2006), it is important to emphasize that we are on a journey of discovery, rather than a day trip, in evaluating what treatment strategies work best for which patients and for which symptoms.

As the general psychiatric research has demonstrated, the combination of psychopharmacologic and psychotherapeutic interventions is often more effective than either cancer populations as well.

Another critical area of research in psychopharmacology is the study of how best to treat co-occurring symptoms—often referred to now as "symptom clusters"—that are frequently experienced by cancer patients. As more and more becomes known about the individual, disease-related, and environmental influences on such clusters of symptoms, it is also becoming clear that to improve treatments of these symptoms, we may need to rethink how we do intervention trials. A "real-world" trial of treatment for the co-occurrence of fatigue and depression in cancer patients, for example, ought to consider multiple modalities that could be effective singly, but perhaps more effective when combined (e.g., drug therapy, psychotherapy, and structured exercise). Consideration of how we define a clinically significant symptom or group of symptoms will be needed for the design of such trials. For example, while the full syndrome of major depression is less common in cancer patients, it appears that there is a significant subgroup who may be experiencing "subsyndromal levels" of depressive symptoms that, while not meeting a cutpoint on a measurement scale, are nevertheless associated with clinically relevant outcomes such as decrements in quality of life (Dunn et al. 2011). These patients may nevertheless benefit from psychopharmacologic intervention, but studies are needed that include well-characterized samples in terms of baseline levels of symptoms and measures and timepoints that are adequate for detecting changes in symptoms.

Finally, studies of specific treatments in specific conditions (e.g., patients with specific high-risk cancers, such as head and neck), subpopulations of cancer patients (e.g., older cancer patients, patients at the end of life), or specific and important symptoms (e.g., treatment-resistant depression; suicidal ideation) are also needed in the psychopharmacology literature.

Conclusion

While a large research literature has emerged in psycho-oncology generally, there remains an important need for psychopharmacologic research in cancer patients. Currently available psychopharmacologic research is limited in the number of studies as well as by certain methodological limitations, making it difficult to draw definitive conclusions about treatment strategies. Training in psycho-oncology should ideally include training in research methods, including the design, conduct, and interpretation of psychopharmacology trials.

▶ Key Points

- There is an urgent and growing need for a larger and more robust evidence base for the use of psychopharmacologic interventions in cancer patients.
- There are a number of important reasons that this research is needed, including that many treatment decisions are made in the absence of an adequate evidence base, as well as to inform our colleagues and reduce stigma.
- Recommendations for future research include multisite collaborative trials, testing of psychopharmacologic interventions against psychotherapy alone and combined treatments, and studies of psychopharmacologic interventions for symptom clusters.

Key References

- Breitbart W, Alici Y. Evidence-based treatment of delirium in patients with cancer. J Clin Oncol. 2012b;30(11):1206–14.
- Hart SL, Hoyt MA, Diefenbach M, Anderson DR, Kilbourn KM, Craft LL, Steel JL, Cuijpers P, Mohr DC, Berendsen M, Spring B, Stanton AL. Meta-analysis of efficacy of interventions for elevated depressive symptoms in adults diagnosed with cancer. J Natl Cancer Inst. 2012b;104(13):990–1004.

- Krystal JH, Sanacora G, Duman RS. Rapid-acting glutamatergic antidepressants: the path to ketamine and beyond. Biol Psychiatry. 2013b;73 (12):1133–41.
- Li M, Fitzgerald P, Rodin G. Evidence-based treatment of depression in patients with cancer. J Clin Oncol. 2012b;30(11):1187–96.
- Rayner L, Price A, Evans A, Valsraj K, Hotopf M, Higginson IJ. Antidepressants for the treatment of depression in palliative care: systematic review and meta-analysis. Palliat Med. 2011b;25(1):36–51.
- Traeger L, Greer JA, Fernandez-Robles C, Temel JS, Pirl WF. Evidence-based treatment of anxiety in patients with cancer. J Clin Oncol. 2012b;30(11):1197–205.

Suggested Further Reading

- Billings JA, Block SD. Integrating psychiatry and palliative medicine: the challenges and opportunities. In: Chochinov HM, Breitbart WS, editors. Handbook of psychiatry in palliative medicine. 2nd ed. New York: Oxford; 2009. p. 13–21.
- Holland JC, Weiss TR. History of psycho-oncology. In: Holland JH, Breitbart W, editors. Psycho-oncology. 2nd ed. New York: Oxford; 2010. p. 3–14.
- Jacobsen PB. Translating psychosocial oncology research to clinical practice. In: Holland JH, Breitbart W, editors. Psycho-oncology. 2nd ed. New York: Oxford; 2010. p. 642–7.
- Johansen C, Grassi L. International psycho-oncology: present and future. In: Holland JH, Breitbart W, editors. Psycho-oncology. 2nd ed. New York: Oxford; 2010. p. 655–62.
- Rosenstein DL, Miller FG. Research ethics in psycho-oncology. In: Holland JH, Breitbart W, editors. Psycho-oncology. 2nd ed. New York: Oxford; 2010. p. 630–5.
- Stefanek M. Basic and translational psycho-oncology research. In: Holland JH, Breitbart W, editors. Psycho-oncology. 2nd ed. New York: Oxford; 2010. p. 637–41.

References

Breitbart W, Alici Y. Evidence-based treatment of delirium in patients with cancer. J Clin Oncol. 2012;30(11):1206–14.
Breitbart W, Poppito S, Rosenfeld B, Vickers AJ, Li Y, Abbey J, Olden M, Pessin H, Lichtenthal W, Sjoberg D, Cassileth BR. Pilot randomized controlled trial of individual meaning-centered psychotherapy for patients with advanced cancer. J Clin Oncol. 2012;30 (12):1304–9.

Bruera E, Valero V, Driver L, Shen L, Willey J, Zhang T, Palmer JL. Patient-controlled methyl-phenidate for cancer fatigue: a double-blind, randomized, placebo-controlled trial. J Clin Oncol. 2006;24(13):2073–8.

Candy B, Jackson KC, Jones L, Tookman A, King M. Drug therapy for symptoms associated with anxiety in adult palliative care patients. Cochrane Database Syst Rev. 2012;10, CD004596.

Carlson LE, Waller A, Mitchell AJ. Screening for distress and unmet needs in patients with cancer: review and recommendations. J Clin Oncol. 2012;30(11):1160–77.

Chochinov HM. Depression in cancer patients. Lancet Oncol. 2001;2(8):499–505.

Dunn LB, Cooper BA, Neuhaus J, West C, Paul S, Aouizerat B, Abrams G, Edrington J, Hamolsky D, Miaskowski C. Identification of distinct depressive symptom trajectories in women following surgery for breast cancer. Health Psychol. 2011;30(6):683–92.

Fann JR, Ell K, Sharpe M. Integrating psychosocial care into cancer services. J Clin Oncol. 2012;30(11):1178–86.

Hart SL, Hoyt MA, Diefenbach M, Anderson DR, Kilbourn KM, Craft LL, Steel JL, Cuijpers P, Mohr DC, Berendsen M, Spring B, Stanton AL. Meta-analysis of efficacy of interventions for elevated depressive symptoms in adults diagnosed with cancer. J Natl Cancer Inst. 2012;104 (13):990–1004.

Hoffman CJ, Ersser SJ, Hopkinson JB, Nicholls PG, Harrington JE, Thomas PW. Effectiveness of mindfulness-based stress reduction in mood, breast- and endocrine-related quality of life, and well-being in stage 0 to III breast cancer: a randomized, controlled trial. J Clin Oncol. 2012;30 (12):1335–42.

Holland JC. History of psycho-oncology: overcoming attitudinal and conceptual barriers. Psychosom Med. 2002;64(2):206–21.

Holland JC, Andersen B, Breitbart WS, Dabrowski M, Dudley MM, Fleishman S, Foley GV, Fulcher C, Greenberg DB, Greiner CB, Handzo RG, Jacobsen PB, Knight SJ, Learson K, Levy MH, Manne S, McAllister-Black R, Peterman A, Riba MB, Slatkin NE, Valentine A, Zevon MA, NCCN. Distress management. J Natl Compr Canc Netw. 2007;5(1):66–98.

Institute of Medicine. Cancer care for the whole patient: meeting psychosocial health needs. Washington, DC: The National Academies Press; 2007.

Irwin KE, Greer JA, Khatib J, Temel JS, Pirl WF. Early palliative care and metastatic non-small cell lung cancer: potential mechanisms of prolonged survival. Chron Respir Dis. 2013;10 (1):35–47.

Jacobsen PB, Ransom S. Implementation of NCCN distress management guidelines by member institutions. J Natl Compr Canc Netw. 2007;5(1):99–103.

Jacobsen PB, Donovan KA, Swaine ZN, et al. Management of anxiety and depression in adult cancer patients: toward an evidence-based approach. In: Chang AE, Ganz PA, Hayes DF, et al., editors. Oncology: an evidence-based approach. New York: Springer; 2006. p. 1552–79.

Jacobsen PB, Holland JC, Steensma DP. Caring for the whole patient: the science of psychosocial care. J Clin Oncol. 2012;30(11):1151–3.

Krystal JH, Sanacora G, Duman RS. Rapid-acting glutamatergic antidepressants: the path to ketamine and beyond. Biol Psychiatry. 2013;73(12):1133–41.

Laoutidis ZG, Mathiak K. Antidepressants in the treatment of depression/depressive symptoms in cancer patients: a systematic review and meta-analysis. BMC Psychiatry. 2013;13:140.

Li M, Fitzgerald P, Rodin G. Evidence-based treatment of depression in patients with cancer. J Clin Oncol. 2012;30(11):1187–96.

Massie MJ. Prevalence of depression in patients with cancer. J Natl Cancer Inst Monogr. 2004;32:57–71.

Northouse L, Williams AL, Given B, McCorkle R. Psychosocial care for family caregivers of patients with cancer. J Clin Oncol. 2012;30(11):1227–34.

Phelps AC, Lauderdale KE, Alcorn S, Dillinger J, Balboni MT, Van Wert M, Vanderweele TJ, Balboni TA. Addressing spirituality within the care of patients at the end of life: perspectives of patients with advanced cancer, oncologists, and oncology nurses. J Clin Oncol. 2012;30 (20):2538–44.

Pirl WF, Greer JA, Traeger L, Jackson V, Lennes IT, Gallagher ER, Perez-Cruz P, Heist RS, Temel JS. Depression and survival in metastatic non-small-cell lung cancer: effects of early palliative care. J Clin Oncol. 2012;30(12):1310–5.

Rayner L, Price A, Evans A, Valsraj K, Hotopf M, Higginson IJ. Antidepressants for the treatment of depression in palliative care: systematic review and meta-analysis. Palliat Med. 2011;25 (1):36–51.

Rush AJ, Trivedi MH, Wisniewski SR, Nierenberg AA, Stewart JW, Warden D, Niederehe G, Thase ME, Lavori PW, Lebowitz BD, McGrath PJ, Rosenbaum JF, Sackeim HA, Kupfer DJ, Luther J, Fava M. Acute and longer-term outcomes in depressed outpatients requiring one or several treatment steps: a STAR*D report. Am J Psychiatry. 2006;163(11):1905–17.

Sheinfeld Gorin S, Krebs P, Badr H, Janke EA, Jim HS, Spring B, Mohr DC, Berendsen MA, Jacobsen PB. Meta-analysis of psychosocial interventions to reduce pain in patients with cancer. J Clin Oncol. 2012;30(5):539–47.

Sood A, Barton DL, Loprinzi CL. Use of methylphenidate in patients with cancer. Am J Hosp Palliat Care. 2006;23(1):35–40.

Temel JS, Greer JA, Muzikansky A, Gallagher ER, Admane S, Jackson VA, Dahlin CM, Blinderman CD, Jacobsen J, Pirl WF, Billings JA, Lynch TJ. Early palliative care for patients with metastatic non-small-cell lung cancer. N Engl J Med. 2010;363(8):733–42.

Traeger L, Greer JA, Fernandez-Robles C, Temel JS, Pirl WF. Evidence-based treatment of anxiety in patients with cancer. J Clin Oncol. 2012;30(11):1197–205.

Trask PC. Assessment of depression in cancer patients. J Natl Cancer Inst Monogr. 2004;414 (32):80–92.

Zabora J, BrintzenhofeSzoc K, Curbow B, Hooker C, Piantadosi S. The prevalence of psychological distress by cancer site. Psychooncology. 2001;10(1):19–28.

Zarate Jr CA, Singh JB, Carlson PJ, Brutsche NE, Ameli R, Luckenbaugh DA, Charney DS, Manji HK. A randomized trial of an N-methyl-D-aspartate antagonist in treatment-resistant major depression. Arch Gen Psychiatry. 2006;63(8):856–64.

Ethics of Psychopharmacological and Biological Treatments in Psycho-oncology

22

Tomer T. Levin and David W. Kissane

Abstract

Ethical frameworks inform the use of psychopharmacological and biological treatment in psycho-oncology. In this chapter we examine ethical aspects of informed consent psychopharmacology, off-label, unproven and "alternative" therapies, pharmacological trials, and the placebo effect. We consider the relationship between the practitioner and the pharmaceutical industry, how to ethically integrate psychotherapy with pharmacotherapy, and common pitfalls in this regard. We describe how to prescribe well and, in this regard examine the challenges of delirium, terminal delirium, terminal sedation, physician assisted suicide and euthanasia. Finally, we review the ethically and clinically challenging subjects of addiction to prescribed medications and transcranial magnetic stimulation.

22.1 Introduction

An ethical framework underpins all medical treatment in oncology and palliative care. The goals of medicine ought not be economic, nor the pursuit of the disease, but rather the relief of suffering through the healing of a person when there is threat to their well-being and integrity (Cassel 1982). We call such a philosophy patient- and family-centered care within a biopsychosocial and spiritual framework.

T.T. Levin (✉)
Department of Psychiatry and Behavioral Sciences, Memorial Sloan Kettering Cancer Center, 641 Lexington Avenue, New York, NY 10022, USA
e-mail: levint@mskcc.org

D.W. Kissane
Department of Psychiatry, Monash Medical Centre, Monash University, Level 3 Building P, 246 Clayton Road, Clayton, VIC 3168, Australia
e-mail: david.kissane@monash.edu

L. Grassi and M. Riba (eds.), *Psychopharmacology in Oncology and Palliative Care*, DOI 10.1007/978-3-642-40134-3_22, © Springer-Verlag Berlin Heidelberg 2014

In this chapter, we firstly consider the ethical frameworks that inform the practice of oncology and palliative care, consider who this person is with their autonomy, dignity, and vulnerability, examine the nature of informed consent in treatment decisions, and consider its particular relevance to psychopharmacology. Challenging ethical domains include the use of unproven therapies and how the clinician responds to a patient's interest in these, the relationship between the practitioner and the pharmaceutical industry, invasive treatments, and complex decisions in end-of-life care.

22.2   Normative Ethical Theories

Ethical principles and caring, viewed through an integrative framework that accounts for the interpersonal, provide the basis for analyzing moral dilemmas.

22.2.1 Principlism

Principlism, the most widely used framework for analyzing bioethical dilemmas, uses four mid-level ethical principles to avoid more polarizing ethical models:

Beneficence This means that the psychotropic medications used in oncology and palliative care should have the patients' welfare as a primary aim, are intended for their good, and have demonstrable effectiveness.

Nonmaleficence This means doing no harm; psychopharmacological medications should not cause damaging side effects such as confusion, or withdrawal, and if side effects do occur, a safety net should allow for efficient treatment and removal of the offending agent.

Autonomy or Respect for Persons This central principle speaks to the respect that clinicians must give to the patient's values, dignity, and sense of self. It incorporates the informed consent process, which requires a dialogue between clinicians and patients about the advantages, disadvantages, and alternatives to a proposed psychotropic treatment, accounting for their needs, values, and tolerance for risk, leading to a choice that is educated and reasonable.

Justice This requires that the patient's voice be heard within psychopharmacologic prescribing. Chemical straitjacketing to keep a disruptive patient quiet without clear beneficence would be considered a travesty of justice. Social justice refers to the fair allocation of medical resources. Excluding mental health from a health insurance plan or not having the resources to manage the behavioral manifestations of delirium with appropriate diagnosis, psychotropic and behavioral therapies would therefore be unjust.

While principlism does lead to exploratory questions, principles can compete with each other.

For example, a patient's autonomy can be in conflict with beneficence in treating the agitation of delirium; balancing these requires good communication and collaborative decision making with involvement of the patient/family and multidisciplinary team. Similarly, justice is compromised when over-extended psychiatrists prescribe psychotropic medications instead of providing psychotherapy or combination psychotropic and psychotherapy, thus lessening the quality of care.

22.2.2 Ethics of Relational Care

Carol Gilligan developed the concept of an ethics of care in the 1980s, noting that moral theories such as utilitarianism or deontological approaches that seek right or wrong answers for ethical problems were based on male perspectives and ignored the importance of caring relationships, an attitude that seemed more feminine (Gilligan 1993). Nel Noddings further developed the notion of ethical caring, extending it to men too, building the now accepted foundation for relationships providing a foundation for ethical care (Noddings 2013).

The ethics of relational care is reflected in the "here and now" of the physician–patient relationship, compassionate care, charity, friendship, love, and altruism and the need to shield the weak and vulnerable. Relational ethics evokes the human condition and the challenges we face as families and communities but has been criticized for its lack of subjective moral rules; for this exact reason it complements the principlism moral framework, and therefore the two ethical approaches work well together.

An ethics of care is seen in the compassionate way that oncologists thoughtfully prescribe psychotropic medications to relieve the anxiety, depression, confusion, fatigue, insomnia, and anguish that accompany cancer treatments and palliative care.

22.2.3 Integrative Ethical Frameworks

There are three main ways that ethical principles are integrated into clinical care. One way is via ethical codes, guidelines, and overviews, such as Pinel and Appelbaum's "Ethical Aspects of Neuropsychiatric Research with Human Subjects" in the American College of Neuropsychiatry's integrative publication, Neuropsychopharmacology—5th Generation of Progress. This provides a forum for applying principlism and an ethics of care to explore specific dilemmas in neuropsychopharmacology research (Pinals and Appelbaum 2002).

A second integrative framework considers the contribution of contextual issues such as interpersonal or institutional factors to ethical problems. Marguerite Lederberg, a psychiatrist–ethicist at Memorial Sloan-Kettering Cancer Center, observed that complicated ethics dilemmas are entangled with confounding personal emotions, which she called the "situational diagnosis" (Lederberg 1997). Consider a daughter, acting as the healthcare agent for her elderly, agitated mother who insists that the patient not receive haloperidol. The daughter may have a fear based on her own experiences or perceived stigma of this medication. This fear superimposes itself on the operant ethical principles of beneficence, non-malfeasance, and caring. Until the daughter's feelings are explored and addressed, the ethical issue will remain unresolved. Similarly, Fins describes a process of ethical problem solving that acknowledges the importance of the interpersonal process of garnering consensus to address ethical problems where there are frequently several ethically defensible solutions (Fins et al. 1997).

22.2.4 Case-Based Ethics

A third integrative framework involves case-centered ethics. Here, moral dilemmas are discussed in ethics committees and case conferences, based on the notion that learning from experience, healthy debate, and sharing knowledge help to understand ethical dilemmas.

Such case-centered ethic approaches are open to criticism because one precedent is not always generalizable, and personal or persuasive opinions can skew the consensus. It can easily conflict with pluralistic societal values. One such example is of a young man who saw it as his right to smoke cannabis, which he considered medicinal and cultural. The problem was that he was admitted to hospital, receiving chemotherapy, and his proposal to visit the park across from the hospital to smoke cannabis would have been illegal in that jurisdiction, although in other states this may be perfectly legal. Case-centered approaches allow healthy debate, promote flexibility and the understanding of the emotions engendered by all sides so that there is more confidence in proposed ethical solutions. In this case, the solution was regular doses of nurse-administered dronabinol (Marinol) while respecting the patient's autonomy to make his own informed medical decisions after discharge.

22.3   Informed Consent

Cancer patients receiving psychotropic medications have the right to receive medications considered to be standard of care, and in this context should be informed of the risks, benefits, and alternatives to these medications. This is known as full disclosure. Decision making should be collaborative with good communication and the chance to ask questions, not paternalistic or coercive.

Patients should be competent to give informed consent. Competence (also called capacity) means that patients are able to evidence a choice that is consistent over time, understand the information presented to them proportional to the risk involved, and can rationally weigh up the information to make a logical decision in the context of appreciating their medical situation. They must also be able to communicate their decision-making process and choice (Pinals and Appelbaum 2002).

The problem in the cancer setting is that patients are often cognitively and physically impaired. Delirium, psychosis, and brain damage can severely impede cognition; anxiety and depression also impair concentration and learning new information. Mild treatment-related cognitive dysfunction, also known as "chemo brain," is frequently seen in cancer patients and affects executive function and memory. Additionally, because cancer and aging intersect, many elderly patients may have varying degrees of dementia that is often underappreciated. Finally, patients who are intubated, for instance, may have undergone head and neck surgery, are very weak, short of breath, or in severe pain (especially of their mouth and throat), and may be unable to communicate well and this impacts true informed consent.

Thus, patients' competence to make decisions must be formally assessed as part of the informed consent process. If they are found to lack capacity, their healthcare agent should make those decisions on behalf of the patient, based on the principles of beneficence, non-maleficence, and substituted decision making. The latter is an ethical principle for decision making whereby the healthcare agents are asked to imagine themselves in the patient's shoes and decide based on how they anticipate the patient would have worked through the problem.

Other troubling problems are low health literacy and patients whom require translators. Communication should be clear and free of jargon, educational material is written at a 5th grade reading level, and interpreters should be readily available.

The complexity of the informed consent process suggests that rather than being viewed as a single conversation or signature at the bottom of the form, it be viewed as a process of information exchange, based on the ethical principles of transparency, respect, beneficence, and non-malfeasance that extends the length of the therapeutic relationship.

22.4 Pharmacological Trials

One the one hand, in complex medically ill patients who may be undergoing treatment with multiple agents, the setting is not optimal for controlled trials of psychotropic medications. Studies of antidepressant and anti-anxiety efficacy are better conducted in cohorts of physically healthy patients where drug interactions and side effects won't be misappropriated to other causes. On the other hand, the level of responsiveness for treatment of specific symptoms is pertinent when agents are known to stimulate appetite and weight gain, reduce nausea, counter fatigue, assist sleep, or have co-analgesic actions.

22.4.1 Design Principles

Initial benefits over side effects should be apparent in open label studies so that there is promise of a therapeutic gain from the medication. Then progression to a randomized controlled trial is desirable to confirm the clinical impression from the open label study.

22.4.2 Explanation of Randomization

Communication studies have shown that patients struggle to understand the concept of randomization, potentially limiting the nature of informed consent in controlled trials. Necessary strategies include the use of a symbol, such as tossing a coin to see whether it comes up as heads or tails, or describing that a computer program makes the selection. These emphasize that the clinician has no ability to influence the outcome of the randomization process.

22.4.3 Equipoise

Patients frequently misunderstand the scientific basis for why a randomized trial is needed, as there is often some suggestion of an expected benefit that motivates them to join the trial. Hence, some explanation of the principle of equipoise is deemed to be important. The study is being done because the clinician does not know if a benefit truly occurs from the medication and so the study has been designed so that either arm of the randomization process may bring benefit, and the study is being done to discover whether one has a clearer advantage over the other. Only through understanding of the principle of equipoise is informed consent truly obtained.

22.4.4 Data Safety Monitoring Committees

Regulatory safety to protect the public from undue danger in any pharmacological study is achieved through the use of an independent monitoring committee that receives periodically mandated reports of the outcomes of the study as it proceeds, thus allowing the early recognition of unacceptable side effects, including deaths or other unanticipated but seriously deleterious side effects, or more rarely, unanticipated benefits that are so powerful that the medication ought ethically to be made available to both arms of the study (Brim and Miller 2013).

22.4.5 Placebo Effect

The use of placebos and sham treatments has been criticized as exposing patients to the risks and burdens of a procedure without the benefits. For example, sham neurostimulation for Parkinsons's disease might involve actual surgical incisions; sham acupuncture uses actual needle pricks. Another example is a RCT drug trial for treating depression in cancer patients—it might be considered unethical to offer a placebo arm if it offered no hope of relieving the patient's suffering. Here, comparison with "established best care" would be the comparison arm against which a new medication would be compared. One difficulty in research design here is when new treatments may not have an adequate standard of best care, necessitating the use of an inactive control.

Another ethical problem is that the placebo effect can produce real improvements in perceived symptoms such as pain and function, with measureable effects on neurotransmitters such as endogenous opioids, endocannabinoids, and dopamine and, the more invasive the procedure, the greater the potential for benefit. A measurable placebo effect can last for years. This has led some researchers to suggest that potential benefit from the placebo effect be listed in the informed consent (Brim and Miller 2013).

22.5   Off-Label Use of Psychotropic Medication

Off-label use of psychotropic medications promotes innovation and seeks to relieve suffering in a field where effective treatments are often evasive. Consider the innovative practice of prescribing of a psychotropic medication prophylactically, such as an antidepressant before starting chemotherapy or an antipsychotic to reduce the risk of delirium before surgery. The potential benefit of dodging or lessening an episode of depression or delirium is enormous, but this must be balanced against the burden and risk of side effects in those people would not have developed these symptoms in the first place.

Cancer-related fatigue or treatment-related cognitive problems (chemo brain) are often treated with off-label stimulants. However, these are not FDA approved for this indication nor are they ever likely to be. Many patients seem to benefit from them in the short term, but others seem to enjoy taking these medications, often using them for many years after the cancer has been cured, raising the question of abuse or what has been more politely termed as cosmetic pharmacology or enhancement therapy, the psychiatric equivalent of plastic surgery (Gutheil 2012).

Polypharmacy is a common approach in all fields of medicine. In psychopharmacology it is based on the premise that numerous receptors and neural circuits are disrupted in different psychiatric conditions. The problem is that data supporting the efficacy of such theoretical approaches are lacking, leaving psychiatrists to find their way by trial and error. For example, should single agent haloperidol be used to manage delirium, or should a cocktail of dexmedetomidine, haloperidol, and valproic acid targeting three different neural circuits be used? There is not enough data to make such a decision and effectively communicating the risks and benefits of managing delirium with psychopharmacology is therefore challenging.

Some medications are prescribed off label because of their side-effects profile: the antidepressant trazodone for a sleep aid, mirtazapine and olanzapine for weight gain, lorazepam as an antiemetic, or olanzapine as an antianxiety agent. This is ethically problematic because data supporting such use are lacking and the side effects, such as the risk of movement disorders from olanzapine or delirium for lorazepam, are often omitted in the informed consent process.

Furthermore, there can be great pressure on prescribers to, for example, prescribe an antipsychotic for a disruptive or noisy patient or an elderly confused patient, without necessarily considering the cardiovascular risks of QTc prolongation and stroke in geriatric patients who are treated with these medications.

Terminal delirium, palliative sedation, and physician-assisted suicide often use psychopharmacological medications such as antipsychotics, benzodiazepines, and barbiturates.

In terminal delirium, often recognized by the presence of multiple organs failing in the setting of advanced and progressive disease such as widespread and terminal malignancy, neuroleptic and sedating medications can ameliorate the symptoms of an agitated delirium (Friedlander and Kissane 2008). The relief of suffering is a core ethical value that can lead to a better death and ease the distress of family members who are accompanying the patient.

In palliative sedation, however, sedating a person for reasons other than pain management can be ethically challenging. The goal is to relieve suffering. The test of this intent is that if the patient reawakens again and the suffering has eased, then sedation need not be re-administered. Fear of death or other sources of existential distress can be dealt with psychologically or with psychopharmacological medications at their usual therapeutic doses.

Similarly, physician-assisted suicide asks the clinician to assist in bringing about death in the noble relief of suffering and promoting patient autonomy, but comprises morality because excellent palliative care should be able to facilitate a "good death" without assigning responsibility for death to a third party. Callahan notes that suffering is not a good indicator of the need to be dead or the desire to be dead (Callahan 1998). Physician-assisted suicide is, of course, a contentious social issue that has been adopted in a small number of countries. In studying the quality of care delivered during a period of legal euthanasia in Australia, a poor standard of palliative care was observed in the actual cases studied (Kissane et al. 1998; Street and Kissane 1999–2000). For the clinician attempting to support the distressed patient, a stance of hope is necessary to counter any loss of morale (Kissane 2002).

Clinicians might be pressured by insurance companies, administrators, nurses, or family members to hasten death or sanitize it for reasons that are the antithesis of good palliative care, blurring the line between assisting death and killing. This is especially true in the absence of data driven support for physician-assisted suicide.

Finally, the ethical doctrine of double effect does allow for using, e.g., a morphine infusion to relieve pain, even if this might risk hastening death by the undesired consequence of suppression of central respiratory drive; dissent to this view calls for more rational and careful medical attention to so-called unintended "side effects" (Mayo 1998).

22.6   Unproven Therapies

Deng and Cassileth state that 40 % of patients use either integrative medicine to complement their cancer therapies or alternative treatments in place of evidence-based treatments. The former are used for psychological and physical symptom management and are more mainstream, often with data supporting their utility (e.g., acupuncture, massage, exercise). Alternative treatments are often politely referred to as miraculous cures (and less politely as quackery). These include laetrile from apricot seeds, also known as vitamin B17, cesium to alkalinize the body, ozone (hydrogen peroxide) and a variety of detoxifying diets, Amazon herbs, supplements, vitamins, enemas (Deng and Cassileth 2013), and medical marijuana. Patients are duped by unethical practitioners who offer false hope and misleading advice at great financial expense and like, the founder of Apple Inc., Steve Jobs, delay evidence-based cancer treatments to their ultimate detriment.

22.7   Ethical Relationships with Pharmaceutical Corporations

Historically, pharmaceutical companies paid medical academics to provide clinical advice, conduct studies, give lectures about, and help market medicines to their clinical colleagues. Initially projected as educational practices, the inherent conflict of interest became apparent when senior university academics in the USA were exposed by Congress as taking millions of dollars annually as honorariums. The lack of integrity of their advice to colleagues about the apparent benefits of medications brought huge disrespect to the medical profession, and quickly demanded separation of the medical discipline from pharmaceutical companies.

The provision of totally unrestricted educational grants by pharmaceutical corporations continues as an approach in many countries, but colleges and professional associations have steadily called for complete distance from "detailing practices" that allow pharmaceutical companies to market products to prescribing clinicians. The resulting challenge is how to educate the professions about new products, and the ethical answer is via peer-reviewed scientific publications—the same method used by all of science to make its discoveries available to its practitioners.

22.8   The Ethical Integration of Psychotherapy and Pharmacotherapy

A major limitation evident unfortunately in the clinical practice of many today is a physician's dependence on pharmaceutically based interventions, without a balanced integration of psychotherapeutic interventions in a complementary and synergistically beneficial manner. Equally of concern is the sole use of counseling techniques when the addition of medication would improve care outcomes. Both of these examples of less than optimal care are sadly common in the world today.

Disciplines are challenged to educate their workforce in comprehensive care delivery, so that when the person presents with their illness, treatment of the whole person results through integrated care that understands the potential of each mode of treatment and refers to relevant specialty disciplines to ensure that comprehensive care of the patient and their family is achieved.

All too often, the balance of this approach is skewered in the direction of the pill that can be so readily prescribed without the associated psychotherapeutic counseling that person-centered care demands. Financial remuneration systems have also contributed to this wrong, exemplified by health insurance corporations that reward cumulative brief consultations over comprehensive models of care and thus induce practitioners to adopt a more pharmacologically driven paradigm of care.

22.9 The Ethics of Prescribing Well

What follows from the limits of knowledge of any one disciplinary group, whether medical oncologist, primary care physician, psychologist, or psychiatrist, is the ethically driven mandate to ask for help when confronted with the limits of one's knowledge. Barriers to such behavior include ignorance, lack of competent skill development, pride and professional ownership of "my patient" in place of the necessary humility, and wisdom to discern when the second opinion is not only clinically required but morally essential.

Mistakes are made in medicine by not knowing, not keeping up-to-date, not practicing with integrity, and not attending to the whole persona and family involved with the illness. Sloppy practice and burnout also contribute towards errors. Lack of clinician well-being can develop through suboptimal work practices, excessive hours, lack of balance between career, family, and leisure, the inability to say "no," or a poor fit between the needs of certain groups of patients and the attributes of the clinician. When clinicians become unwell, abuse alcohol or drugs, are overwhelmed and demoralized by personal stress, patient care can be neglected. The medical, nursing, and allied health professionals carry a moral self-responsibility to maintain competence and fitness to practice; their disciplines are bound to provide continuous medical education and to recertify competencies in a regular manner that safeguards the community from the dangerous practitioner. For example, prescribing an antidepressant such as paroxetine or fluoxetine that inhibits CYP 2D6 can negatively impact the effectiveness of tamoxifen in breast cancer treatment (Holzman 2009). Although initially controversial, this interaction is now established and highlights the ethical importance of considering drug–drug interactions when prescribing.

Cosgrove reviewed the literature associating antidepressants with breast and ovarian cancer and found that authors reporting negative studies were significantly more likely to have pharmaceutical industry affiliations (Cosgrove et al. 2011), suggesting that physicians need to be aware of the potential for research funding to bias their data [a more recent meta-analysis did not find an association between long-term use of antidepressants and cancer; Eom et al. (2012)]. Biased science is obviously unethical, but even an appearance of bias can compromise the science and subsequent confidence in prescribing.

22.10 Addiction to Prescribed Medications

While no clinician should feel coerced into prescribing, consider a common case: a male cancer patient in his thirties, his cancer in remission, and he is left with significant vertebral damage. He asks his pain management physician, oncologist, and psycho-oncologist for ultrashort acting narcotics instead of a Fentanyl patch, which he complains is less effective and, when his request is declined, he protests loudly.

Many cancer patients and survivors become addicted to their pain, anxiety, and stimulant medications, and their physicians may feel pressured into continuing them indefinitely. One strategy is to transition these patients to less addictive, long acting opioids or benzodiazepines, and another strategy might be to wean them off these drugs altogether. Certainly, it is ethically acceptable not to prescribe an opioid, benzodiazepine, or stimulant that is not indicated and to clearly state the management strategy that is suggested in place of this. Ethically, saying "no" exists in tension with a physician's duty to relieve pain and suffering. This is why such cases are so challenging. The solution lies in working with a multidisciplinary team to crystallize an acceptable management plan that is well communicated to all parties involved with the ethical adage, *primum non nocerum*, first do no harm, at the forefront.

22.11 Transcranial Magnetic Stimulation

Electroconvulsive therapy (ECT) is rarely used in advanced cancer because of firstly the risk of anesthesia and secondly the risk of bleeding, or bleeding into a tumor, especially in those patients with low platelets or clotting abnormalities. Transcranial magnetic stimulation (TMS) presents a noninvasive option that might be helpful for patients with resistant depression or those taking medications such as linezolid that preclude prescribing antidepressants because of the risk of serotonin toxicity.

ECT's history is such that it is used as a last resort for patients who have exhausted other options, and there is a similar ethical danger that TMS will be applied to broad off-label conditions for which there is not clear data supporting its efficacy. Desperate patients are an ethically vulnerable group.

Furthermore, TMS is not a single therapy. Theta burst stimulation, different coil shapes and pulse characteristics, stimulation sites, and power levels build a picture of a modality that is both broad and nuanced. This implies the ethical need for training and certification and device licensing. While consensus guidelines and FDA approval have helped to ensure morally defensible use of this modality, therapeutic indications are still narrow. There is no FDA approval for long-term maintenance TMS and its effect might wear off after 4–6 months forcing patients to undergo a full treatment course again. Additional concerns relate to insurance not reimbursing the treatment, limiting its positive effects to the wealthy. Another issue is how to ethically advertise TMS when FDA approved indication criteria are limited. Finally, there is little long-term safety data for this modality in general (Horvath et al. 2011).

Despite these doubts, it seems likely that such noninvasive brain stimulation will be helpful to many cancer patients with resistant depression or contraindications to antidepressants, and we are likely to see its off-label use for the variety of neurocognitive disorders that are seen in psycho-oncology. Genetic predictive models may help guide the choice of which patients are more likely to respond to this treatment in the future.

Conclusion

Attention to ethical care is the basis for patient and family centered care, but this is particularly challenging in psycho-oncology because of the common practice of using medications for off-label treatments, highlighting the moral importance of informed consent in clinical care and rigorous research ethics in this often vulnerable population. Relationships with pharmaceutical companies should be transparent, and psychopharmacology should not be considered an easy substitute for psychotherapy. Addiction to prescribed medications and newer modalities such as TMS remain ethically and clinically challenging.

▶ Key Points

- Informed consent involves full disclosure and an assessment of capacity; patients with low health literacy or foreign language speakers are at a disadvantage.
- Ethically designed research is paramount and the concepts of randomization and equipoise need to be carefully explained to patients.
- Off-label prescribing can promote innovation but attention to informed consent is vital.
- Desperate patients are ethically vulnerable to exploitation when they agree to unproven cancer "cures."
- Undisclosed honorariums and relationships with pharmaceutical companies create an ethical conflict of interest.
- It is unethical to prescribe psychopharmacological treatment without considering efficacious psychotherapies, or vice versa, and it is worthwhile considering the potential synergistic effect of one on the other.
- Maintaining professional standards is essential for ethical prescribing.

- Addiction to prescribed medication creates an ethical dilemma for clinicians whose duty it is to relieve suffering.
- Transcranial magnetic stimulation is not a single treatment because it can be applied in different ways at different strengths; this challenges informed consent especially when used off label.

Suggested Further Reading

- Beauchamp TL, Childress JF. Principles of biomedical ethics. 7th ed. New York: Oxford University Press; 2012.
- Bloch S, Green S. Psychiatric ethics. 4th ed. Melbourne: Oxford University Press; 2009.
- ten Have H, Clark D, editors. The ethics of palliative care. Buckingham: Open University Press; 2002.
- Steinberg MD, Youngner SJ, editors. End-of-life decisions. A psychosocial perspective. Washington, DC: American Psychiatric Press; 1998.

References

Brim RL, Miller FG. The potential benefit of the placebo effect in sham-controlled trials: implications for risk-benefit assessments and informed consent. J Med Ethics. 2013;39:703–7.

Callahan D. Physician-assisted suicide: moral questions. In: Steinberg M, Youngner SJ, editors. End-of-life decisions. A psychosocial perspective. Washington, DC: American Psychiatric Publishing; 1998. p. 283–95.

Cassel EJ. The nature of suffering and the goals of medicine. N Engl J Med. 1982;306(11):639–45.

Cosgrove L, Shi L, Creasey DE, Anaya-McKivergan M, Myers JA, Huybrechts KF. Antidepressants and breast and ovarian cancer risk: a review of the literature and researchers' financial associations with industry. PLoS One. 2011;6(4):e18210. doi:10.1371/journal.pone.0018210.

Deng G, Cassileth BR. Complementary or alternative medicine in cancer care-myths and realities. Nat Rev Clin Oncol. 2013;10:656–64. doi:10.1038/nrclinonc.2013.125.

Eom CS, Park SM, Cho KH. Use of antidepressants and the risk of breast cancer: a meta-analysis. Breast Cancer Res Treat. 2012;136(3):635–45. doi:10.1007/s10549-012-2307-y.

Fins JJ, Bacchetta MD, Miller FG. Clinical pragmatism: a method of moral problem solving. Kennedy Inst Ethics J. 1997;7(2):129–45.

Friedlander M, Kissane DW. The contribution of delirium to prognosis. In: Glare P, Christakis NA, editors. Prognosis in advanced cancer. Oxford: Oxford University Press; 2008. p. 381–95.

Gilligan C. In a different voice: psychological theory and women's development. Cambridge, MA: Harvard University Press; 1993.

Gutheil TG. Reflections on ethical issues in psychopharmacology: an American perspective. Int J Law Psychiatry. 2012;35:387–91.

Holzman D. Tamoxifen, antidepressants, and CYP2D6: the conundrum continues. J Natl Cancer Inst. 2009;101(20):1370–1. doi:10.1093/jnci/djp366.

Horvath JC, Perez JM, Forrow L, Fregni F, Pascual-Leone A. Transcranial magnetic stimulation: a historical evaluation and future prognosis of therapeutically relevant ethical concerns. J Med Ethics. 2011;37(3):137–43. doi:10.1136/jme.2010.039966.

Kissane DW. Deadly days in Darwin. In: Foley K, Hendin H, editors. The case against assisted suicide. Baltimore, MD: Johns Hopkins University Press; 2002. p. 192–209.

Kissane DW, Street A, Nitschke P. Seven deaths in Darwin: case studies under the Rights of the Terminally Ill Act, Northern Territory, Australia. Lancet. 1998;352:1097–102.

Lederberg MS. Making a situational diagnosis. Psychiatrists at the interface of psychiatry and ethics in the consultation-liaison setting. Psychosomatics. 1997;38(4):327–38.

Mayo D. Termination-of-treatment decisions: ethical underpinnings. In: Steinberg M, Youngner SJ, editors. End-of-life decisions. A psychosocial perspective. Washington, DC: American Psychiatric Publishing; 1998. p. 259–81.

Noddings N. Caring. A relational approach to ethics and moral education. 2nd ed., updated ed. Berkley, CA: University of California Press; 2013.

Pinals DA, Appelbaum PS. Ethical aspects of neuropsychiatric research with human subjects. In: Davis KL, Charney D, Coyle JT, Nemeroff C, editors. Neuropsychopharmacology: fifth generation of progress. Philadelphia, Pennsylvania: Lippincott, Williams, & Wilkins; 2002.

Street AF, Kissane DW. Dispensing death, desiring death: an exploration of medical roles and patient motivation during the period of legalized euthanasia in Australia. Omega. 1999–2000;40:231–48.

Index

A

AAA. *See* Auricular acupuncture for anxiety (AAA)
AAR. *See* Auricular acupuncture for relaxation (AAR)
Aberrant drug taking behaviors, 274, 275
Acetaminophen, 339
Acetominophen, 353
Acetylcholine, 20, 204, 352
Acupuncture
    anxiety, 106
    fluoxetine, 108
    and hypnosis, 88
    sham acupuncture, 105–107
    sleep disorders, 259–260
    traditional, 105
    treatment, 259
Acute stress disorder
    amnesia and emotional paralysis, 135
    children, 333
    diagnosis, 135
    leukemia, 135
    PTSD, 136
Addiction
    behaviors, aberrant drug, 274, 275
    current/remote histories, patients, 275–276
    definition, 275
    differential diagnosis, 275, 276
    economic and insurance, 268
    personality disorders, 275
    pseudoaddiction, 273
    risk, misuse, 268–269
    and substance abuse, 272–273
ADEs. *See* Adverse drug events (ADEs)
Adjustment disorder
    anxiety, 136
    diagnosis, 41, 135
    distress, 50
    pediatric, 333, 335

prevalence, 132, 139
psychological assessment, 50
Adverse drug events (ADEs), 350, 352, 354–356, 365
Aging
    pharmacodynamics, 352–354
    pharmacokinetics, 350–352
Agomelatine, 154–155, 256
Agoraphobia, 134
Albumin levels, 351
Alcohol
    DTs, 272
    prevalence, 271
    screening, 272
    socioeconomic barrier, 271–272
    withdrawal
        administration, vitamin-mineral solution, 280
        delirium tremens, 279
        early stages, 280
        guidelines, 280, 281
        hydration, 280
        neuroleptics, 280, 281
        preventing and minimizing, 280
        risk, 279, 280
        symptoms, 279
        therapeutic impacts, 281
        thiamine, 280
        types and characteristics, benzodiazepines, 280, 281
        Wernicke–Korsakoff's syndrome, 279–280
ALS. *See* Amyotrophic lateral sclerosis (ALS)
Amantadine, 325
American Society of Clinical Oncology, 340
Amyotrophic lateral sclerosis (ALS), 373
Anaesthetics, 376
Anorexia
    antidepressant effect, 154

Anorexia (*cont.*)
   cancer-related symptoms, 147
   insomnia, 384
   physical/emotional symptoms, 341
   psychostimulants, 155
Anticholinergic delirium, 325, 352, 353
Anticipatory anxiety, 132, 248, 297, 305, 307
Antidepressant medication
   acute treatment, 149
   adverse effects, 150–151
   atypical, 154–155
   choosing, 149
   cyclophosphamide, 156
   discontinuation syndrome, 147–148
   effects, period of time, 147
   hypothyroidism and vitamin B12
      deficiency, 149
   impacts, 158
   meta-analyses, effectiveness, 151–152
   prominent anxiety, 149–150
   psychostimulants, 155–156
   randomised controlled trials, 151
   side effects, 147
   SNRIs, 153–154
   SSRIs, 153
   suicidality risk, 148–149
   tamoxifen, 156
   tricyclic, 155
Antidepressants (ADs)
   breast cancer, 179
   dopamine, 20–21
   dose effects, body system, 23
   interactions, cytochrome P450 system, 22
   psychotropic drugs, 6–7
   sleep disorders
      amitriptyline, 255
      doxepin, 255
      mianserin, 255
      mirtazapin, 255
      paroxetine, 256
      side effects, 255
      trazodone, 255
      venlafaxine, 256
   SNRIs, 19
   SSRIs, 18–19
Antiepileptics, 375–376
Antihistamines, 376–377
   diphenhydramin, 251
   doxylamine, 251
   efficacy, 251
   hydroxyzine, 251
   hypothalamus regulation, 251
   promethazine, 252

Antipsychotic medications, 327, 364, 365, 366
   and dosages, 213–215
   evidence-based recommendations, 207, 212
   FDA, 213
   open-label and randomized controlled
      trials, 206, 208–211
   postoperative care, 213
   prevention, 216–218
   psychotropic medications, 205
   QTc, 213
   recommendations, 213, 216
   side effects, 213
   typical and atypical, 206
Antipsychotics
   advanced cancer patients, 232
   and anticonvulsants, 139
   and antidepressants, 18, 352
   and anxiolytics, 6
   atypical, 138, 171, 257, 357, 364
   atypical, higher and lower potency, 23
   benzodiazepines, 231
   BPAD treatment, 196–197
   cancer setting, 233
   cardiovascular, 23–25
   causes, 23
   characteristics, 231
   childhood and adolescence, 338
   cytochrome P450, 23, 24
   cytochrome P-450 enzyme, 232
   delirium (*see* Delirium)
   dopamine deprivation, 23
   drug interactions, 23
   elderly patients, 365, 366
   first-and second generation, 231
   generation, 232
   generation of, 7
   hallucinations and delusions, 23
   hepatic, 24, 25
   insomnia, 384
   lapatinib, 232
   mood stabilizing medications, 191
   neuroleptics, 23
   overdose/intoxication, 327
   pharmacotherapy, 231
   psychiatric disorders, 5, 6
   sedation, 374
   side effects, 232
   tardive dyskinesia, 356
   treatment, psychotic disorders, 233
   typical, 353
Anxiety, 332–333, 339, 362–364
Anxiety disorders
   acupuncture, 106

and adjustment disorders, 52, 136
advanced lung cancer, 133
alcoholism, 279
cancer (see Cancer)
cognitive dysfunction, 132
DSM-5 and ICD-10, 40
evaluation, 132
generalized, 134
identification, 384
non-pharmacotherapy, 136–138
organic/substance-induced, 132
pathophysiology
    GABA, 131–132
    mechanism, 130, 131
    noradrenaline regulation, 130, 131
    noradrenergic and serotonergic nerve
        activity, 130, 131
    serotonergic nerve activity, 131
pharmacotherapy, 138–139
prevalence, 132–133
psychological and physical, 130
screening scales, 386
symptoms, 132
treatments, elderly patients, 362
uncomfortable emotional phenomena, 130
Atypical antipsychotics (AP), 257
Auricular acupuncture for anxiety (AAA), 106
Auricular acupuncture for relaxation
    (AAR), 106

B
Barbiturates, 255
BDZ-H. See Benzodiazepine hypnotics
    (BDZ-H)
Benzodiazepine hypnotics (BDZ-H)
    actions, 252, 254
    flurazepam, 252
    management, insomnia, 252
    precautions, 252, 253
    temazepam, 252
    triazolam, 252
Benzodiazepines (BZPs), 323, 326, 333, 340,
        341, 343, 362–363, 365, 366
    anxiety, 138
    and lorazepam, 17
Bipolar affective disorder (BPAD)
    anticonvulsants
        antipsychotics, 196–197
        CBZ, 194–195
        FDA approval, 193
        lamotrigine, 195–196

valproic acid/valproate/VPA, 193–194,
        200–201
data, randomized placebo-controlled
        trial, 200
drug interactions
    CYP450 enzymes status, 197–198
    effects, chemotherapy agents, 198–199
lithium, 192–193
and MDD, 190–192
risk–benefit assessment, 200
symptoms, 190
BPAD. See Bipolar affective disorder (BPAD)
Bromocriptine, 323, 325
Bupropion, 7, 20, 154, 178, 328, 336
Buspirone, 131, 363–364
BZPs. See Benzodiazepines (BZPs)

C
Caffeine, 342
Cancer
    anxiety
        chemotherapy, 133
        generalized anxiety disorder, 134
        life-threatening condition, 130
        panic disorder, 134
        phobias, 134
        social anxiety disorder, 134–135
    CAM, 102–103
    distress, 103–104
    and sleep disorders
        BDZ-H, 251–252
        chemotherapy, 248–250, 258
        delirium, 248
        depression and anxiety, 247–248
        distress, 247
        DORA, 257–258
        fatigue, 246–247
        glucocorticoids, 250
        HD, 243
        immunotherapy, 250
        impacts, 243
        insomnia, 243
        non-pharmacological treatment,
            258–260
        OSA, 245
        pain, 246
        pharmacotherapy, 251
        psychotropic drugs (see Psychotropic
            drugs)
        radiotherapy, 248
        RLS, 243–244

Cancer (*cont.*)
    surgery, 248
    treatment procedures, 251
    somatoform disorders (*see* Somatic
        symptom disorder/somatization)
    survival outcomes, 102
Cancer care
    adherence, 72
    clinician-patient alliance, 73
    communication process, 70–72
    interpersonal relationship ingredients,
        72, 73
    psychopharmacological treatment, 72, 73
Cancer-related fatigue (CRF)
    acupuncture/acupressure and moxibustion,
        177–178
    acupuncture benefit, 105
    ADs, 7
    in adults, 342
    anemic, 178
    antidepressant, 178
    CBT, 177
    disease-free survivors, 175
    drugs, 178
    erythropoietin and darbepoetin, 178
    exercise, 176
    hatha yoga, 113
    insomnia, 246
    modafinil, 178
    NCCN guideline, 178
    off-label stimulants, 399
    oral Withania somnifera, 178
    parameters, 176, 177
    pathophysiological factors, 175–176
    psycho-educational strategies, 177
    psychostimulants, 385
Cancer survivors, 306
Cancer treatment
    anxiety, women, 88
    chemotherapy, 88
    trauma-related memories, 89
Cannabanoids, 340
Carbamazepine (CBZ)
    BPAD, 194–195
    mood stabilizers, 7, 28, 191
Cardinal symptoms, 324
Cardiotoxic chemotherapy drugs, 333
Cardiovascular, antipsychotics
    Cochrane review, 24
    dementia, 23–24
    QTc intervals, 23
CBT. *See* Cognitive behavioral therapy (CBT)
CBZ. *See* Carbamazepine (CBZ)

CDI. *See* Children's Depression Inventory
    (CDI)
Children's Depression Inventory (CDI), 335
Cholinergic hypothesis, 364
Chronic pain, 166, 172, 246, 268, 271, 340
Citalopram
    fluoxetine and fluvoxamine, 22
    head and neck cancer, 152
    venlafaxine, 91
Clitoral therapy device (CTD), 301
Clonidine, 91, 131, 179, 335, 338, 376
Clonus, 151, 320, 321
Cognitive behavioral therapy (CBT), 171, 174,
    176, 177, 249–250, 258–259, 336
Cognitive restructuring, 298, 309
Colorectal cancer, 258, 296
Communication process
    clinical psychiatry, 71
    components, 70
    interview techniques, 71–72
    psychological distress, 70
    reciprocal trust promotion, 70
Cytochrome P450 system
    3A4,4 substrates, 22
    2C9 and 2C19, 22
    2D6, 22
    interactions, 22
    psychotropic medications, 22

D
Dantrolene, 323, 325
Delirium, 337–338, 354, 364–366
    causes, 204
    clinical features, 203–204, 206
    diagnosis, 204
    dysfunction, 204
    etiologies, 205, 207
    metabolic abnormalities, 204–205
    morbidity and mortality, 205
    neuropsychiatric symptoms, 203–205
    predisposing risk factors, 204
    prevalence, 205, 206
    treatment
        cancer patients, 205
        non-pharmacologic management,
            218–219
        pharmacological (*see* Pharmacological
            treatment)
        predisposing risk factors, 205
        prevention, 216–218
        psychostimulants, 213–215
        psychotropic medications, 205

Depression, 335–337
  antidepressant treatment, 361
  in cancer
    adverse effects, drug interactions, 158
    antidepressants (*see* Antidepressant
        medication)
    anxiety, 146
    clinical activity, 158
    diagnosis, 146, 148
    and dysthymia, 145
    quality of life, 145–146
    randomised controlled trials, 158
    screening tools and scales, 146
    symptoms, 147
  psychostimulants, 361
  SNRIs, 360
  SSRIs, 358–260
  TCAs, 360–361
Diagnostic issues
  acceptable, normal and abnormal
      experiences, 32
  clinical, 39
  evaluation, psychological reactions, 32
  ICD and DSM
    adjustment disorders, 41
    clinical attention, 44
    common disorders observation, 40
    depressive disorders, 41–42
    psychological factors influence, medical
        condition, 42–43
    psychosocial disorders, 41
    psychosomatic research, 43–44
    signs and symptoms, 40
    somatization, 42
  psychiatric (*see* Psychiatric interview and
      examination)
  psychopharmacological intervention, 39
Diazepam, 259, 280, 351–354, 362
Diphenhydramine, 21, 251, 340, 342–343
Dopamine
  advantages and disadvantages, 20
  anti-α1 adrenergic effects, 21
  anticholinergic effects, 20, 21
  antihistamines, 20, 21
  antipsychotics, 23
  bromocriptine and amantadine, 325
  bupropion, 360
  complications, 20
  dosing, 20
  drug interactions, 21
  muscarinic/nicotinic acetylcholine
      receptors, 20
  neuroleptic malignant syndrome, 25

reuptake inhibitors, 20–21
DORA. *See* Dual Orexin 1 and 2 receptor
    antagonists (DORA)
Doxylamine, 251
Drug absorption, 351
Drug addict, 339
Drug-induced movement disorders, 357
Dual Orexin 1 and 2 receptor antagonists
    (DORA), 257
Dyspareunia, 297

E
ED. *See* Erectile dysfunction (ED)
Edmonton symptom assessment system
    (ESAS), 56–57, 59, 132, 177
Educational and psychosocial intervention
    techniques
  anticipatory anxiety, 305
  body awareness and relaxation, 307
  cancer survivors, 306
  cognitive restructuring techniques, 309
  problem-solving techniques, 308
  self-stimulation, 307–308
  sexual arousal, 306
EEG. *See* Electroencephalography (EEG)
Electroencephalography (EEG), 116–117, 204,
    241, 336
Emotion thermometers (ET), 57
Encephalopathy, 23, 335, 337, 370
EPS. *See* Extrapyramidal symptoms (EPS)
Erectile dysfunction (ED), 302–304
  and depression, 296
  penile injections, 302
  radical prostatectomy, 301–302
ESAS. *See* Edmonton symptom assessment
    system (ESAS)
Escitalopram, 6, 153, 332–334, 336
Eszopiclone, 253
Ethics, medical treatment
  attention, 404
  case-centered, 396
  framework, 393–396
  informed consent, 396–397
  integration, psycho and pharmacotherapy,
      401–402
  off-label usage, psychotropic medications,
      399–400
  prescription (*see* Prescription)
  principlism
    analysis, bioethical dilemmas, 394
    beneficence, 394
    justice, 394–395

Ethics (*cont.*)
    nonmaleficence, 394
    patient's autonomy, 394, 395
    relational care, 395
    relationships, pharmaceutical
        corporations, 401
    TMS, 403–404
    trials, pharmacological (*see*
        Pharmacological trails)
    unproven therapies, 401
Euthanasia, 373–374
Extrapyramidal symptoms (EPS)
    cancer setting, 233
    delirium treatment, 209
    olanzapine, 257
    side effects, 232

F
Fatality, 327
Fatigue
    anxiety, 134
    cancer treatment, 94
    hypnosis intervention, 89
    insomnia, 246
    modafanil, 342
    pain, 104
    paroxetine, 178
    psychiatric disorders, 166
Flumazenil, 326
Fluoxetine's drug, 336

G
GABA. *See* γ-Aminobutyric acid (GABA)
γ-aminobutyric acid (GABA)
    anxiety and depression, 113
    anxiety disorder, 131–132
    BDZs, 252
    level, asana practice, 113
    neurotransmission, 193
    non-benzodiazepines, 27
    positive allosteric modulators (PAMs), 253
    sedative hypnotics, 25
Gastrointestinal (GI) bleeding, 355, 356
Generalized anxiety disorder, 134, 332
Glomerular filtration rate, 17, 351–352
Granisetron, 340
Guanfacine, 338

H
Haloperidol
    chlorpromazine, 212
    delirium, 327, 399

    lorazepam, 27
    risperidone, 24
Hatha yoga
    GABA, 113
    Iyengar yoga, 113–114
    RCT, 113
HD. *See* Hypersomnolence disorder (HD)
Hepatic dysfunction, 320
5-HT receptor antagonists, 323
Hunter Serotonin Toxicity Criteria
    (HSTC), 321
Hydroxyzine, 251
Hyperreflexia, 320
Hypersomnolence disorder (HD), 243
Hyperthermia, 320, 323–325
Hypoactive delirium, 221, 337–338
Hyponatraemia, 151, 352, 358
Hypotension, 20, 323, 327, 338, 384

I
Ibuprofen, 339, 353
"Ideal" antidepressant, 357, 358
Illicit drugs, 270–273, 275, 288, 318, 320
Inflatable penile prostheses (IPPs), 303–304
Insomnia
    antihistamines, 251
    diagnostic criteria, 243, 244
    literature, 243
    prevalence, 243, 245
    symptoms, 243
    syndrome and sleep complication, 243, 244
Interpersonal psychotherapy (IPT), 336
Intraurethral suppositories, 303
IPPs. *See* Inflatable penile prostheses (IPPs)
IPT. *See* Interpersonal psychotherapy (IPT)
IV haloperidol, 338
Iyengar yoga, 113–114

J
Jutong theory, 106, 107

L
Lamotrigine, 191, 195–196
Linezolid, 320, 322–323, 332, 403
Lithium, 17, 28, 192–193, 352
    BPAD, 27, 191–194
    dose maintenance, 28, 84
    kidneys, 17, 352
    serotonin syndrome, 19
    water-soluble drugs, 351
Lorazepam, 6, 17, 26, 95, 280, 321, 326, 363,
    374, 375, 399–400

M

Major depressive disorder (MDD)
  antidepressants, 191
  and BPAD
    antidepressants, 191
    lamotrigine and quetiapine, 191
    management, mood disorders, 190–191
    mania treatment, 191–192
    non-pharmacologic treatments, 190
    pharmacotherapies, 192
  chronic pain, 172
  and DSM5, 52
  DSM-5 diagnostic criteria, 335
  somatic symptoms, 24
MAO inhibitors. *See* Monoamine oxidase
    (MAO) inhibitors
Mastectomy, 88, 165, 353
MBSR. *See* Mindfulness-based stress reduction
    (MBSR)
MDD. *See* Major depressive disorder (MDD)
Medication
  drug interactions, antipsychotic, 24
  insomnia, 92–93
  lorazepam, 95
  physician-patient relationship, 96
  polypharmacology, 94
  prescription and management, 97
  psychostimulants, 27
  SSRIs, 95–96
Medication administration errors/non-
    adherence, 354–355
Meditation
  components, 115
  description, 114–115
  EEG, 116–117
  mantra meditation, 115
  MBSR, 115
  mindfulness meditation, 115
Melatonergic agents, 256
Melatonin, 154, 205, 218, 256, 342
Memorial Symptom Assessment Scale
    (MSAS), 335
Mental health, 84–85
Mental status examination (MSE)
  attachment style, 33–34
  oncology settings, 33, 34
  patient and family relationship, 33
  personality traits, 35–36
  psychological
    and behavioral symptoms, 33, 35
    tools, 38
  risk factors, cancer and palliative care, 37
  therapeutic relationships, 34

Metabolism, 16, 17, 21, 197, 351
Metaclopromide, 325
Methadone, 22, 25, 282–284, 338
Mindfulness-based stress reduction (MBSR)
  breast and prostate cancer patients, 115
  mental health, cancer patients, 116
Mirtazapine, 20, 23, 138, 150, 154, 180, 255,
    336, 360
Monoamine oxidase (MAO) inhibitors, 322,
    336, 355
Morphine, 17, 22, 333, 334, 378, 400
MSAS. *See* Memorial Symptom Assessment
    Scale (MSAS)
MSE. *See* Mental status examination (MSE)

N

Nasal continuous positive airway pressure
    (CPAP), 258
Nausea/vomiting, 340–341
Neuroleptic malignant syndrome (NMS)
  antichlinergic delirium, 325
  bromocriptine and amantadine, 325
  cardinal symptoms, 324
  dantrolene, 325
  dopamine, 324
  metaclopromide and promethazine, 325
  serotonin syndrome, 325
  serotonin toxicity, 325
Neuroleptics
  chlorpromazine, 375
  delirium, 24, 375
  haloperidol, 375
  malignant syndrome, 24, 25, 232
  methotrimeprazine, 375
  phenothiazine, 25
  quetiapine, 343
Nonbenzodiazepine hypnotics, 253
Non-pharmacotherapy
  anxiety disorders, 136–138
  trauma and stressor-related disorders,
    136–138
Noradrenergic and specific serotonergic
    antidepressant (NaSSA), 154
Norepinephrine reuptake inhibitor (NRI), 154

O

Obstructive sleep apnea (OSA), 245
Olanzapine, 257
  atypical antipsychotics, 212
  quetiapine, 27, 191, 364
Ondansetron, 340

OSA. *See* Obstructive sleep apnea (OSA)
Overdose/intoxication, 326–328

P

Pain/hypoxia, 332
Palliative sedation therapy (PST)
  and ALS, 373
  classification, 370–371
  definition, 370
  and euthanasia, 373–374
  guidelines, 372–373
  pharmacology, 374–377
  psychological/existential suffering,
    371–372
  refractory symptoms, 369, 370
Panic disorder, 134
PDE5 inhibitors, 302
Pelvic floor and Kegel exercises, 299
Penile injections, 302–303
Pharmacodynamics
  antidepressants (*see* Antidepressants)
  antipsychotics, 23–25
  mood stabilizers, 27–28
  psychostimulants, 27
  reactions, medications, 17, 18
  rule of thumb, 18
  sedative hypnotics, 25–27
  side effects, 17–18
Pharmacokinetics
  bioavailability
    determinants, volume of distribution, 16
    drug delivery to systemic circulation,
      14, 15
    impacts, gut metabolism, 14, 15
    protein binding on drug toxicity, 16
  drug metabolism and excretion, 16
  physiological mechanisms, medications,
    14, 15
Pharmacological trails
  data safety monitoring committees, 398
  description, 397
  design principles, 398
  equipoise, 398
  explanation of randomization, 398
  placebo effect, 398–399
Pharmacological treatment
  antipsychotics (*see* Antipsychotic
    medications)
  cholinesterase inhibitors, 215–216
  FDA, 206
  prevention, 216–218

psychostimulants, 213, 215
psychotropic medications, 205
Pharmacology, sedation
  alpha-2-adrenergics agonists, 376
  anaesthetics, 376
  antiepileptics, 375–376
  antihistamines, 376–377
  anxiolytic sedatives, 374–375
  neuroleptics, 375
Pharmacotherapy, 349–366
  anxiety disorders, 138–139
  depression (*see* Depression)
  stressor-related disorders, 138–139
Phototherapy/light therapy, 258
Polypharmacy, 354
Post-traumatic stress disorder (PTSD),
    135–136
  benzodiazepines, 335
  breast cancer patients, 136
  chronic illness, 333
  citalopram, escitalopram/sertraline, 334
  clonidine and propranolol, 335
  delirium, 334
  dopamine, 334–335
  morphine, 334
  psychopathology, 136
  SSRI, 334
  trauma-and stress-related disorders, 333
  trauma symptoms, 333
  treatment, 138
Posttreatment/survivorship phase, 89–91
Pramipexole, 257
Pranayama, 111–114, 117, 118
Pregabalin, 17, 179, 354, 363
Prescription ethics
  addiction, 403
  confidence, 403
  knowledge and behavior, physician, 402
  mistakes, 402
  pharmaceutical industry affiliations, 402
  unwell, abuse alcohol/drugs, 402
Primary psychiatric disorders, 24, 338
Procarbazine, 21, 156, 320, 322
Promethazine, 252, 325, 376
PST. *See* Palliative sedation therapy (PST)
Psychiatric emergencies, 317–329
Psychiatric interview and examination
  attachment styles, coping and defense
    mechanisms, 35, 36
  clinical formulation, 33
  liaison with referring physicians, 33
  medical and psychosocial assessment, 39

mental functioning areas, 37–38
MSE (*see* Mental status examination
    (MSE))
oncology and palliative care, 32
psychopharmacological treatment, 32, 33
psychosocial attention, 33
Psychological assessment
    adaptation, disease, 61
    classification, 51
    clinical approach, 51
    clinicians accuracy, 53
    communication, 52
    operational criteria, mental disorder, 52
    QoL, 50
    screening (*see* Screening, psychological
        assessment)
    supportive care, 50
Psychopharmacology, oncology and
        palliative care
    anxiety and depression diagnosis, 4–5
    cancer, 4
    literature, 4
    psychiatric disorders, treatment, 7–8
    psychotropic drugs
        ADs, 6–7
        advanced stages of cancer,
            antipsychotic agents, 5
        BDZ, 7
        guidelines, 6
        hypnotics, antipsychotics and
            antianxiety agents, 5
        psychiatric disorders and of cancer-
            related symptoms, 6
    PSYCOG outcomes, 5
    treatment, psychiatric disorders, 7–8
Psychopharmacology research
    limitations, 385–386
    oncology and palliative care, 382
    rationale
        cancer patients management, 384–385
        clinical practice guidelines, 382
        definition, "caseness", 382
        dispel myths, 383
        effectiveness, 383–384
        identification, syndromes, 384
        lack of evidence, 384
        NCCN, 382–383
        RCTs, antidepressants, 382
        side effects, 384
        stigma, psychotropic medications, 383
        systematic review, 382
    recommendations
        awareness, 386–387

control, confounding variables, 387
        co-occurring symptoms, 387–388
        drug treatment algorithms, 387
        RCTs, 387
Psychostimulants
    adverse effects, 155
    antidepressant medications, 156, 157
    modafinil, 155
    reduction, 155
    research, 155
Psychotherapy
    anxiety, 83
    chronic heart failure, 85
    disease phase and stage, 86
    distress, cancer patients, 84
    medication, 81–82
    preexisting psychiatric conditions, 84
Psychotic disorders
    antipsychotics (*see* Antipsychotics)
    consultation and communication, 233–234
    diagnosis, DSM-5, 230, 231
    drug–drug interaction, 232, 234
    meaning, 230
    primary and secondary, 230
    risk, 234
    schizophrenia, 230, 234–235
    side effects, 232
Psychotropic drugs
    antidepressants, 255–256
    antihistamines, 251–252
    atypical antipsychotics (AP), 257
    barbiturates, 255
    BDZ-H, 252–253
    dopaminergic agents (DA), 257
    melatonergic agents, 256
    nonbenzodiazepine hypnotics, 253
PTSD. *See* Post-traumatic stress disorder
        (PTSD)

Q
Quetiapine, 257
    antipsychotics, 196
    anxiety/delirium, 343
    metabolism, 197
    olanzapine, 27, 191, 327

R
Radical prostatectomy (RP), 304–305
Radiotherapy, 353
Ramelteon, 256
Randomized control trials, 340

Reboxetine, 154
Restless legs syndrome (RLS), 243–244
Risk factors, suicide attempts, 335–336
Risperidone, 197, 338
Ropinirole, 257
RP. *See* Radical prostatectomy (RP)

S
SARI. *See* Serotonin antagonist and reuptake inhibitor (SARI)
Schizophrenia, 230, 234–235
Screening, psychological assessment
  cognitive impairment, 55–56
  depression/anxiety, 54–55
  distress, cancer care, 55
  emotional disorders, 58
  emotion thermometers, 57
  ESAS, 56–57
  PTSD, 57
  tools, 59–60
  unmet needs tools, 57
  well-being, 56
Sedative antihistamines (AHs), 251
Sedative hypnotics medications
  alcohol, 26
  alprazolam and clonazepam, 26
  benzodiazepines, 25–26
  CYP P450, 26–27
  lorazepam, 26
Selective serotonin reuptake inhibitors (SSRIs), 18–19
  antidepressant medications, 152, 157
  antidepressants, 362
  bone mineral density, 358
  cognitive-behavioral therapy, 334
  CYP2D6 inhibition, 95
  cytochrome P450, 153
  depression and anxiety, 153
  elixir formulations, 358
  fluoxetine, 358
  fluoxetine and escitalopram, 336
  fluoxetine/paroxetine, 95
  fluvoxamine, fluoxetine and sertraline, 332
  hyponatraemia, 352, 358, 360
  and irinotecan, 156
  linezolid, 332
  pediatric cancer/palliative care, 336
  platelet aggregation, 23
  QT prolongation and arrhythmias, 358
  serotonin toxicity, 332
  sertraline, citalopram and escitalopram, 153
  side effects, 153

and SNRIs, 18, 20
and steroids, 95
upper gastrointestinal (GI) bleeding, 355, 356
venlafaxine, 360
Sequenced Treatment Alternatives to Relieve Depression Trial (STAR_D), 361
Serotonin antagonist and reuptake inhibitor (SARI), 154
Serotonin-norepinephrine reuptake inhibitors (SNRIs)
  bupropion, 360
  desvenlafaxine, 153
  duloxetine, 153
  milnacipran, 153–154
  mirtazapine, 360
  and SSRIs, 18
  and TCAs, 19
  venlafaxine, 153
  venlafaxine and duloxetine, 360
Serotonin syndrome, 318–323
Serotonin toxicity, 318, 320
Seva, 112–113
Sexual dysfunction
  men, 301–305
  women, 297–301
Sexual function, 296
Side effects
  antipsychotics
    EPS, 232
    TD, 232
    ziprasidone and sertindole, 232
  neuroleptic malignant syndrome, 232
Sleep disorders
  biological function, 240
  and cancer (*see* Cancer)
  chart or diary, 241–242
  classifications, 242
  clinical interviews, 241
  etiology
    oncologic treatment, iatrogenic factors, 248–250
    tumor-related factors, 246–248
  pattern of sleep, 241
  quantity and quality measures, 240–241
  REM and non REM, 241
  screening, 241
  treatment
    acupuncture/acupressure, 259–260
    antidepressants, 255–256
    antihistamines, 251–252
    AP, 257
    barbiturates, 255

BDZ-H, 252–254
CBT, 258–259
CPAP, 258
DA, 257
DORA, 257–258
melatonergic agents, 256
nonbenzodiazepine hypnotics, 253
phototherapy/light therapy, 258
procedures, 251
wake-promoting drugs/
psychostimulants, 257
wake cycle regulation, 241
Sleep disruption, 86–87
Sleep disturbance, 342–343
SNRIs. *See* Serotonin-norepinephrine reuptake
inhibitors (SNRIs)
Social anxiety disorder, 134–135
Somatic symptom disorder/somatization
abnormal illness behavior, 165
amplification, somatosensory, 166
attribution style, 165–166
catastrophizing, 166
depression, 164, 385
diagnosis, 166–167
effectiveness, 181–182
emotional, 164
physical/somatic symptoms, 164
psychiatric disorders, 166
somatization condition, 164, 165
treatment, cancer
anorexia and weight loss, 181
antidepressants, 169–170
CBT, 171–172
CRF (*see* Cancer-related fatigue (CRF))
depressive disorder, 169
educational interventions, 172
glucocorticoids and glutamate, 169
hormonal hypothesis, 169
hot flashes, 179
inflammation and immune
response, 170
low-dose antidepressants, 167–168
nausea and vomiting, 181
neurotransmitterrelated hypothesis, 169
non-Hodgkins lymphoma, 168
pain and chronic pain, 172–175
pruritus, 180
psychotropics, 170–171
somatizing process, 170
symptoms, 168
therapeutic management, 168, 169
SPIKES Rx protocol, cancer settings
component, 75, 76
emotions, 78
invitation, 77
knowledge, 77–78
perception, 76–77
psychotropic medications, 78–79
trusting relationship, 75
SSRIs. *See* Selective serotonin reuptake
inhibitors (SSRIs)
Steroids, 336
Substance abuse
aberrant drug-taking behaviors and
severity, 274, 275
and addiction (*see* Addiction)
alcohol (*see* Alcohol)
assessment, 277–278
cancer and non-cancer pain, 268
control, 268
creation of structure, therapy, 278
current/remote histories, patients, 275–276
defining abuse and addiction, 272–273
definition, 275
drug-related behaviors, 274
drugs selection and administration
aberrant drug-taking behaviors, 284
anxiety and depression, 285
development, coping skills, 284–285
education and programs, 285
high doses, 284
inpatient management plan, 285–286
long-acting analgesics, 284
outpatient management plan, 286–287
evaluation and treatment, comorbidity of
personality disorders, 279
guidelines, prescription
evaluation, 287
family sessions and meetings, 288–289
procedures, 287
12-step programs, 287
UDT, 288
literature, 268
management
anxiety, 269
risk, 278
symptom, 277
opioid, 268
pain, 269, 277
prescription drug abuse, 270–271
prevalence, 269–270
pseudoaddiction, 273
psychiatric assessment, 275
psychopharmacology
buprenorphine and naltrexone, 283
disulfiram/antabuse, 282
MMT, 282–283
requirements, therapy, 278
risk stratification, 278
symptom management, 277

Succinylcholine, 323
Symptom cluster, 321, 322

T
Tai Chi Chuan (TCC)
    Chinese martial arts tradition, 109–110
    "moving meditation", 109
    outcomes, 109
    Qigong, 108–109
Tardive dyskinesia (TD)
    atypical antipsychotic, 357
    and EPS, 232
    examination, abnormal movements, 356
    and extrapyramidal symptoms, 357
    parkinsonian symptoms, 24
    side effects, 232
    susceptibility, 232
TCAs. See Tricyclic antidepressants (TCAs)
TD. See Tardive dyskinesia (TD)
TDM. See Treatment decision-making (TDM)
Testosterone therapy, 300–301
TMS. See Transcranial magnetic stimulation
        (TMS)
Torsades de pointes (TdP), 327
Traditional Chinese medicine (TCM)
    AAA, 106
    AAR, 106
    acupuncture, 105
    applications, clinical oncology, 110
    insomnia, anxiety and depression, 106
    Jutong theory, 106, 107
    pain and fatigue, 104
    TCC, 107–110
    and WM, 110
    Zang-Fu organs, 106
Transcranial magnetic stimulation (TMS),
        403–404
Trauma and stressor-related disorders
    acute, 135
    and adjustment disorder, 136
    early stage breast cancer, 135
    non-pharmacotherapy, 136–138
    pharmacotherapy, 138–139
    PTSD, 135–136
Trazodone, 94, 154, 255, 321, 343, 399–400
Treatment
    cancer-related symptoms
        anorexia, 341
        fatigue, 341–342
        nausea/vomiting, 340–341
        pain, 339–340
        sleep disturbance, 342–343
    psychiatric symptom
        anxiety, 332–333

    delirium, 337–338
    depression, 335–337
    primary psychiatric disorders, 338
    PTSD (*see* Post-traumatic stress
        disorder (PTSD))
Treatment decision-making (TDM), 120
Tricyclic antidepressants (TCAs)
    cardiovascular system, 23
    cyclophosphamide, 156
    desipramine/lofepramine, 361
    neuropathic pain syndromes, 360–361
    urinary retention and central
        anticholinergic effects, 360

V
Vacuum devices, 303
Vaginal dilator therapy, 299
Vaginal estrogen therapy, 299–300
Vaginal moisturizers and lubricants, 298
Vaginismus, 297
Valeriana officinalis, 257–258
Valproic acid/valproate/VPA
    cancer patients, 28
    glucuronidation, 196
    targeting neural circuits, 399
    treatment, BPAD, 193–194

W
Wake-promoting drugs/psychostimulants, 257
Water-soluble drugs, 351
Wedding communication, 74–75
Wernicke–Korsakoff's syndrome, 279–280
Western medicine (WM), 110
WHO ladder, 339–340

Y
Yoga
    description, 111
    hatha yoga, 113–114
    meditation, 114–117
    pranayama, 114
    psychology, Indian philosophy, 111–112
    psychotherapeutic yoga practices, 112
    RCT, 117
    seva, 112–113

Z
Zaleplon, 253
Ziprasidone, 191, 216, 232, 327
Zolpidem, 253, 321